Second Opinions

＊＊＊＊

Second Opinions

SIXTY PSYCHOTHERAPY PATIENTS
EVALUATE THEIR THERAPISTS

Lee D. Kassan, M.A.

JASON ARONSON INC.
Northvale, New Jersey
London

Production Editor: Elaine Lindenblatt

This book was set in 10 pt. Stone Serif by Alpha Graphics of Pittsfield, NH and printed and bound by Book-mart Press, Inc. of North Bergen, NJ.

Library of Congress Cataloging-in-Publication Data

Kassan, Lee D.
    Second opinions : sixty psychotherapy patients evaluate their
therapists / by Lee D. Kassan.
        p.   cm.
    Includes bibliographical references.
    ISBN 0-7657-0205-3
    1. Psychotherapist and patient.   2. Psychotherapy patients—
Attitudes.   3. Psychotherapy.   I. Title.
RC480.8.K37   1999
616.89'14—dc21   98-53683

Printed in the United States of America on acid-free paper. For information and cata-log write to Jason Aronson Inc., 230 Livingston Street, Northvale, NJ 07647-1726, or visit our website: www.aronson.com

All professions are conspiracies against the laity.

George Bernard Shaw,
The Doctor's Dilemma

Contents

Part III—The Ending

Acknowledgments

I could not have written this book without the cooperation and willing participation of the sixty individuals who spoke so candidly and revealed so many of their experiences, reactions, and opinions. I thank them all.

I want also to thank Bob Hack and Peter Kassan for their careful and thoughtful editing, Dr. Rena Subotnik for her help with the references, all the staff at Jason Aronson for their attention to my books, and C. B. for patience and understanding.

Introduction

Imagine this scenario: a new patient comes to a psychotherapist's office. She finds the waiting room a little dark and the furniture a little shabby. The magazines are two years old. A few minutes after the appointed time, the therapist opens the door, asks the patient inside, and offers a chair. They sit down and the therapist, after sipping from a cup of tea, invites the patient to tell the therapist why she is there. After about twenty minutes the phone rings. The therapist says, "Excuse me," and picks up the phone. He speaks briefly to another patient and hangs up. He apologizes and asks the patient to continue.

She reveals what is bothering her and describes something of her background and present situation. They discuss briefly some of the possible issues. Toward the end of the session, the therapist says that he thinks they can work together. He announces his fee, and describes his rules: the patient is responsible for all sessions and is expected to take her vacation when he does. They make an appointment for the following week.

The next day he discovers that the patient has left a phone message saying that she has changed her mind and decided that she needs to "think about it" before she starts therapy. How will the therapist understand what has happened? Will he think about his own behavior, or simply assume that the patient got scared and ran away?

Psychotherapists want to believe that they are doing what is best for their patients, and that treatment is organized to achieve this goal. They may think that patients will tell the therapist when they find a remark or a behavior objectionable but, as we will see, this does not always happen.

This book is a companion volume to *Shrink Rap: Sixty Psychotherapists Discuss Their Work, Their Lives, and the State of Their Field,* in which I interviewed psychotherapists of many different theoretical persuasions and levels of experience about what they do and why they do it. For this book I interviewed 60 patients about their experiences in psychotherapy, and I found that they often told me things they never told their therapists.

Originally I intended to interview only nonprofessionals, educated and uneducated, about the therapeutic process. Later, I thought that it would be useful to have a comparison group of professionals, therapists as patients themselves. As a result of this decision, there are two interview subgroups: the professionals—practicing psychotherapists themselves—and the nonprofessionals. In order to keep the emphasis on the experience of the general public, there are 40 subjects in the nonprofessional group and 20 in the professional group. None of the psychotherapists in the *Shrink Rap* group are among the 20 professionals interviewed here.

Many of the people interviewed for this book have had more than one therapist (see Question 2). To make the material manageable, subjects were asked only about their most recent experience, the last therapy they had completed. Therapies had to have been completed no more than 10 years ago and at least 3 months prior to the interview (one subject, at the end of the interview, was discovered to still be in treatment after 20 years, and his answers were also included). In most cases the therapist being discussed was not identified to me.

Although the majority of the therapists interviewed for *Shrink Rap* were from New York City, the subjects of this book are spread over the country and come from New York, New Jersey, Connecticut, Florida, California, Maryland, Massachusetts, and Washington, D.C. As a result of the geographic distribution, interviews were conducted mostly by telephone, from September 1996 to March 1998. Interviews usually lasted between 45 minutes and an hour. In general, the interview questions parallel those in the *Shrink Rap* interviews.

The subjects for this book are not a random sample, and again no claim is made for statistical validity. There were 18 men and 42 women overall, 5 men and 15 women in the professional group and 13 men and 27 women in the nonprofessional group. The age range of the participants overall was 26 to 62; the professionals ($N = 20$) ranged from 30 to 62 with a mean of 50, and the nonprofessionals ($N = 40$) ranged from 26 to 52 with a mean of 46. Because quotations without attribution are hard to evaluate, I have identified each speaker by sex and age, and indicated whether the individual is a mental health professional or not. Since informal speech is so different from written prose, some quotations have been lightly edited for readability, but nothing has been substantially altered.

Because I will be talking a lot about patients and therapists, I have reserved these terms for the psychotherapeutic situation. Subjects who happen to be therapists themselves will be referred to as "professionals" to distinguish them from their therapists. While I have problems with the medical model implied by the term, I will use "patient" throughout to identify persons from either group when they are in a therapist's office talking about themselves.

Material is organized in the same way as in *Shrink Rap*. The book is divided into three main sections. Part I, The Beginning, covers the decision to enter treatment, the selection of the therapist, and the initial sessions. Part II, The Treatment, deals with patient and therapist behavior in the course of psychotherapy. Part III, The Ending, covers the reasons for stopping, what happened afterward, and feelings about the overall experience as seen with some hindsight.

Within each question, I present the range of responses as objectively as possible, and this range is organized in the **Numerical Distribution** section. I reserve my personal opinions for the **Comments** section, in which I point out significant differences between the professional and nonprofessional groups, and try to highlight some of the issues addressed in the question from the points of view of both the therapist and the patient.

As with *Shrink Rap*, a list of all the relevant books and articles about all these topics would itself fill a thick volume. In the **Related Reading** sections I have listed a few recent articles or books pertinent to the question. In some cases there were thousands to choose from; in others it was difficult to find any at all.

This book, like *Shrink Rap*, is directed at both therapists and their patients. Patients, even in this day of media therapists and appearances by mental health professionals on almost every daytime talk show, are often terribly ignorant about what is supposed to happen in a therapist's office. Therapists themselves need to rethink their behaviors, their methods, and their rationales, and to consider the possibility that they are acting in ways counterproductive to effective treatment. Some therapists may find me presumptuous in telling them how to work, but perhaps they will listen more readily to the patients in this book.

I want to thank all the people, professional and nonprofessional, who took the time to tell me about their experiences in psychotherapy, good and not so good. All those who responded sounded quite candid and authentic to me, and I hope they all like what I have done with their stories. As with my earlier book, I hope that anyone who reads this one, therapist or patient, will come away more knowledgeable about what constitutes good therapy.

The Beginning

This section covers the start of the process: the decision to enter treatment, the selection of the therapist, the initial impressions, the hopes and expectations, and the first few sessions. Many people admitted they knew almost nothing about the process, and had no idea what to expect. It might be hard to imagine such a patient challenging or questioning anything the therapist might do.

▧▧▧▧

Question 1: How did you select your therapist?

Once the decision is made to seek therapy, a good therapist has to be identified and selected. How does one choose a therapist? Who does one ask for suggestions?

Many of the professionals got their therapists through their training institute. Sometimes there is a choice available.

> I had begun training at an institute, and there was a list of analysts to choose from, and I chose her because she was close to where I lived.
>
> [Female, 62, Professional]

> The last one was required because I was in analytic training, so I selected from a list of analysts that were associated with my institute and approved by them.
>
> [Male, 42, Professional]

> I was at an institute, and I selected her because she was part of the institute and I had to be in therapy.
>
> [Female, 55, Professional]

> I was at an institute and some people there talked about how good she was.
>
> [Female, 56, Professional]

> She had been a trainer where I was training.
>
> [Female, 45, Professional]

And sometimes there is no choice.

> I went to a training institute, and she was assigned to me.
>
> [Male, 44, Professional]

> I went through the referral service at an analytic institute, and I was assigned to him.
>
> [Male, 53, Professional]

Selecting a therapist while in training can sometimes involve changing roles.

7

> He was my instructor at one of the analytic institutes I was attending.
> I then hired him to be my supervisor, and then he became my analyst.
>
> [Female, 57, Professional]

Professionals had greater resources in consulting colleagues or selecting from therapists whose work they were familiar with in some way.

> My supervisor gave me the name of his former supervisor.
>
> [Female, 48, Professional]

> I had seen him do a presentation at a conference, and I was very impressed with how he worked.
>
> [Female, 59, Professional]

> I had had a very bad experience with my first therapist, and I worked with a psychiatrist who was fabulous, but I couldn't see her because I worked with her. I asked her for a referral and the person she thought would be perfect for me. I knew her husband because I worked with him professionally too. So I was referred to someone else for an evaluation.
>
> [Female, 50, Professional]

> I had met her at the house of a colleague. I practice a particular kind of therapy and I knew that she did too. I liked her manner.
>
> [Female, 62, Professional]

Many people from both groups asked someone they knew for a recommendation.

> I found her through a friend who was also seeing her.
>
> [Female, 45, Professional]

> It was a referral from my cousin, who had visited her during her divorce and found her to be very helpful.
>
> [Female, 45, Nonprofessional]

> I thought about which of my friends I really liked and felt close to at the time and asked her who her therapist was, figuring that someone I liked would probably be going to a therapist I would like.
>
> [Female, 50, Nonprofessional]

> My neighbor referred me to her.
>
> [Female, 40, Nonprofessional]

I was referred through a friend who had been seeing her for a number of years. She recommended her highly.

[Male, 45, Nonprofessional]

I got a referral from someone I work with, whose husband had been seeing her.

[Male, 49, Nonprofessional]

I found her through a friend of mine who was seeing her colleague.

[Female, 47, Nonprofessional]

Sometimes the person making the referral has a particular role.

I got him through my church. The priest made a referral.

[Female, 42, Nonprofessional]

It was a referral from my physician.

[Female, 48, Nonprofessional]

Several people got their therapists through an agency, either at work or privately.

I went to the phone book and looked under "Psychological Services" and I made a couple of phone calls, and some of them said they would have somebody call me back, or I had to make an appointment for an intake interview, and one place gave me an initial interview over the phone and was able to give me an appointment the very next day for a more intensive intake interview, so that's the one I went with.

[Female, 48, Nonprofessional]

We have an Employee Assistance Program where I work. They advertise it.

[Female, 48, Nonprofessional]

I called [name of agency] because I had been involved with a group there around the death of my friend, and that person recommended her.

[Female, 26, Nonprofessional]

I saw a poster on a community bulletin board for people with anxiety and panic attacks. I contacted the group, and it was a small group of five or six psychologists. I told them I could only afford a certain amount and they said there was only one person I could see for that fee. I had an intake interview.

[Female, 28, Nonprofessional]

She was recommended to me by an agency that supports Americans overseas. This occurred while we were living in Europe.

[Female, 53, Nonprofessional]

I went through Health Services, who gave me a list. I chose her from the list because her name sounded like it was the same ethnic background as me. They suggested I see more than one person and then choose, which I did.

[Female, 39, Nonprofessional]

Sometimes using an agency is complicated.

I found him through work, an employee assistance program (EAP). You call up and they do a brief phone interview, and then they give you your choice of people, and I chose someone who was close to where I work. The deal was that you got to see this person free for three sessions, and then if that person decided that you needed further therapy then he would assign you to someone else. I guess they didn't want the fox in charge of the chicken coop. I saw him for three sessions, and I really liked him, but then he had to assign me to someone else. He was not allowed to continue seeing me, so I saw another person for four or five sessions, and we did not hit it off. At the time I was traveling a lot, and I had told her that. I said she had to factor that in somehow. She said that her philosophy was that if she couldn't fill the slot she would have to charge me for the session. I said that wouldn't work. I said I could give her lots of notice, and she said let's try it. The first time I had to travel I gave her eight days' notice, and at the end of the month when I went to pay the bill, she had charged me for the session, so I chose not to go back to her. A year later I went back to the first guy and said I'd still like to see him, and they had changed the rule and I could see him.

[Female, 41, Nonprofessional]

I knew of a clinic in [name of town] so I just went there on my own. I had an intake interview, and they assigned me to someone I didn't like, so I requested the woman who did the intake interview, and waited three months to start with her.

[Female, 48, Nonprofessional]

Therapists with an existing connection to the family are sometimes the choice.

> She was recommended by my older brother, who was seeing her, and the reason we both saw her is she's the daughter of my mother's psychiatrist.
>
> [Female, 45, Nonprofessional]

> He had seen my father, who had stopped seeing him, but I thought that since my father was kind of central to my problems it would be useful to see someone who knew him. I also knew he was a hypnotherapist and I hoped he could help me control my weight.
>
> [Male, 53, Nonprofessional]

Prospective patients sometimes became aware of the therapist through books, classes, or workshops.

> My girlfriend bought me a book he had written about combining Eastern and Western psychotherapy. I was inspired by the book and I called him up.
>
> [Male, 30, Professional]

> I had read a book of his. He was connected to a church I was in. I wasn't in a circle of friends who were going to therapy, so I couldn't ask anyone for a referral.
>
> [Male, 48, Nonprofessional]

> I took a course with her about letting go and moving on and I liked her. She seemed gentle and she knew her stuff.
>
> [Female, 50, Nonprofessional]

> I had been with him in a workshop, and he agreed to take me on as an individual patient.
>
> [Male, 46, Nonprofessional]

The selection process often involves "shopping around."

> When my husband and I decided to go for therapy, we saw three or four people and picked the one we liked best.
>
> [Female, 44, Nonprofessional]

I called a friend who is also a therapist and she recommended several people. I called each of them and got the best feeling from the person I chose. We were looking for couple counseling and my wife had the same feeling and we agreed to see this person.

[Male, 49, Nonprofessional]

People occasionally had criteria other than the therapist's competence.

I tried to find someone in my neighborhood, so I went from name to name to name. I needed someone who could see me in the middle of the day. I finally found someone.

[Female, 39, Professional]

My therapist in the last city I was in knew someone whose wife had gone on a marathon with this man. So I when I came here he gave me two names. One was someone he knew, and the other was this person he had heard about. He was geographically more convenient so I looked him up first.

[Male, 50, Professional]

Recently, choice of a therapist has been restricted by health maintenance organizations (HMO) and managed care insurance companies.

I was in an HMO and I selected him from a list that gave some vague background information.

[Male, 50, Nonprofessional]

NUMERICAL DISTRIBUTION

Professionals: Eight people said they got their therapist at a training institute; 6 were referred by a friend or colleague; 3 were referred by their previous therapist; 2 from a book or workshop; 1 chose based on location.

Nonprofessionals: Twenty-two people said they had been referred by a friend; 6 said they went through a clinic or institute; 6 through an employee assistance program or HMO; 3 said they were referred by a previous therapist or physician; 3 said they chose the therapist based on a workshop, class, or book.

COMMENTS

I think the best way to find a therapist is to ask the person who seems to be getting the most out of therapy. Sometimes that therapist will not take on as a patient a person close to the one already in treatment, but it's a good place to start. Picking a name out of the phone book is probably not the best way to find a therapist, but even that method may work if the prospective patient trusts his or her feelings, and stays in treatment only if it feels good to be there.

Many patients may find it useful to consult a number of therapists before making a decision. This process, while it may become expensive, can show the wide array of different styles and personalities, and can be especially valuable for someone new to treatment.

As the therapist, I probably would want to know a little about where the prospective patient is coming from, so a referral from a colleague or a former patient identifies the new person somewhat.

As the patient, I'll ask my friends for recommendations, especially those whose lives seem to be improving as a result of therapy. I'm put off by ads in the paper with a long list of "specialties" and am even a little suspicious of why anyone good would need to advertise.

RELATED READING

Alexander, L. B., Harber, J. P., and Luborsky, L. (1993). On what bases do patients choose their therapists? *Journal of Psychotherapy Practice and Research* 2(2):135–146.

Michaels, A. S. (1990). How women patients choose women therapists. In *Women as Therapists: A Multitheoretical Casebook,* ed. D. W. Cantor, pp. 20–32. New York: Springer.

Ruben, D. H. (1993). Selecting therapies and therapists. In *Handbook of Managed Care for Inpatient to Outpatient Treatment,* ed. D. H. Ruben and C. E. Stout, pp. 19–48. Westport, CT: Praeger/Greenwood.

Saunders, S. M. (1993). Applicants' experience of the process of seeking therapy. *Psychotherapy* 30(4):554–564.

Tillett, R. (1996). Psychotherapy assessment and treatment selection. *British Journal of Psychiatry* 168(1):10–15.

🖾🖾🖾🖾

Question 2: How many therapists have you had?

While this book focused only on their most recent experience in treatment, most of the subjects had seen more than one therapist, at different times for different reasons. Professionals may be required to have additional therapy or analysis in the course of training, and sometimes want more after training, when the training institute is no longer involved. Nonprofessionals may see more than a single therapist for many reasons: dissatisfaction with the first experience, therapist or patient relocation, a new problem or situation, or the desire for a different point of view.

NUMERICAL DISTRIBUTION

Professionals: N = 20; Range: from 1 to 10; Mean = 4.20
Nonprofessionals: N = 40; Range: from 1 to 8; Mean = 2.98

COMMENTS

Once the process of self-examination begins, many people find it hard to stop. Only 1 of the professionals and only 7 of the nonprofessionals had just a single therapist. Since every therapist has blind spots or areas of difficulty, seeing a different therapist can bring a new perspective. Therapists of different genders can be especially useful in eliciting new material and stimulating fresh discussion.

As the therapist, I welcome patients who have had previous therapy, because they will probably be more knowledgeable and may appreciate what I offer even more. Since there is probably a reason they aren't returning to the earlier therapist, I may also get the ego gratification of being better than the previous therapist.

As the patient, I like the variety of experiences possible with different therapists. I discover new things about myself and about the process of therapy with each new therapist.

RELATED READING

Cummings, N. A. (1991). Brief intermittent therapy throughout the life cycle. In *Psychotherapy in Managed Health Care: The Optimal Use of Time and Resources,* ed. C. S. Austad and W. H. Berman, pp. 35–45. Washington, DC: American Psychological Association.

Gabbard, G. O. (1995). When the patient is a therapist: special challenges in the psychoanalysis of mental health professionals. *Psychoanalytic Review* 82(5):709–725.

Halgin, R. P., and Caron, M. (1991). To treat or not to treat: considerations for referring prospective clients. *Psychotherapy in Private Practice* 8(4):877–896.

Ruben, D. H. (1993). Selecting therapies and therapists. In *Transitions:
Handbook of Managed Care for Inpatient to Outpatient Treatment,* ed.
D. H. Ruben and C. E. Stout, pp. 19–48. Westport, CT: Praeger/
Greenwood.

𝕽𝕽𝕽𝕽

Question 3: Was there any requirement you had for the therapist?

People considering therapy may have an image in mind of the person
they want to talk to, and try to match it up with the actual therapist.
Such factors as gender, age, or orientation can be significant to prospective patients. Do prospective patients focus on some characteris-
tic, in hopes of finding a sympathetic understanding? Or does some
other factor predominate?

A match in gender is often the primary consideration.

> I really wanted to talk to a woman. Age didn't matter, although I
> think I needed someone closer to my age than to my mother's age.
>
> [Female, 40, Nonprofessional]

> I must have hoped it would be a female, because I was disappointed
> that it was a male [assigned by EAP].
>
> [Female, 48, Nonprofessional]

> I wanted a woman because some of my issues had to do with a very
> powerful father, and lack of connection to my mother, and I felt that
> I needed a connection to a woman. I didn't want to get into my
> pattern with authoritative men.
>
> [Female, 46, Nonprofessional]

> All my other therapists had been women, and I normally have a strong
> preference for a woman, but I was so impressed with him in the
> workshop.
>
> [Male, 46, Nonprofessional]

> I wanted a woman, someone who had been a mother and was in a
> healthy relationship.
>
> [Female, 39, Professional]

> I suppose in the back of my head I was looking for a woman.
>
> [Female, 45, Nonprofessional]

> At that time I was interested in seeing a woman. It was the politically correct thing to do.
>
> [Female, 47, Nonprofessional]

Sometimes the preference is for the opposite gender.

> I did want an analyst, and I wanted a man.
>
> [Female, 48, Professional]

> I requested a female therapist, because I thought I'd be more comfortable with a female therapist.
>
> [Male, 42, Nonprofessional]

Sometimes gender was specified as a complement to a previous therapist.

> I wanted a woman because I had had a male therapist before.
>
> [Female, 55, Professional]

> I very specifically wanted a man because I had already seen a female and the issues I have are generally not with females.
>
> [Female, 50, Nonprofessional]

> I wanted a woman, because I had seen a man before. She was older than me but not too much older. We came from the same ethnic background.
>
> [Female, 45, Professional]

> I wanted a woman. I'd had a man first, and I felt that my problems at that point would be better served by a woman. I also wanted someone to whom I wouldn't have to travel very far.
>
> [Female, 53, Nonprofessional]

Age and experience were also mentioned as important.

> I wanted somebody older, who was calm and comfortable.
>
> [Female, 48, Professional]

> I didn't want anyone who was younger than I was. Somebody who had more experience.
>
> [Male, 52, Professional]

I wanted an older woman.

[Male, 44, Professional]

A particular expertise was sometimes specified.

Not gender, age, or background, but I wanted someone who had experience working with people in the creative arts.

[Male, 48, Nonprofessional]

Sometimes people were looking for a particular style, a way of working.

I wanted someone who was very related, more active and involved. I also wanted someone who ran a group.

[Female, 59, Professional]

At the time, I felt more comfortable with a man, and I was looking for someone with skill in a certain incisive exploratory way of asking questions and then making a summary reflection of what he heard me saying. Someone who was analytically trained, and who had a flexible open approach to bringing different points of view to bear on an issue, not someone who was rigidly locked into a particular model just because he was trained in that model.

[Male, 42, Professional]

I didn't want the kind of therapy where the relationship with the therapist becomes the subject of the therapy.

[Female, 39, Nonprofessional]

I didn't want a long analytic process so I wanted someone who was willing to work with me for a briefer therapy.

[Female, 51, Professional]

I wanted someone who was sharp, sharper than me. Someone who could get into emotional content, not just intellectual stuff.

[Female, 50, Professional]

I wanted someone who practiced the kind of therapy I do myself.

[Female, 62, Professional]

I just wanted someone who was empathetic.

[Female, 42, Nonprofessional]

Some people mentioned a particular background, or at least some familiarity with it.

> At that time I was thinking more about someone who was familiar with my religious upbringing.
>
> [Male, 48, Nonprofessional]

> I wanted to see a smart New York Jewish guy, because that was the kind of man I had just left, my husband.
>
> [Female, 50, Nonprofessional]

Many people said they had no preference in mind, and a few said why.

> I don't think I knew enough then to have an educated preference.
>
> [Male, 50, Nonprofessional]

> I didn't know enough to have any requirement. I didn't care about male or female. I felt that a reference from someone I knew was the best start.
>
> [Female, 46, Nonprofessional]

NUMERICAL DISTRIBUTION

Professionals: (Some people gave more than one answer.) Ten said they wanted a particular gender; 5 said they wanted a specific type of therapy; 3 said they wanted a level of experience, intelligence, or skill; 3 said they wanted a specific age range; 2 said they wanted a particular style; 2 said they wanted a specific personal background or situation; 6 said they had no preference in mind.

Nonprofessionals: (Some people gave more than one answer.) Fifteen said they wanted a particular gender; 3 said they wanted a specific age range; 2 preferred a particular style; 2 said they wanted a specific professional or personal background; 2 said they chose partly on the basis of location; 1 said she wanted a specific type of therapy; 19 people said they had no requirements.

COMMENTS

Patients need to be comfortable and have a certain level of trust in the therapist, especially at the beginning of treatment, and they come with certain requirements in mind that they believe will create that environment. It makes no sense to try to dismiss these preferences, even though we may think them irrelevant, and try to talk the patient into seeing someone who doesn't fit the bill.

As the therapist, I want to know what the patient envisions the therapist to be, and why certain qualities are significant and others irrelevant. I don't want to have to convince anyone that I am what they're looking for, so if a patient wants a woman, I'm not going to argue but will just make a referral.

As the patient, I think I know what I need to be comfortable and to open up to someone. I'm open to discussion but it may not change my mind. There's no point in starting from a place of dissatisfaction with the therapist.

RELATED READING

Beutler, L. E., Clarkin, J. F., Crago, M., and Bergan, J. (1991). Client–therapist matching. In *Handbook of Social and Clinical Psychology: The Health Perspective,* ed. C. R. Snyder and D. R. Forsyth, pp. 699–716. New York: Pergamon.

Dorken, H., and VandenBoa, G. (1986). Characteristics of 20,000 patients and their psychologists. In *Professional Psychology in Transition: Meeting Today's Challenges,* ed. H. Dorken, B. E. Bennett, L. G. Carpenter, et al., pp. 20–43. San Francisco: Jossey-Bass.

Person, E. S. (1986). Women in therapy: therapist gender as a variable. In *Between Analyst and Patient: New Dimensions in Countertransference and Transference,* ed. H. C. Meyers, pp. 193–212. New York: Analytic Press.

Pikus, C. P., and Heavey, C. L. (1996). Client preferences for therapist gender. *Journal of College Student Psychotherapy* 10(4):35–43.

Stamler, V. L., Christiansen, M. D., Staley, K. H., and Macagno-Shang, L. (1991). Client preference for counselor gender. *Psychology of Women Quarterly* 15(2):317–321.

ছঞ্চছঞ্চ

Question 4: What was your therapist's degree?

There are four major categories of professional background: psychiatry, psychology, social work, and other assorted disciplines such as rehabilitation or nursing. The nonprofessionals appear to have seen more M.S.W.s than the professionals, who saw more Ph.D.s.

NUMERICAL DISTRIBUTION

Therapists: Seven said they saw an M.S.W.; 8 saw a Ph.D. or D.S.W.; 5 saw an M.A.; no one saw an M.D.

Nontherapists: Twenty-two said they saw an M.S.W.; 11 saw a Ph.D.; 3 saw an M.D.; 3 saw an M.A. or M.S.; 1 person didn't know what the therapist's degree was.

COMMENTS

The days when psychiatry was the most prestigious and dominant discipline in the field of psychotherapy and psychoanalysis appear to be over, and more people appear to be seeing therapists with a nonmedical background, especially the M.S.W. None of the professionals and only 3 of the nonprofessionals saw an M.D. Many prospective patients seem to want to avoid psychiatrists, with their medical orientation and perceived preference for drugs as treatment. Several people said that they didn't care what the therapist's degree was; they cared only about competence, skill, and ability.

As the therapist, I know that I am well trained and experienced. If people want a therapist with a particular degree as an assurance of competence, they can have him, but they ought to know that credentials are no guarantee of good treatment.

As the patient, I want some way of assessing professionalism and competence before I start treatment, and facts about training and academic degree are one way of getting that. Once the minimum standards are met, however, the personality and style of the person become far more important.

RELATED READING

Murstein, B. I., and Fontaine, P. A. (1993). The public's knowledge about psychologists and other mental health professionals. *American Psychologist* 48(7):839–845.

Richardson, P., and Handal, P. (1995). The public's perception of psychotherapy and counseling: differential views on the effectiveness of psychologists, psychiatrists, and other providers. *Journal of Contemporary Psychotherapy* 25(4):367–385.

Strom, K. (1994). Social workers in private practice: an update. *Clinical Social Work Journal* 22(1):73–89.

🔊🔊🔊🔊

Question 5: What did you know about therapy before you started?

Only nonprofessionals were asked this question, since we can assume that professionals would know a great deal about how the process works (although this was not always the case with professionals who started treatment early in their training).

Because the nonprofessionals were asked only about the most recent treatment that they had completed, and only a few of them had never been in treatment before, even the nonprofessionals were fairly educated by the time of this interview.

> I knew a great deal.
>
> > [Male, 48, Nonprofessional]

> I had been in therapy several times before, so I knew a lot.
> > [Female, 48, Nonprofessional]

> I'd been in therapy before for several years, so I had some idea of what it could do or should do.
> > [Female, 45, Nonprofessional]

Some people said that in spite of previous experience they knew very little.

> I had been in therapy before for 2 years, but I really knew nothing.
> > [Female, 45, Nonprofessional]

There were some who acknowledged that they did not know much about therapy when they started the most recent treatment.

> I knew nothing about therapy. I had no notion of what it was about. I was a complete blank slate about it.
> > [Male, 49, Nonprofessional]

> I knew the pop stuff.
> > [Female, 40, Nonprofessional]

> I had seen a therapist a year before for a month. I didn't know much about the different schools of therapy.
> > [Female, 42, Nonprofessional]

Even when they knew only a little, they still knew that therapy could be helpful.

> I had been to a couple of therapists briefly, but I never felt like I really connected. I had never had satisfying experiences with therapists, but somehow I felt the value of it.
>
> [Female, 41, Nonprofessional]

> I had been in family therapy before, so I knew it was supposed to be helpful to talk to someone.
>
> [Female, 26, Nonprofessional]

> My mother and father used to say that they thought it was a good idea when people would go to therapists, and that it was a shame that more people didn't.
>
> [Male, 42, Nonprofessional]

Some people said they knew bits and pieces.

> I knew that you talk to the person and they ask you questions and give you feedback.
>
> [Female, 50, Nonprofessional]

> I knew there were lots of different kinds of therapists and lots of different theories, and I didn't want somebody heavily analytical in the Freudian sense. At the same time, I knew that it wasn't the school or the theory of the therapist but your feeling about the person.
>
> [Female, 50, Nonprofessional]

> I knew some from general reading, from literature, and I had read a little Freud.
>
> [Female, 46, Nonprofessional]

> I knew it helped people but I didn't know how.
>
> [Female, 44, Nonprofessional]

> I knew there was someone you were supposed to talk to and she would help you.
>
> [Female, 41, Nonprofessional]

A few people had studied psychology earlier in their lives.

I had actually planned to be a therapist once upon a time. After taking some psych courses I changed my mind. I guess I knew what anyone would know.

[Male, 52, Nonprofessional]

I had seen several people previously. I also did part of a training that people who are becoming therapists do.

[Male, 49, Nonprofessional]

I knew quite a bit because I had been in before and I had also studied psychology.

[Female, 48, Nonprofessional]

Some knew a lot because of experience in the family or with friends.

I knew quite a bit because my wife was becoming a therapist herself.

[Male, 46, Nonprofessional]

My mother saw a psychiatrist most of my life, so I grew up in a household that was pro-therapy.

[Female, 45, Nonprofessional]

I had seen a psychiatrist when I was in my early teens, and I was somewhat familiar with the routine.

[Male, 53, Nonprofessional]

I knew a fair amount. I have several friends who are therapists and was close to them while they were doing their training. It's also been something that I've always been interested in and done a lot of reading in.

[Female, 46, Nonprofessional]

NUMERICAL DISTRIBUTION

Nonprofessionals: Seventeen people said they thought that they knew a lot about therapy going into this treatment; 18 said they knew only a little; 4 said they knew nothing at all. Twenty-one people said they had been in therapy prior to the treatment discussed in these interviews.

COMMENTS

About half this group of nonprofessionals had been in therapy and were fairly knowledgeable. But many knew little or nothing about the process. One of my purposes in doing this book and its partner, *Shrink Rap*, was to create more educated patients. The more the patient knows about what creates good therapy, the less likely he or she is to settle for bad or mediocre therapy. In the past, patients were often advised not to read in the field or discuss their treatment. The fear that the educated patient will be more resistant or difficult is not borne out; in fact, the educated patient is less likely to question the process or challenge the therapist who is working well.

As the therapist, I want a knowledgeable patient, one who understands what I'm doing and why, one who isn't thrown when I talk about our own relationship, one who sees the value of working with dreams, one who appreciates my skill and experience.

As the patient, I like knowing as much as I can about the process: what to expect, how to work most effectively, whether my therapist is doing what he or she is supposed to be doing. The more I know, the more I feel like an equal partner.

RELATED READING

Kotin, J. (1995). *Getting Started: An Introduction to Dynamic Psychotherapy*. Northvale, NJ: Jason Aronson.

Murstein, B. I., and Fontaine, P. A. (1993). The public's knowledge about psychologists and other mental health professionals. *American Psychologist* 48(7):839–845.

Rothstein, A. (1995). *Psychoanalytic Technique and the Creation of Analytic Patients*. Madison, CT: International Universities Press.

Walborn, F. S. (1996). *Process Variables: Four Common Elements of Counseling and Psychotherapy*. Pacific Grove, CA: Brooks/Cole.

▧▧▧▧

Question 6: What were you told about the therapist before you started?

When asking for a referral, the person considering therapy is usually told something about the recommended therapist. What kinds of information are imparted to prospective patients about the therapist?

Patients are often told about the competence or experience of the therapist.

> I was told that she had very good diagnostic skills and that she was able to go very deep into the therapy process.
>
> [Female, 47, Nonprofessional]

> The person who referred me to him said he was wonderful. I was definitely told how great he was.
>
> [Female, 48, Professional]

> I was told that she was wise, and that she was quite a bit older, and that I could learn a lot from her.
>
> [Female, 52, Professional]

> I was told that she was very smart, and I remember the person who referred me said that there weren't a lot of therapists that he trusted, and he trusted her, and I thought, "That's it."
>
> [Female, 40, Nonprofessional]

> I was told that she was sharp, that she was a gestalt therapist, and was adept at getting out of the intellectual stuff into emotional material, and that she would not get seduced by me.
>
> [Female, 50, Professional]

> I was told only that he was very good.
>
> [Male, 51, Nonprofessional]

Sometimes a specific area of expertise is emphasized.

> I was told that she was good working with couples, and that she could actually help me bring in my spouse.
>
> [Female, 44, Nonprofessional]

> Basically I was told that she was experienced with couples situations, and issues about being able to connect.
>
> [Male, 52, Nonprofessional]

> I was told that she had an M.S.W., that she had training in some psychoanalytic institute, that a professional colleague had recommended her highly, and that she did have experience with people in the creative arts.
>
> [Male, 48, Nonprofessional]

I was told that she had a lot of experience dealing with my particular problem.

[Female, 28, Nonprofessional]

I was told she was extremely helpful in getting my cousin through a really bad divorce. She found her very supportive.

[Female, 45, Nonprofessional]

Patients are sometimes told about the personal background of the therapist.

I was told that he was excellent, and very bright, and that he understood social work school, which I was in at the time.

[Female, 50, Professional]

I knew he had a kid about my age.

[Female, 50, Nonprofessional]

I was told that she was very spiritual, and that she did a lot of work with children. Since I worked with children also, we would have a common ground to start with.

[Female, 42, Nonprofessional]

Patients are sometimes told about the personality or style of the therapist.

I was told she was very nice.

[Female, 45, Nonprofessional]

I was told that he was a very compassionate person and very good at what he did, and that I would feel comfortable, which was my main concern.

[Female, 48, Nonprofessional]

I was told that she was very smart, and that she lived her personal life with dignity.

[Female, 51, Professional]

I was told just that he was a nice guy and that he had helped other people.

[Female, 53, Nonprofessional]

Occasionally patients are told details that might seem irrelevant.

> I was briefly told something of a slightly flattering, almost sexually provocative nature. I don't remember the exact words. It was enticing but disturbing.
>
> [Male, 44, Professional]

Often patients are told virtually nothing, except the recommendation.

> I knew nothing about her, only her name.
>
> [Male, 49, Nonprofessional]

> I was told nothing, except his location, and that he was acceptable to the EAP.
>
> [Female, 41, Nonprofessional]

> I was just told that the person who had gone on a marathon weekend with him was very impressed with him.
>
> [Male, 50, Professional]

> I was told only that she had gone to the same analytic institute as the person making the referral.
>
> [Female, 50, Professional]

> I was told just that the person who referred me to her liked her and thought she was good.
>
> [Female, 45, Professional]

NUMERICAL DISTRIBUTION

Professionals: Six people were told about the therapist's skill or ability; 4 were told the therapist was smart; 3 were told something about his or her background. Six said they were told nothing.

Nonprofessionals: Eight people said they were told about the skill or ability of the therapist; 6 were told something about his or her personal qualities; 3 were told about his or her professional background or expertise; 1 was told about his intelligence. Twenty-two were told nothing about the therapist.

COMMENTS

Is it better to know something about the therapist, or to know nothing and form one's own opinion? A recommendation that includes endorsement of the therapist's expertise, competence, or style may help get the new patient into treatment, but may create expectations that interfere with spontaneous experience. Revealing details of the therapist's personal life or background is probably not a good idea, because it prevents the therapist from making the choice of what to reveal, and risks letting the patient know something he would prefer not to know (see also Question 77).

As the therapist, I want the patient to know whatever he wants about my professional self. I don't want personal details from my private life revealed, because then I'm not in control of when or whether I reveal them to this particular person.

As the patient, all I really need to know is that someone I respect has a high opinion of the therapist. Beyond that, I'm capable of coming to my own conclusions about whether this is the right therapist for me.

RELATED READING

Coles, D. (1995). A pilot use of letters to clients before the initial session. *Australian and New Zealand Journal of Family Therapy* 16(4): 209–213.

Eissler, K. E. (1993). The maligned therapist, or an unsolved problem of psychoanalytic technique. *Journal of Clinical Psychoanalysis* 2(2): 175–217.

Jacobs, T. J., and Rothstein, A., eds. (1990). *On Beginning an Analysis.* Madison, CT: International Universities Press.

ᘔᘔᘔᘔ

Question 7: Was there anything you were worried or concerned about before entering therapy?

When embarking on a commitment like therapy, people sometimes have concerns about the process, and what might happen there, or what might be required of them. What kinds of things are on people's minds as they consider entering treatment?

Many people were concerned about the quality or effectiveness of the treatment.

> I wanted to be sure that I wasn't going to have another bad experience.
>
> [Female, 50, Professional]

> I was concerned about whether it would be effective. I had been in therapy before where a lot of surface issues came up, but it didn't affect my basic personality and hadn't affected me in an emotional way. I was concerned that this would be glossing over the surface, and hoped that some deeper thing was going to happen.
>
> [Male, 52, Nonprofessional]

> I was concerned that it would be like the experience I had had earlier and I would get nothing from it.
>
> [Female, 42, Nonprofessional]

> I had been concerned because when I looked back on my previous therapists, I felt that a lot of them were not very good. I know a lot of people in the profession and I didn't respect them. Because I knew so much I figured I'd probably be a difficult patient. So I was concerned about competence.
>
> [Female, 59, Professional]

> I had some basic negative feelings about therapy in the past but I didn't see any other way. I knew I was having panic attacks from some books that I had picked up, and it seemed the only way I would get over them was to go back into therapy. Although I had gone to a therapist and I knew what my problem was, they didn't seem to address that. I never felt like it was ever addressed in the past.
>
> [Female, 28, Nonprofessional]

> I wanted it not to be like the first one. I wanted it to be really good.
>
> [Female, 50, Professional]

This is not always a worry about the therapist.

> I was afraid of making the same mistakes as I had made with my prior therapist, of having kept things back.
>
> [Female, 45, Professional]

I was unsure about how easily I would take to the process involved. Because I knew a lot about the theory I was concerned that knowledge would get in the way of the process, which did not happen. I was worried that the purpose of therapy was to "normalize" me.

[Male, 50, Nonprofessional]

Others, both professionals and nonprofessionals, were concerned about the skill of the therapist.

My biggest concern was that with previous therapists I had felt that I was smarter than they were, and I needed someone who I couldn't fool or put one over on, and someone who could keep pace with me.

[Female, 46, Nonprofessional]

I was worried that I might be able to outmaneuver the therapist.

[Female, 50, Professional]

Some people said they were concerned about the fit with the therapist, and whether they would get along well.

There's always some concern about whether I'm going to like the therapist, or if I'm going to be afraid of the therapist. Is it going to be easy or hard? What's his approach and how will I react to it?

[Female, 48, Nonprofessional]

Some people were concerned about the way the therapy would be set up, the structure and mode of treatment.

This was back in 1977, when encounter groups were the big thing, and I was concerned that there was going to be too much touchy-feely stuff.

[Male, 50, Professional]

I was worried about a situation where you talk the whole time and they don't say a word.

[Female, 50, Nonprofessional]

I wasn't sure what it was going to be like. I knew it would be nontraditional, and I was concerned about that, about how far out it was going to get.

[Male, 30, Professional]

I was not interested in doing anything on the couch. I had done that for many years and felt that I didn't accomplish very much.

[Female, 53, Nonprofessional]

I was nervous about opening myself up to a complete stranger. I had some anxiety about that. I had very rarely confided in anybody, so I was a little leery about talking to a stranger about personal things.

[Male, 45, Nonprofessional]

I was a little concerned because I had heard she was a real Freudian, and I wasn't sure I agreed with Freud. Also, for some reason, I had a big fear of being on the couch.

[Female, 42, Nonprofessional]

Others said they were concerned about confidentiality and boundaries, especially those in training.

Confidentiality was my biggest concern, because I knew that he was involved with the institute, on a number of committees, and I wanted to be perfectly assured that anything I talked about would stay within the confines of the therapy and not be discussed in any way.

[Male, 42, Professional]

It was great to be referred by a colleague, but then I was a little concerned about having some distance and privacy.

[Female, 51, Professional]

I was concerned a little bit whether it would be weird to be seeing a therapist that my cousin had seen, since my cousin and I had a close relationship, and though my cousin was not in therapy at that time, it always made me wonder what this therapist might or might not know about my family.

[Male, 45, Nonprofessional]

Many people said they were worried about what might be discovered or revealed.

It's terrifying. I was in therapy for a year and a half, which I realize is not a long time, and you get used to it. But I used to tell my therapist that I'd rather be going to the dentist for root canal.

[Female, 40, Nonprofessional]

> I was concerned with the possibility of the revelation that I was much crazier than I had feared, and that there was a seething mass of neurosis underneath an apparently placid functional exterior.
>
> [Male, 48, Nonprofessional]

Several people said they were concerned about the fit with the therapist, and how they would get along.

> I was concerned about the general question of whether he was going to be what I was looking for.
>
> [Female, 48, Professional]

> I was fairly resistant because I had completed a therapy that I thought was quite good and successful, but they made me do it again.
>
> [Female, 55, Professional]

Several nonprofessionals were concerned about the length of treatment.

> My main worry was that it wasn't going to do anything, and it would go on forever.
>
> [Female, 46, Nonprofessional]

> I had a basic distrust of people in the profession. I didn't want it to go on forever. I had seen too many people who were strung out for too many years that weren't getting anywhere. I was leery of paying money for nothing.
>
> [Male, 52, Nonprofessional]

Several nonprofessionals were worried about the meaning of being in therapy.

> I remember feeling that whatever was going on was something that I should be able to fix on my own. I also remember a sense of it not being very significant. So I remember being very shocked at the end of my first session because I expected her to say something like "You know, what you're going through is typical," and so on, and instead she said she wanted to see me twice a week. It upset me because it meant that I was going through something very serious that I couldn't handle by myself.
>
> [Female, 48, Nonprofessional]

Others were worried about the cost, especially of long-term treatment.

I was concerned about the expense.

[Female, 44, Nonprofessional]

I was worried about how I was going to pay for it.

[Female, 47, Nonprofessional]

Other individuals mentioned some specific worries.

I was concerned about my family's reaction to it, that they would make me an outcast.

[Female, 52, Nonprofessional]

He was my supervisor for 8 years before he was my therapist, and I was concerned about the transition. As my supervisor he was extraordinarily helpful, and my practice flourished because of his work with me. I was pretty sure because he was so insightful and helpful with all the various types of people I was working with that he would have no problem working with me.

[Female, 57, Professional]

I was going into couples therapy with my wife and it was a female therapist and I was concerned that the women would gang up on the man. That fear seemed to materialize in the first session, but it was quickly dispelled.

[Male, 49, Nonprofessional]

Many people said they had no worries or concerns going into therapy.

I was too naive to have any concerns.

[Female, 45, Nonprofessional]

It was covered by my company so I thought that there was no downside.

[Male, 42, Nonprofessional]

NUMERICAL DISTRIBUTION

Professionals: Four people were concerned about the quality of the treatment; 2 were concerned about confidentiality; 2 were worried about what might go on in the therapy; 2 were concerned about their use of the process; 1 person each was concerned about fit with the therapist, about the skill of the therapist, and about the transition from supervisor to therapist. Seven people said they had no worries or concerns about the treatment when starting.

Nonprofessionals: (Some people gave more than one response.) Nine people said they were worried about the effectiveness; 5 said they were worried about what might be revealed or uncovered; 4 said they were worried about the financial cost; 2 said they were concerned about the length of treatment; 2 said they were worried about whether they would like the therapist; 1 said he was worried that he might see a silent therapist; 1 was concerned about her family's negative reaction to her going; and 1 was concerned about the therapist's fairness and objectivity. Sixteen people said they had no worries or concerns.

COMMENTS

Most patients, especially those who have thought about therapy for a long time before actually beginning, come in with fears, worries, fantasies, and concerns, and it is important for the therapy that these be understood, addressed, and relieved as soon as possible. Patients who have had previous therapy that was less than terrific will be worried about the effectiveness of the new treatment.

As the therapist, I expect patients to be afraid of the process and unsure of me. I know I have to demonstrate my skill and my effectiveness, and my ability to create a space safe enough for them to look at themselves. This can take a few sessions or even a few years.

As the patient, I am worried about trusting the therapist and about trusting myself to handle whatever comes up. It will take me some time, and fears apparently relieved may reemerge later. I will tolerate all of this if I feel progress is being made.

RELATED READING

Jacobs, T. J., and Rothstein, A., eds. (1990). *On Beginning an Analysis.* Madison, CT: International Universities Press.

Kushner, M. G., and Sher, K. J. (1989). Fear of psychological treatment and its relation to mental health service avoidance. *Professional Psychology: Research and Practice* 20(4):251–257.

Levine, J. L., Stolz, J. A., and Lacks, P. (1983). Preparing psychotherapy clients: rationale and suggestions. *Professional Psychology: Research and Practice* 14(3):317–322.

Melnick, J. (1978). Starting therapy: assumptions and expectations. *Gestalt Journal* 1(1):74–82.

꧁꧁꧁꧁

Question 8: When you first contacted the therapist, what was he or she like on the phone?

For most patients, the phone call to the new therapist is the first impression of that person. How did therapists come across in this initial contact?

Most people had a positive experience in this area.

> He sounded warm, concerned, and interested, but not overly enthusiastic or presssuring.
>
> [Male, 51, Nonprofessional]

> We exchanged voice mail messages and I thought she had such a soothing voice, very soft, and I was impressed with that.
>
> [Female, 40, Nonprofessional]

> He was very nice, very engaging.
>
> [Male, 50, Professional]

> Her voice sounded very strong, and I liked that.
>
> [Female, 47, Nonprofessional]

> He had a very good phone manner.
>
> [Female, 41, Nonprofessional]

> He was very good on the phone, very nice and friendly but not too friendly, warm and welcoming.
>
> [Female, 48, Professional]

> He was a soft-spoken guy, and he was informative and answered all my questions. It was an encouraging conversation.
>
> [Female, 46, Nonprofessional]

> She seemed very calm. She had a very calming voice, and reassuring, and approachable.
>
> [Female, 40, Nonprofessional]

A few had some negative reactions.

> She was very businesslike and officious, as most of them are. It always puts me off.
>
> [Female, 42, Nonprofessional]

> She was tough. It was a little daunting.
>> [Female, 52, Professional]

> She was hard to understand because of her accent.
>> [Female, 55, Professional]

> He had somewhat of a flat affect, not much emotion, which actually scared me a little bit because I wanted someone who would be enthusiastic to see me.
>> [Female, 46, Nonprofessional]

> He was rather businesslike, a little formal.
>> [Male, 53, Nonprofessional]

Others felt differently about formal, professional behavior by the therapist.

> She was cool, and that was reassuring. Anyone who was too enthusiastic would have put me off.
>> [Female, 50, Professional]

> She's always got a neutrality that I like.
>> [Male, 49, Nonprofessional]

> She was pretty chatty, more than I was expecting. She was a little too chatty.
>> [Female, 51, Professional]

> She was not very talkative, a little distant, but sympathetic. I remember thinking that maybe she had to be that way because of the kind of people she was dealing with.
>> [Male, 42, Nonprofessional]

A quick reply is probably a good idea, as this response suggests.

> I left a message and he called back. He seemed gentle and concerned. By the time he called back I was ready to not do it, but he invited me to come in and I did.
>> [Female, 52, Nonprofessional]

As these responses imply, a strong negative reaction to the initial contact would probably mean no further pursuit of that therapist.

He was quite nice, so I did make the appointment with him.

[Female, 48, Nonprofessional]

I felt good enough about him that I showed up for my appointment.

[Female, 50, Nonprofessional]

I don't remember clearly, but it must have been a reasonably positive contact or I wouldn't have continued. I think she was professional, and I think she had a pleasant phone manner.

[Male, 48, Nonprofessional]

Several people did not make the initial contact by phone.

I already knew him.

[Female, 57, Professional]

The EAP director gave me his name. I don't think I ever talked to him on the phone, I was just scheduled to see him by the EAP.

[Female, 48, Nonprofessional]

My parents made the call—I don't know.

[Female, 26, Nonprofessional]

There was no phone contact. I had been assigned an appointment and she met me in the waiting room.

[Male, 44, Professional]

I called and made an appointment with the clinic. I had to wait to see the person I wanted, so she called me when she had an opening. She was fine on the phone, but that wasn't my first contact with her because she had done the intake.

[Female, 48, Nonprofessional]

NUMERICAL DISTRIBUTION

Professionals: Nine said the therapist was warm or friendly; 4 said he or she was businesslike in a positive way; 2 said he or she was cold or remote; 1 said her therapist was too friendly. Two people said there was no phone contact before the first session, and 2 said they had no recollection of the first call.

Nonprofessionals: Twenty-three said the therapist was warm or friendly; 10 said the therapist was businesslike or professional; 3 said he or she was too cold or remote. Two people said there was no phone contact before the first session, and 2 said they had no recollection of the first call.

COMMENTS

Some patients call for the first appointment wanting to express a lot of feelings and concerns, or ask a lot of questions. Others only make the appointment and save the questions for the actual meeting.

As the therapist, I try to be friendly without being seductive, and make the phone call as brief as possible while still making it clear that whatever the patient wants to ask or discuss will be addressed. Long discussions about fees, schedules, and the nature of therapy are best had in person.

As the patient, since I already have some confidence in the therapist (otherwise I wouldn't be calling), I'm able to wait until the first session to ask my questions, although I do have a problem with a therapist who refuses to tell me what the fee will be.

RELATED READING

Budman, S. H., Hoyt, M. F., and Friedman, S., eds. (1992). *The First Session in Brief Therapy.* New York: Guilford.

Grossen, M., and Apotheloz, D. (1996). Communicating about communication in a therapeutic interview. *Journal of Language and Social Psychology* 15(2):101–132.

Kantrowitz, J. L. (1995). The beneficial aspects of the patient–analyst match. *International Journal of Psycho-Analysis* 76(2):299–313.

Speck, A., and Stitz, S. (1987). A study of the verbal interaction in the initial phase of therapeutic discourse. In *Neurotic and Psychotic Language Behavior,* ed. R. Wodak and P. Van de Craen, pp. 95–124. Clevedon, England: Multilingual Matters.

℞℞℞℞

Question 9: What was your reaction to the waiting room?

Patients often spend significant periods of time in the waiting room, and often have strong feelings about and reactions to that space. Often the space is shared with other people waiting to see other therapists in the same suite of offices.

Many people reported feeling perfectly comfortable in the waiting room.

> It was a woman's therapy group office, and there were lots of things in the waiting area about women's issues, supportive to women, and as I walked in there was a couch exactly like my best friend's couch, where we had spent years talking about things, so I immediately felt safe and at home. It was a comfortable place to sit and be and organize my mind before I went in for therapy.
>
> [Female, 46, Nonprofessional]

> It was very small, but it was neat and clean, with good magazines. I felt comfortable even though it was such a small space.
>
> [Female, 40, Nonprofessional]

The reading material provided is a particular feature that may have special meaning to the patient, positive or negative.

> I liked it because even though it was another city, it had *New York* magazine in it.
>
> [Female, 39, Nonprofessional]

> It was just a room, with only *New Yorker* magazines and gardening magazines, which also told me something about her.
>
> [Female, 62, Professional]

> It was interesting, because she had art books there.
>
> [Female, 42, Nonprofessional]

> I didn't feel that comfortable there. It was kind of gray and bland, with old magazines.
>
> [Female, 26, Nonprofessional]

> I found it very pleasant. There were interesting magazines.
>
> [Female, 41, Nonprofessional]

> It was a typical therapist's waiting room, with outdated furniture and even more outdated magazines.
>
> [Female, 45, Nonprofessional]

Many others do not feel comfortable, for various reasons. Often, the layout of the space is disturbing.

It was more like a porch that was converted, so it was long and narrow. I was glad I didn't have to face anybody. You just faced a wall.

[Female, 50, Professional]

I had been warned that her waiting room was inadequate. Her waiting room was basically a chair in the first-floor lobby of a row tenement building, and sometimes even the chair was missing and I had to sit on the stairs. This was not ideal.

[Male, 48, Nonprofessional]

I didn't like it. All the chairs faced in one direction, like in a bus depot. It was a long narrow hallway.

[Female, 45, Professional]

I didn't like the environment—it was shoddy, and that made me think her practice was that way too. She eventually moved to a much nicer space.

[Female, 42, Nonprofessional]

It was very small, not a real room.

[Female, 44, Nonprofessional]

Over time, I was concerned that I could hear people outside, and I told him that it upset me, so he got a white noise machine.

[Female, 48, Nonprofessional]

Sometimes the way the room is decorated is upsetting to the patient.

The room was more or less shoddy. I knew that his vision had become poorer and I chalked it up to the fact that he couldn't see very well.

[Female, 57, Professional]

It was a little dinky, and very middle class. It looked like she had decorated it a long time ago.

[Female, 62, Professional]

I saw him at an office in his home, and the waiting room was the foyer, walled off from the rest of the apartment. I wasn't happy with that—I didn't care for his taste. I thought it was sort of seedy-looking and unattractive.

[Male, 42, Professional]

Patients often have strong feelings about a shared waiting area.

> There was a problem because there was another therapist in the same suite, and it turned out to be his wife.
>
> [Female, 48, Professional]

> The chairs were very close together, and there was more than one person in the practice so there were lots of people sitting around. So there was some discomfort. The people, because they were waiting for their therapists, were in various states of neurotic agitation, and every time the door would open I would wonder who they were coming for. So it wasn't a place where I wanted to start chatting and making friends. I had to make believe that I was alone. You don't make eye contact.
>
> [Female, 48, Nonprofessional]

> I didn't know what kind of place I was going to. When I got to her office I realized there was another therapist sharing the suite and another session going on. I was always curious about what was going on. The first time I went I heard somebody crying.
>
> [Male, 42, Nonprofessional]

> It was institutional, and there were a number of people. I was aware of a mixture of curiosity and embarrassment, since everyone knows why the others are there.
>
> [Male, 50, Nonprofessional]

> It made me nervous because she shared an office with her father, who was my mother's psychiatrist, and I didn't want to run into him.
>
> [Female, 45, Nonprofessional]

> It's in the place where I work, so I was uptight about two things: one was seeing anybody I knew, and the other was that one of the therapists in the EAP had worked with someone I knew with whom I'd had a bad relationship, and I felt awkward that she knew about me.
>
> [Female, 48, Nonprofessional]

> She shared it with two other therapists, and I guess their style was not to show any recognition, even after I had been sitting there for year after year seeing them, and they pretended they had never seen me before. The room itself wasn't too bad, but this kind of feeling that I was anonymous after all that time was too much.
>
> [Female, 50, Nonprofessional]

Sometimes a professional building can feel like a shared space.

> I saw him in a building where there are a lot of therapists practicing, and I had a jolt when I first went to see him, because I saw two people I knew just coming into the building and was uncomfortable having a therapist where a lot of my friends were going for supervision or their own therapy.
>
> [Female, 58, Professional]

An open waiting area doesn't always feel safe.

> It was in a house, so it was the living room. A group of therapists shared the house, so you just walked into the living area. I was concerned because it was in a residential area and anyone could just walk in.
>
> [Female, 39, Professional]

When the therapist practices from home, patients often have a strong reaction.

> It was in her house, which made me a little uncomfortable, because you had to go through some living space to get to her office, which was upstairs. The waiting area was one of the vestibules of the house, in front of the fireplace. I never met a family member, but I would have preferred to be a little more distant from the family.
>
> [Female, 53, Nonprofessional]

> It was a little strange because it was in his apartment, so it was a little bit unprofessional.
>
> [Male, 53, Professional]

Sometimes patients deliberately avoid the waiting area.

> It was a crummy upstairs suite. Downstairs was another business, and there were some offices upstairs, and it was like an apartment that had been made into offices. It was kind of weird, very low-budget. I wasn't comfortable there so I timed it so I wouldn't have to wait there.
>
> [Female, 48, Nonprofessional]

> I never sat in it; I always sat in the staff area, because I didn't want to feel like a client.
>
> [Female, 45, Professional]

Sometimes there is no waiting area.

There was no waiting room—she saw me in her living room. I showed up at the exact time and called up from the lobby. If someone was still with her, she would ask me if I could wait a few minutes.

[Female, 50, Nonprofessional]

There was no waiting room. It was her apartment and she used her living room. It looked like she didn't spend a lot of time there. If I was early I would wait downstairs. She seemed to space her appointments out enough so that if I did come a little early I could wait in the space where we would be meeting.

[Female, 44, Nonprofessional]

NUMERICAL DISTRIBUTION

Professionals: Eight said they were comfortable with the waiting room; 6 said they were not; 3 said they had no feelings about it; 4 said there was no waiting room.

Nonprofessionals: Fourteen said they were comfortable in the waiting room; 15 said they were not; 6 said they had no feelings about it; 5 said there was no waiting room.

COMMENTS

Almost half of the nonprofessionals whose therapist had a waiting room said they were not comfortable there, which suggests that therapists need to pay more attention to this aspect of their office arrangement. There is almost nothing in the professional literature about the waiting area: how to set it up, how patients might feel about it, or the kind of interaction with other patients and other therapists that may go on there. Most therapists seem to do whatever their own therapist did, or change whatever they found objectionable about that experience.

As a therapist who shares a waiting area with two other therapists, I have become aware of what kinds of events can occur there and how important that space can be. I try to keep the magazines interesting and recent, and the space clean and comfortable. I also try to be aware of who has adjacent hours and may meet in the waiting room between sessions.

As a patient, I want a relaxing space without a lot of noise or distraction, with some privacy if I feel like it, and something interesting to read if I need to wait. I don't want to have to wait in the lobby, and I don't want to be in the private space of the therapist, such as his living room. I want some boundaries, because otherwise I'm going to wonder how well the therapist keeps the other professional and personal boundaries of the therapy.

RELATED READING

Addison, D. (1996). Message of acceptance: "gay-friendly" art therapy for homosexual clients. *Art Therapy* 13(1):54–56.

Astrom, J., Thorell, L., and D'Elia, G. (1991). Psychotherapists' attitude toward observations of nonverbal communication in a greeting situation: I. Psychometrics of a questionnaire. *Psychological Reports* 69(3, pt. 1):963–975.

Norman, S. L. (1982). Nonverbal communication: implications for and use by counselors. *Individual Psychology Journal of Adlerian Theory, Research and Practice* 38(4):353–359.

Rotholz, T. (1985). The single session group: an innovative approach to the waiting room. *Social Work with Groups* 8(2):143–146.

ᛤᛤᛤᛤ

Question 10: What was your reaction to the office itself?

The office space sets the background for what happens there. The furnishings, the lighting, the arrangement, the colors, the noise level all contribute to creating an environment. Patients have many different feelings about the offices of their therapists.

Some people liked the office and felt comfortable there.

> I thought it was beautiful. She does everything very carefully, I know that, and even the pieces of artwork were perfect. Nothing was distracting, yet there were things that were interesting to look at.
> [Female, 40, Nonprofessional]

> I liked his office a lot. He had a good sense of color, good taste. It was not chaotic, it was restful.
> [Female, 58, Professional]

> I remember that when I walked in I was struck by how it was very small but very cozy, so it seemed like a nice place.
> [Female, 45, Nonprofessional]

I really liked it. I loved all his books—he had a whole wall of books—and it was very comfortable, but it was noisy from the street.

[Female, 48, Professional]

The office was very nice: dark wood, and books. Not antique but old-fashioned cushiony furniture and it was very comfortable.

[Male, 51, Nonprofessional]

She had a very nice office. It was very tastefully done. It wasn't her home, but it was very homey. You had a choice of where you wanted to sit. There were artwork and plants.

[Female, 50, Professional]

Several people mentioned that they liked being able to choose where they sat.

It had a couch and a chair, so I got to choose.

[Female, 39, Nonprofessional]

It was big, spacious, plenty of windows, and plenty of seating so you could choose and feel comfortable wherever you sat.

[Female, 41, Nonprofessional]

Some aspect of the office furnishings may have special meaning for a patient.

There were posters on the wall that were also about women's issues, and that also made me feel safe.

[Female, 46, Nonprofessional]

I was very impressed when I went in. It had many Japanese ornaments, a Buddha and bamboo wallpaper, and I have many such things in my own apartment.

[Female, 59, Professional]

He had a very nice Persian rug, and lots of books, which means a lot to me.

[Female, 50, Nonprofessional]

It was very nice, and I responded because when I looked at his desk there was a rose quartz and an amethyst geode, and those are things I'm interested in. I felt that there must be some point of sympathy or empathy with him.

[Female, 48, Nonprofessional]

Many others did not like the therapist's office. A number of these people found the furnishings run-down, old, and unappealing.

> The office was a little shabby. His couch was in disrepair. I thought perhaps he wasn't doing well financially. But I thought more that he couldn't see well.
>
> [Female, 57, Professional]

> It was dowdy and drab.
>
> [Female, 45, Nonprofessional]

> I didn't like the environment—it was shoddy, and that made me think her practice was that way too.
>
> [Female, 42, Nonprofessional]

> Janet Malcolm said that shrinks' offices are furnished with the furniture that used to be in the living room. That was the way it felt.
>
> [Male, 50, Professional]

> It seemed kind of standard—what I expected. It had a couch and some overstuffed chairs. It seemed like a bedroom that had been turned into an office, which is what it was.
>
> [Male, 53, Nonprofessional]

A few people mentioned other specific complaints.

> It was filled with books and papers and seemed a little disorganized. He also had a couple of cats there. I can't imagine how he finds anything.
>
> [Female, 52, Nonprofessional]

> He shared the office with another therapist who worked a lot with children, so there were a lot of children's drawings on the wall. The furniture was old and looked sort of thrown together. Not very pleasant.
>
> [Female, 48, Nonprofessional]

> There were a lot of pillows around, so it was very casual, and I was a little uncomfortable physically sitting in the arrangement she had. I felt unsupported.
>
> [Female, 53, Nonprofessional]

> It showed some kind of sentimental cute quality, which I don't really care for.
>
> [Male, 49, Nonprofessional]

It was not to my personal taste. It was too overstuffed. The furniture was too big for my liking and for her size.

[Female, 51, Professional]

Several people mentioned windows, or the lack of them.

It was conducive to the therapy. The furnishings were nice, she had plenty of fresh air and light. I was very comfortable in the office.

[Male, 42, Nonprofessional]

It was very comfortable, the seats were comfortable. It had windows at street level, and for some reason I liked that. My previous therapist's office was on the thirtieth floor, and it had a spectacular view, but I felt more comfortable in the ground-level office.

[Female, 41, Nonprofessional]

At first I was somewhat taken aback by the space. It didn't have any windows—it was an interior room. It was somewhat cavelike. Eventually I grew to like it.

[Female, 45, Professional]

When the therapist practices out of his or her house, patients may have complicated feelings.

It was his living room. It was weird. It was at once comfortable and awkward to be in someone's living room.

[Male, 30, Professional]

It was her house, and I was not as comfortable with that. I would have liked it to be an office space, a space that was a little more professional.

[Female, 44, Nonprofessional]

Some people noticed very little about the physical space.

I had no reaction at first, but later on it felt very comfortable.

[Male, 43, Nonprofessional]

It was all right, nothing special.

[Female, 44, Nonprofessional]

I came to feel very much at home in the office, because it became a very safe place, the only safe place I had in my life at the time. At the time I started, I was so consumed with my own stuff that she could have had anything in there and I would have said, "Oh, that's nice."

[Male, 49, Nonprofessional]

Some people noticed almost everything.

The office was fine. It was a front room with wooden shutters, and I remember being a little bit concerned that I might be visible from the street, although I wasn't really. Of course, I was curious about everything in the office. There were the books—I was always scanning the bookshelf for book titles, and her pile of current reading, and where she had her clocks and the tissue box, and the couch and the chair. I was very interested in all the decor.

[Male, 48, Nonprofessional]

Very warm, filled with a lot of personal knickknacks and treasures. A lot of interesting things to look at. There was a poster that I always disliked.

[Male, 46, Nonprofessional]

NUMERICAL DISTRIBUTION

Professionals: Fourteen said they liked the office and were comfortable there; 4 said they did not like the office; 2 said they had mixed feelings about the office.

Nonprofessionals: Twenty-seven said they liked the office and were comfortable there; 9 said they did not like the office; 4 said they had no feelings about the office.

COMMENTS

The office space is significant for most patients, whether it registers consciously or not. Almost a quarter of the total sample said they were not at ease in the office space. It's easy for the therapist not to notice the furnishings deteriorating, since they may fade into the background for someone who is there all day, every day, but patients—especially new patients—will notice. Offering the patient the choice of where to sit is perhaps a good idea, if the office has room for several options. Artwork and knickknacks may have meaning to individual patients, who may read some significance into them.

As the therapist, I'm always surprised when a patient remarks on a feature of the office, and asks if it was just added, when it has actually been there since the beginning of treatment. This can signal less anxiety, less self-absorption, or more relatedness—all positive signs.

As the patient, I want a space that's neither too small nor too large, one that is clean and well lighted, with comfortable furniture. I don't want it too spartan and bleak, which might suggest a therapist who isn't going to give me much, but I don't want it cluttered with personal objects either, which might make me wonder how much room there will be for my own material. I want to feel at ease, and believe it's up to the therapist to create such a space. An office lacking these basic qualities may lead me to wonder how well the therapist is going to take care of me.

RELATED READING

Bloom, L. J., Weigel, R. G., and Trautt, G. M. (1977). Therapeugenic factors in psychotherapy: effects of office decor and subject–therapist sex pairing on the perception of credibility. *Journal of Consulting and Clinical Psychology* 45(5):867–873.

Cantor, D. W. (1983). Independent practice: minding your own business. *Psychotherapy in Private Practice* 1(1):19–24.

Greenson, R. R. (1992). The preliminary contacts with the patient. In *The Technique and Practice of Psychoanalysis, vol. 2: A Memorial Volume to Ralph R. Greenson,* ed. A. Sugarman, R. A. Nemiroff, and D. P. Greenson, pp. 1–41. Madison, CT: International Universities Press.

Weinrach, S. G. (1980). Part-time private practices for the reluctant entrepreneur. *Counseling Psychologist* 9(1):87–89.

🕭🕭🕭🕭

Question 11: What was your reaction to the therapist's appearance and dress?

Therapists have many options in how to dress, from business clothing to casual and beyond. What kind of impression do they want to convey? Patients notice hair style, jewelry, clothing, and general demeanor in forming an opinion about the new therapist.

Most people had a positive reaction to the appearance of the therapist. Many people liked his or her professional appearance.

He looked about my age. He was nice looking, he dressed very hand-somely, he was clean and tidy. He presented himself very well.

[Female, 48, Nonprofessional]

He was very meticulously dressed, very well kept. Every hair was in place. I liked that, although I don't think I would have cared if he had been more casual.

[Female, 41, Nonprofessional]

She was dressed impeccably, very well, and she looked good, like someone I could identify with.

[Female, 39, Professional]

She was an older woman, and she wore good clothes and was more or less dressed up.

[Female, 62, Professional]

Some liked that the therapist was casually dressed.

He was unconventional, compared to the image I expected of a professional in a suit and tie. He wore flannel shirts, and was relaxed. It made him more real to me.

[Female, 52, Nonprofessional]

She was very informally dressed, and I was surprised. I think she had jeans on, and I thought she would be more businesslike. It was good, because I was more comfortable, more relaxed, than if she had a suit on.

[Female, 45, Professional]

He always dressed casually, in jeans, and he had a taste for Western wear, cowboy boots and such. He was always casual, never business-like, and I found that to be welcoming because that's how I dress.

[Male, 46, Nonprofessional]

She was not intimidating by being too stylish. She was pretty natural, but not frumpy.

[Female, 50, Professional]

A few people had a mixed reaction to a more formal appearance.

She was very professional, the way she dressed and her demeanor too, which was both reassuring and slightly off-putting. You kind of want someone warm and fuzzy, but you don't want someone unprofessional.

[Female, 39, Nonprofessional]

Some people had a negative reaction to the therapist's appearance. Sometimes this was because the therapist was too casual.

He was at times very casual—T-shirt, old chinos, untied shoes. It varied a lot. If he came from teaching, which I eventually found out he did, he would be dressed in a much more conventional way. It was a little disturbing and I remember mentioning it. He said he works best when he's comfortable.

[Male, 53, Professional]

He dressed very informally. When he used to come to the office right after a tennis game, he would be wearing a high-class warm-up suit. At one point, he felt that I was showing aggression toward him because I would comment on the way he was dressed, and he changed as a result.

[Male, 50, Professional]

Sometimes patients were a little disturbed because the therapist seemed too formally dressed.

She was a little bit conservative, which I'm not, so I wasn't sure that she would know what I was feeling because she was such a different person from me.

[Female, 28, Nonprofessional]

Some strong reactions to the therapist's style or taste occurred.

I noted to myself that she sometimes had dreadful taste.

[Male, 49, Nonprofessional]

She dressed very nicely, and that was fine. Sometimes I felt I was paying for her shoes.

[Female, 44, Nonprofessional]

She was a little glitzy, she way she dressed and carried herself was bordering on flamboyance.

[Female, 44, Nonprofessional]

> It's funny, because I once confronted her about it. She always wore black, and I told her she was a blank slate, and she just smiled.
>
> [Female, 40, Nonprofessional]

The therapist's physical appearance—age, stature, weight, coloring—can elicit strong reactions. Some are positive.

> He seemed like a grandfatherly person at ease with himself.
>
> [Female, 59, Professional]

> He was older than me by about 20 years, and he seemed like a wise person.
>
> [Male, 48, Nonprofessional]

> He was very tall, and very nice looking. He was very soft, gentle, and I felt very safe.
>
> [Female, 57, Professional]

> He looked more elderly than I was expecting, gray hair, tall and thin, but nice-looking and friendly.
>
> [Male, 51, Nonprofessional]

> He seemed like a wise old man.
>
> [Male, 30, Professional]

The therapist's appearance can be reassuring.

> I liked her right away because she looked like an academic. She was an attractive woman who was not glossy. She looked attractive but she also looked warm, which was very appealing to me.
>
> [Male, 52, Nonprofessional]

> He dressed very appropriately. He sort of reminded me of Woody Allen. I thought he looked like a safe person, like a man that I could talk to.
>
> [Female, 50, Professional]

> I remember thinking that she was very unthreatening and very kind, and that turned out to be true.
>
> [Male, 49, Nonprofessional]

> She was physically very plain, which was probably purposeful on her part, but she had a smile like an angel, a very gentle demeanor, and

it felt like the world lit up when she smiled. It was wonderful. I felt totally like she was nonthreatening and that there was an incredible warmth coming from her that made her very appealing to be sitting with.

[Female, 46, Nonprofessional]

Sometimes physical features or characteristics over which the therapist has no control can elicit strong reactions.

She was a little too skinny, but she dressed fine.

[Female, 51, Professional]

She had a very interesting face. She looked like my mother when my mother was young.

[Female, 47, Nonprofessional]

I'm tall, and she was even taller than me, and I liked that.

[Female, 62, Professional]

She had black hair, and much of my life I've been afraid of women with black hair. I'm not any longer.

[Female, 50, Nonprofessional]

Sometimes the therapist's appearance raises some doubt or other hesitation.

Sometimes I felt that she was frumpy, and I felt self-conscious about that, and then I talked to her about it.

[Female, 51, Professional]

I remember I was surprised by what she looked like. I'm not sure what I expected but she didn't look like what I expected. She had very red hair, and I remember that took me aback. And she was very small, a small, thin, slender woman. On the phone I got the feeling that she was going to be larger. I expected her physical being to be more impressive.

[Female, 45, Nonprofessional]

She looked too young and too attractive.

[Male, 44, Professional]

I was surprised that she was so old, and she was tough-looking.

[Female, 52, Professional]

He actually reminded me a little of Freud, like the consummate conservative Freudian analyst. He was different from me—he seemed more conservative, more tentative, more cautious, more muted, more moderate. But I got a sense of warmth and empathy and clinical skill that came through and those were the more important things.

[Male, 42, Professional]

He had a very deep voice on the phone, so I was a little surprised because he's not a big guy. He's short and thin, and had a very boyish look, which surprised me because I expected him to be older. He's not that much younger than me, but he looks a lot younger. Once we talked I didn't feel that way, he was fine.

[Female, 58, Professional]

NUMERICAL DISTRIBUTION

Professionals: Fifteen said they had a positive reaction to the therapist's appearance; 4 said they had a negative reaction; 1 said he had no reaction.

Nonprofessionals: Thirty-three said they had a positive reaction to the therapist's appearance; 4 said they had a negative reaction; 3 said they had no particular reaction.

COMMENTS

There isn't much a therapist can do about his or her physical appearance: age, height, weight, or coloring. How to dress is another question, one that sends a message to the patient about how to regard what goes on in the office, although it may not be as simplistic as "the more formal the dress, the more serious the approach." A casual style may raise questions about the professionalism of the therapist, but may also be reassuring and welcoming. We can see from the array of responses that there is tremendous variation among individuals, and whatever style of dress and presentation the therapist selects, it is important to discover any meaning it may have to the patient.

As the therapist, I try to dress in a relaxed but not too casual way: no jacket and no tie, but no shorts and no sneakers either. I need to be comfortable when I work, but I realize that I am working. I seem to be meeting the expectations of my patients, because no one has ever remarked on the way I dress.

As the patient, I don't really care what the therapist wears, although I might have a reaction if I thought they were dressing in some outlandish or bizarre way. A suit and tie has always signaled to me a formality that I don't want, a kind of stiffness, but I realize that to others it signals professionalism.

RELATED READING

Lukavsky, J., Butler, S., and Harden, A. J. (1995). Perceptions of an instructor: dress and students' characteristics. *Perceptual and Motor Skills* 81(1):231–240.

Roach-Higgins, M. E., and Eicher, J. B. (1992). Dress and identity. *Clothing and Textiles Research Journal* 10(4):1–8.

Ross, G. M., Shoham, A., Kahle, L. R., and Batra, R. (1994). Social values, conformity, and dress. *Journal of Applied Social Psychology* 24(17):1501–1519.

Tham, S. W., and Ford, T. J. (1995). Staff dress on acute psychiatric wards. *Journal of Mental Health UK* 4(3):297–299.

🔊🔊🔊🔊

Question 12: How long did you expect to see the therapist? How long did you actually stay in therapy?

Sometimes people start therapy with a specific time frame in mind for meeting their goals, and sometimes they have no definite length of time in mind.

Most people with an anticipated time frame stayed longer than they expected.

> I wanted it to be short-term, but I was with him 6 years.
> [Female, 58, Professional]

> I expected to be in a group a year or two, to facilitate my relocating and getting settled here. I was in 20 years, and I was very surprised.
> [Male, 50, Professional]

> I didn't have any strong expectations, but I did think it was helpful to have a length of time in mind, and I had a consultation before I saw him and I was comforted by the idea that certain diagnoses took

certain amounts of time. I stayed about 25 years. I never would have guessed that in advance; that's an unfathomable amount of time.

[Male, 53, Professional]

When I started, about a year or so. I stayed 6. I became an analyst in the course of it, and he became my training analyst.

[Female, 48, Professional]

I thought about 1 or 2 years. I stayed 5 years.

[Female, 59, Professional]

Professionals in training had expectations of a longer treatment.

I had to be in therapy as a training requirement, but I stayed for 8 years.

[Male, 44, Professional]

I expected I'd be seeing her for 4 years at least, because of the institute. I stayed 5 years.

[Female, 62, Professional]

I expected it would be a rather lengthy analysis. I stayed 8 years. I did expect to see him longer than the 4 years of analytic training.

[Male, 42, Professional]

Some people thought that therapy would be brief.

I expected a month or two. I stayed about 26 years. I was very surprised. I'm not sure at what point it occurred to me that it was going to take longer than I thought.

[Female, 52, Nonprofessional]

I expected to see her for 3 or 4 months, and she said that there was a commitment of at least a year, and I was taken aback, and thought, "A year? I don't know about a year. Well, all right." But I was thinking I could leave before a year if I didn't want to stay. I stayed almost 10 years. I was surprised by that.

[Female, 45, Professional]

A relatively short amount of time. I actually stayed about 12 years. I was surprised, but it was okay.

[Female, 48, Nonprofessional]

I thought it was going to be fairly short-term, dealing with a work issue. I stayed almost 20 years, on and off. I was surprised at what the process was like, that it's not like talking to a friend.

[Female, 45, Nonprofessional]

Sometimes people accepted the revised length of treatment.

I thought I would see her for 6 months to a year. I stayed about 5½ years. It seemed very natural and very worthwhile.

[Female, 45, Nonprofessional]

I expected to do it maybe a couple of years. I stayed for most of 8 years. I would have stayed longer but I couldn't afford both individual and group.

[Female, 42, Nonprofessional]

I went in to discuss a specific issue and come to terms with that issue, and I wanted to be there for a couple of months and just get it over with. I stayed 2 years, and went back to see her two or three times a year and accessed her by phone two or three times a year for a couple of years after that. I wasn't surprised, because I know that it takes a long time.

[Female, 42, Nonprofessional]

I told her at the beginning that I wasn't there for the duration, that I expected to do something and then get out. I stayed 5 years. I probably could have stayed longer, but I think you have to figure it out sooner or later and then get on with it.

[Male, 52, Nonprofessional]

I knew I wanted to work on some very specific issues, and I probably thought it would be about a dozen sessions. I stayed a full year. I was happy with how fast we were working, and she cautioned me occasionally about going too fast.

[Female, 41, Nonprofessional]

I thought it would take about 6 weeks, 2 months maximum. I actually stayed 12 years. Once I got into it I realized that no superficial answer was going to work.

[Male, 49, Nonprofessional]

And sometimes they were upset that treatment lasted so long.

> I expected to stay maybe a couple of years. I stayed about 10 years. I wasn't surprised, but annoyed. I didn't want to be in therapy that long.
>
> [Female, 50, Professional]

Sometimes people stay longer than they expected because of pressure from the therapist.

> I had no time frame. I stayed 9 years. In retrospect I think I was ready to leave after 7 years, but he didn't think I should.
>
> [Female, 45, Nonprofessional]

> I thought it would be a year or two. It was 10 years. I think I wanted to stop earlier, but I thought she was against that.
>
> [Female, 50, Nonprofessional]

Others expected to be in therapy for some time.

> I had some specific short-term objectives that I wanted to resolve, and I was prepared to go for as long as it would take to resolve them. I actually stayed a year and a half, but that was only because she relocated. I'm sure I would have been there a while.
>
> [Male, 48, Nonprofessional]

Occasionally treatment is briefer than the patient expects.

> I was just expecting to see her till I didn't need to see her anymore. I was expecting a year or 2 years, but that didn't happen. She wasn't able to do anything about the fee, which was very high, so it stopped after 6 months.
>
> [Female, 28, Nonprofessional]

> I expected a couple of years, at least. I stayed until he left town, about a year and a half.
>
> [Male, 30, Professional]

> I always think that it's going to be short-term, but I don't know exactly what that means. I stayed just a few months. Nothing much was happening, and he ended it.
>
> [Female, 48, Nonprofessional]

Many people started therapy with no expectation of its length, and were open to seeing where it went.

I came with some problems initially, and I knew that was where we were going to start. I didn't know if we would go on to talk about some other problems that I had. We ended up doing that. I was there for longer than I thought, for 2 years. I was a little surprised.

[Male, 45, Nonprofessional]

I didn't have a time in mind. It was free so I could just "go with the flow." I stayed 2½ years. I wasn't surprised, because other friends of mine who use the service had gone for years.

[Female, 48, Nonprofessional]

How long it would take was one of my concerns, but I don't think I had any expectation at all. I stayed for 6 years, including a break. Throughout there were periods where I'd be having a lot of frustration and be wanting to leave, like this is going nowhere, and then there'd be periods where I wouldn't feel that way.

[Female, 46, Nonprofessional]

I was open to any length. I stayed about 3 years. Once I got started I was willing to stay for quite a time.

[Male, 52, Nonprofessional]

NUMERICAL DISTRIBUTION

Professionals: Six said they had no expectations; 3 said less than a year; 6 said 1 to 2 years; 5 said as long as the institute training lasted. Of the 14 who had expectations, 10 said they stayed longer than they expected, and 7 of those people said they were surprised at how long they actually stayed in treatment. Average length of treatment was about 7 years.

Nonprofessionals: Nineteen said they had no expectations; 12 said less than a year; 9 said 1 to 2 years. Of the 21 who had expectations, 16 stayed longer than they expected and 11 of them were surprised at how long. Average length of treatment was about 4½ years.

COMMENTS

Professionals seem to stay longer in treatment, which is not surprising since they probably have somewhat different goals. Patients often have a time frame in mind, whether they mention it or not. Long treatment can represent to patients that their problems are deeper and more serious, and they may hope for brief treatment as a sign of mental health. Therapists have to be open to any length of treatment, and not make the patient feel as if he or she is signing a lifetime contract.

As the therapist, I have to respect the patient's plans and not indicate that I expect him to stay forever. If the therapy is going well, the patient is not likely to stop suddenly.

As the patient, how long I plan to stay in treatment depends on why I'm there. If I have a specific complaint I want it to be addressed and treated directly. If I'm there for self-exploration and understanding I probably don't care how long it takes.

RELATED READING

Koss, M. P. (1979). Length of psychotherapy for clients seen in private practice. *Journal of Counseling and Clinical Psychology* 47(1):210–212.

Meyer, W. S. (1993). In defense of long-term treatment: on the vanishing holding environment. *Social Work* 18(5):571–578.

Punter, J. (1995). Report on psychotherapy audit in the NHS: How long do patients stay in therapy? *British Journal of Psychotherapy* 12(2): 251–254.

Westbrook, D. (1991). Can therapists predict length of treatment from referral letters? A pilot study. *Behavioural Psychotherapy* 19(4):377–382.

◈◈◈◈

Question 13: What were your expectations of therapy? Were those expectations met?

What the patient expects from therapy depends a lot on how much he knows about the process. Most of our sample, both professionals and nonprofessionals, had been in a number of treatments.

> I knew what therapy was about, and I was a pretty aggressive worker, ready to get into it. I expected to do some really good work, to go in and deal with the shit that was inside me.
>
> [Male, 46, Nonprofessional]

> I had a lot of expectations, because I had had a lot of prior experience with other therapists, and so—to use a phrase we sometimes use in business—I had the utmost confidence coupled with deep misgivings.
>
> [Male, 48, Nonprofessional]

I expected this to be different, because the therapist I had seen before practiced cognitive therapy, and it was very specific. I expected that I was going to emerge in some way a whole, non-neurotic person.

[Female, 45, Nonprofessional]

Most people expected some insight or understanding of their own behavior and inner dynamics.

I expected to understand more about how I got to be depressed, and what there was about me that did this more than once, and what I was doing in interaction with my environment that led to circumstances that would be depressing.

[Male, 51, Nonprofessional]

I expected to get some help, to figure out what was happening with my marriage and why things went the way they did.

[Male, 48, Nonprofessional]

I expected to find the master key to my own peculiar development, that I would uncover something from earliest childhood that would unlock the mystery.

[Male, 49, Nonprofessional]

I expected to get some insight into why I had gotten so depressed, and why I wasn't recovering.

[Female, 51, Professional]

I expected insight and awareness, so that I could begin to cope better and make better choices.

[Female, 45, Nonprofessional]

I expected that I would understand why I was doing things and feel a lot better.

[Female, 45, Professional]

Several people focused on the emotional aspect of the therapy experience.

I expected to get more than insight—I already had a lot of insight—but to be touched more emotionally, and to maybe deal with some earlier preverbal issues that might have been interfering with being in a relationship.

[Female, 59, Professional]

Some people expected an improvement or alteration in performance or functioning.

> I expected to feel like I wasn't carrying a lot of baggage from childhood, like I could get on with my life.
>
> [Female, 46, Nonprofessional]

> I wanted to get through the crises that I started with, and then after a while it became, "Let me learn about myself, let me learn about this process, let me become a better therapist."
>
> [Male, 53, Professional]

> I remember an overwhelming feeling of not being able to make a decision about anything. I couldn't decide on the simplest things anymore, and I thought that I would be given assistance that would enable me to find clarity in my life. My expectations were definitely met.
>
> [Female, 48, Nonprofessional]

> My hope was that I would have a different outlook on life, that I wouldn't see it as so hard, like it was just work.
>
> [Female, 50, Professional]

> I wanted some kind of relief from the obsessiveness of the pain I was going through. But I also had a lot of anxieties and worries. I'd be excessively concerned if my husband was late, way beyond what is appropriate for someone being late.
>
> [Female, 46, Nonprofessional]

Many people just wanted to feel better.

> I was hoping that I wouldn't feel as bad as I felt.
>
> [Female, 48, Nonprofessional]

> I expected to feel better, less anxious and less depressed.
>
> [Female, 50, Nonprofessional]

> I expected to calm down, feel less anxious, and be able to meet women as a result.
>
> [Male, 50, Professional]

Some expected emotional support.

I was in such crisis, I was looking for a sanctuary and for some wisdom.
[Female, 45, Professional]

I needed some support, and I needed someone to clear some ideas with. Maybe I wanted to be able to handle some situations better.
[Female, 50, Professional]

In the beginning I just wanted to be saved.
[Male, 44, Professional]

Some expected an improvement in self-image, and a diminution of negative attitudes toward themselves.

I wanted to have an enhanced sense of self.
[Female, 57, Professional]

Several people said that they expected to work on a particular issue.

I expected to sort out the relationship and get out of it if I chose to. That was most of my focus and most of what I talked about.
[Female, 50, Nonprofessional]

I expected to be able to work out my issues about commitment in a relationship, and certain work inhibitions that I had.
[Male, 42, Professional]

I expected to come to terms with how I felt about my divorce. I had already decided to get divorced; I wanted to clarify how I was feeling about it.
[Female, 42, Nonprofessional]

I hoped to deal with issues about mothering, about my child. I also wanted to have a clearer sense of direction in my work.
[Female, 48, Professional]

I very much did not want deep psychotherapy. I wanted concrete help—that's why I went to a social worker, because I thought I would get concrete help with my mother's illness.
[Female, 48, Nonprofessional]

I expected to have a clearer understanding of myself and get past the hurdle of the intimacy issue. I thought I had worked it out and then in subsequent relationships I recognized that I was still choosing inappropriate people and the problem had not been solved.

[Female, 41, Nonprofessional]

Limiting the therapy to a particular issue is not always possible, and the focus often widens out to other areas and conflicts.

I expected to be helped with the job issues that brought me in. It went so far beyond that. Once I started talking about that it led into everything else.

[Female, 45, Nonprofessional]

I saw it as going to the orthopedist for a broken ankle, that they would take care of it. I didn't know how, but I didn't need to know. I soon learned that there was a lot more to it.

[Male, 49, Nonprofessional]

I was expecting to have some help losing weight, but it turned out to be more traditional psychotherapy. We did continue with the hypnosis, or at least the attempts with hypnosis. We both decided that the weight was not a simple, vestigial symptom. My eating problems were more complicated. I never did succeed in losing weight.

[Male, 53, Nonprofessional]

Initially I expected it to fix my marriage, and I soon got away from that. I learned that it doesn't work that way. Then I started working on me.

[Female, 40, Nonprofessional]

Several people said they expected a brief therapy, a simple repair of simple problems, and were often surprised that this was not possible.

I expected something that was different from what I got. I underestimated how many of the things that were going on were actually deeply unresolved issues for me. I felt, based on all my previous therapy, that it would be easier to just hook things in and do a little extra work around them. In fact, issues were coming up that I had never dealt with before.

[Female, 58, Professional]

A few people expected education or training in specific skills.

I expected to learn something about Eastern perspectives, and how to meditate.

[Male, 30, Professional]

NUMERICAL DISTRIBUTION

Professionals: Six people said they expected some emotional or intellectual insight; 6 said they expected to feel or function better; 4 said they expected to work on a specific issue; 3 said they expected emotional support; 1 said he expected training in a particular skill. Seventeen said expectations were met or mostly met; 3 said they were disappointed.

Nonprofessionals: Sixteen people said they expected to feel or function better; 15 said they expected to work on a specific issue; 7 people said they expected some emotional or intellectual insight; 1 said he expected emotional support. One person said he had no expectations. Twenty-nine said their expectations were met or exceeded; 11 said they were disappointed.

COMMENTS

Patients with more experience in treatment know that what you expect is not always what you get. Focusing on a specific issue in the present may be difficult when the issue is connected to historical material and unconscious conflicts. It's unfortunate that so many people were disappointed in their treatments; almost a quarter of the total group said they were unhappy in some way with the results.

As the therapist, I know that patients have many kinds of expectations, some of which may not even be conscious. Uncovering all the different expectations, hopes, and wishes is an important part of the process.

As the patient, I expect to see some progress sometime soon, a sense that we are on the right track, a new insight or understanding that leads to some behavioral change, something concrete and specific that confirms the feeling that this therapy is the right thing to be doing.

RELATED READING

Cramer, D., and Takens, R. J. (1992). Therapeutic relationship and progress in the first six sessions of individual psychotherapy: a panel analysis. *Counselling Psychology Quarterly* 5(1):25–36.

Gaston, L., Marmar, C. R., Gallagher, D., and Thompson, L. W. (1989). Impact of comfirming patient expectations of change processes in behavioral, cognitive, and brief dynamic psychotherapy. *Psychotherapy* 26(3):296–302.

Kirsch, I. (1990). *Changing Expectations: A Key to Effective Psychotherapy.* Pacific Grove, CA: Brooks/Cole.

Martin, P. J., Friedmeyer, M. H., Moore, J. E., and Claveaux, R. A. (1977). Patients' expectancies and improvement in treatment: the shape of the link. *Journal of Clinical Psychology* 33(3):827–833.

11
The Treatment

This section covers the course of therapy—sometimes a few months, often many years. The focus throughout is on therapist behavior and patient reactions. Many patients indicated that they had negative feelings about certain therapist practices but often said nothing, out of fear or lack of knowledge. These patients instead may have withdrawn or even quit treatment.

∾∾∾∾

Question 14: Why did you start going?

The reasons a person enters therapy are as varied as the people themselves. Yet there are some things in common: unhappiness or dissatisfaction with current life circumstances; reactions to traumatic events, present or past; and the wish to understand oneself better.

Some people had a very specific goal.

> At the time I was concerned with why I wasn't able to successfully finish a novel.
>
> [Male, 48, Nonprofessional]

> I started going specifically because I had a lot of trouble controlling my weight.
>
> [Male, 53, Nonprofessional]

> I think it was to help me extricate myself from a bad relationship.
> [Female, 45, Nonprofessional]

> I wanted to get divorced.
>
> [Female, 42, Nonprofessional]

> I was having difficulty changing jobs.
>
> [Female, 45, Nonprofessional]

Many people began therapy to deal with a problem in the area of relationship.

> I started because I was leaving a relationship of 14 years and getting involved with another. I was a little concerned about what I was doing.
>
> [Female, 50, Professional]

> I had been in a relationship that was very volatile, and that man broke up with me and I was very depressed. I wasn't sleeping at night.
> [Female, 42, Nonprofessional]

> I started because of the abrupt ending of an important relationship. I was dumped.
>
> [Male, 44, Professional]

I was trying to break up my first marriage at the time, but I didn't have the nerve to do it, and I thought if I got a therapist the therapist would reinforce my feelings and encourage me to do it.

[Male, 49, Nonprofessional]

I was very lonely. I had no dating success for about a year. I was becoming very hopeless and despondent about the possibility of ever meeting anyone who I could relate to. I dated a lot but I couldn't relate to anyone.

[Female, 51, Professional]

It was because of my separation and divorce from my wife. I was so upset and stressed out at the time that I thought I was risking my well-being and stability if I didn't see someone.

[Male, 42, Nonprofessional]

I was at a point where I was suddenly behaving in ways that I had never behaved before. I had always been monogamous, and was in a new relationship and wasn't being monogamous at all and didn't understand why I was behaving that way.

[Female, 45, Professional]

It was relationship disappointment, having had very high expectations for a relationship. I thought I was totally on top of it, and it fell apart in a very explosive manner, and I was totally unprepared, and had no structure to understand it or analyze it or put it in perspective, and I thought I needed someone to help me do that. I thought, "If I can't do this now, when am I ever going to be able to do it?" So I was willing to let someone help me do that.

[Male, 52, Nonprofessional]

I started therapy because I had recognized that I had a history of getting involved with people who weren't very good for me, and I wanted to break that pattern.

[Female, 41, Nonprofessional]

Some began treatment due to depression.

I had recognized myself for the first time as being depressed. I'm pretty extroverted, but a lot of that is facade. I didn't feel a lot of joy in life.

[Female, 50, Professional]

The immediate events that triggered it for me were that I had lost a pregnancy. I had a mid-term abortion for anomalous genetic problems. Then I had years of infertility. That was the most devastating thing that ever happened, and I was at a very high level of depression.

[Female, 46, Nonprofessional]

Some started treatment to deal with anxiety.

I was having panic attacks.

[Female, 28, Nonprofessional]

I wanted to work on a very specific area of anxiety.

[Female, 56, Professional]

I was anxious about the transition to a new city. I had been out of social work school a year, working in another city, and I was anxious about getting settled and meeting people, and my therapist in the old city thought that being in a group would help with those anxieties.

[Male, 50, Professional]

Some people were unhappy with the way they were functioning.

I felt like I couldn't tell why I was doing things.

[Female, 39, Nonprofessional]

I didn't have a grasp on my life: I was unhappy, I didn't know what was wrong, I'd lose my temper very easily, I didn't have a direction, I didn't know how I was going to get anywhere I wanted to.

[Female, 52, Nonprofessional]

It was just feeling that I was out of control, not having a grasp on things that were going on.

[Female, 26, Nonprofessional]

I've always been a moody person, and at the time I was facing the inevitability of an organ transplant. I was walking around with a lot of bottled-up stuff. I had always been a people pleaser. I never gave myself much comfort.

[Male, 46, Nonprofessional]

I was having some kind of breakdown. I really didn't want therapy, I wanted to be hospitalized. I felt so desperate, and the psychiatrist I saw to get some tranquilizers, or to be hospitalized so that I could be taken out of the world and be told I didn't have to work on this, said that I had to work on this, that it was the only thing I could do. He said that it wasn't chemical, it was psychogenic, and I had to work on it. In a sense, I didn't have a choice. I wasn't that eager to go, except that I was desperate.

[Female, 50, Nonprofessional]

A few people mentioned a difficult family situation as the main reason for starting therapy.

I had just left my husband, and was a single mother with a 2-year-old.

[Female, 50, Nonprofessional]

I was a young mother, and I was having a lot of problems with my little girl. It was hard to be home—it was boring, understimulating.

[Female, 48, Professional]

I was having trouble dealing with who am I now that I'm a mother and I'm not working full-time. I needed a sounding board.

[Female, 39, Professional]

My husband was going through a crisis with his business and was relying on me for support. I had a brand-new baby, and we were living in a foreign country. The combination of all those things caused me to feel I needed support.

[Female, 53, Nonprofessional]

I had lost one parent, and the other was dying.

[Female, 45, Professional]

My mother was sick and I started needing advice on how to help deal with her and how I could feel better about dealing with her.

[Female, 48, Nonprofessional]

A traumatic incident, past or present, can sometimes be the stimulus for starting therapy.

It was right after having the man I was living with simply disappear, never to be heard from again, so I was in a kind of post-traumatic shock.

[Female, 48, Nonprofessional]

I grew up with a crazy father, who killed himself and my brother when I was in my early twenties. I walked around for about 15 years after that worrying that I was crazy, because I felt so much like him. When I realized that I wasn't crazy but that I did have some stuff to work on, I went into therapy.

[Female, 46, Nonprofessional]

Professionals often began treatment as a part of training.

I was in training, and graduate school was very stressful. I wanted to have the experience of being in therapy, more than I had been. I wanted to learn to do the kind of therapy that my therapist had written about in his book.

[Male, 30, Professional]

I started because I was required to as part of my training.

[Female, 55, Professional]

I started analytic training and it was required.

[Male, 42, Professional]

I was in social work school, and I had had a bad experience with another therapist. I thought that when seeing patients, which is what you immediately start doing in school, I wanted to have someone to help me through that—and everyone else in school was in therapy. I felt that it was important in doing this kind of work to make sure that you don't have any of your own craziness.

[Female, 50, Professional]

Several people said that they were told to start therapy.

I went because the woman I was with said I needed to.

[Male, 52, Nonprofessional]

I didn't feel a need to go, but other people around me said I needed to go. This was right after the breakup of my marriage.

[Male, 43, Nonprofessional]

NUMERICAL DISTRIBUTION

Professionals: Six started the most recent therapy as a training requirement; 6 started because of relationship problems; 3 started because of anxiety; 3 started because of depression; 2 began due to family or parenting issues. Average age at start of treatment was 39.4 years.

Nonprofessionals: Twenty said they started due to relationship problems or difficulties; 8 because they were unhappy with their level of functioning in a specific area or in general; 5 because of depression; 4 because of anxiety; 3 due to a problematic family situation. Average age at start of treatment was 36.2 years.

COMMENTS

The main difference here is that so many professionals began therapy as a training requirement. Of course, someone can use this professional requirement as a way to start treatment without having to admit that problems exist. With the exceptions of professionals who start therapy because of a training requirement and those who are told to go by a spouse, almost everyone begins treatment because he is unhappy with some aspect of his own functioning. The situation that pushes the patient into that state can be almost anything, but at some point things reach a critical mass and action is taken. Some patients begin with relief, some with reluctance or resentment, but all recognize the need to do something.

As the therapist, I don't really care why someone starts, except as it sheds light on the issues. The work is the same no matter what the reason.

As the patient beginning treatment, I'm nervous about the new situation but relieved to finally be doing something about whatever has been bothering me. I have probably realized that, whatever the problem, I have been creating or contributing to it in some way, and want enough insight and understanding to be able to change my own part of the situation.

RELATED READING

Cornell, W. F. (1986). Setting the therapeutic stage: the initial sessions. *Transactional Analysis Journal* 16(1):4–10.

Garfield, S. L. (1989). The prediction of outcome in psychotherapy. In *Psychotherapy*. Directions in Psychiatry Monograph Series, No. 5, ed. F. Flach, pp. 30–42.

Saccuzzo, D. P. (1975). What patients want from counseling and psychotherapy. *Journal of Clinical Psychology* 31(3):471–475.

🎑🎑🎑🎑

Question 15: How often did you go each week?

The original therapy, psychoanalysis, was conducted 4, 5, even 6 times a week. How often do people normally go now?

Most people, professionals and nonprofessionals, simply said they went once a week; a smaller number said they went twice a week; and a few said they went 3 times a week. Once the frequency was set, it was normally maintained until the end of treatment.

A few patients said the schedule varied quite a bit.

> I started twice a week, moved to 3 times a week after about 2 or 3 years. Two years later, I joined his group and dropped one of the individual sessions.
>
> [Male, 53, Professional]

> I started going once a week, then I quickly went to twice a week, and then 3 times a week.
>
> [Female, 48, Professional]

> Generally I went once a week. There were times when I was going twice a week, and group as well.
>
> [Male, 49, Nonprofessional]

> I went at least once a week, but often twice for long periods of time, and occasionally 3 times a week. It was always at my request.
>
> [Male, 44, Professional]

> I started at once a week, went up to 3 times a week, and then back down.
>
> [Male, 52, Nonprofessional]

Several people said the frequency changed over time in response to crisis situations.

> I went once a week, but during times of crisis twice a week.
>
> [Female, 45, Professional]

There may be more sessions in the beginning of treatment, until the precipitating crisis has died down.

> For the first 4 weeks I went twice a week. After that it was once.
>
> [Male, 42, Nonprofessional]

> In the beginning I went twice a week, maybe even 3 times.
>
> [Female, 48, Nonprofessional]

Often patients are in a group as well as individual therapy.

> For a while, I was just in group, then group plus individual once a week, then just group, then group plus 1, 2, or 3 times a week.
>
> [Male, 50, Professional]

> I went once a week for about a year, and then I joined his group too. At some point I added a second individual session.
>
> [Female, 50, Professional]

Occasionally a patient's schedule is less frequent for financial reasons, or because the therapy is tapering off.

> For a while I went every other week because I couldn't afford more. Then I got a job that enabled me to go weekly.
>
> [Male, 30, Professional]

> Toward the end when I was weaning off I went about once every 2 months.
>
> [Female, 48, Nonprofessional]

> In the beginning I went 3 times a week, then 2 times, and the last few years just once a week.
>
> [Female, 45, Nonprofessional]

NUMERICAL DISTRIBUTION

Professionals: Twelve people said once a week; 4 said twice a week; 4 said three times a week. Seven people said it sometimes varied, or changed over time. Some people also had a group session each week.

Nonprofessionals: Thirty-two people said they went once a week; 7 said twice a week; 1 said three times a week. Ten of them said it varied over time, usually from fewer to more sessions.

COMMENTS

How often the patient sees the therapist varies widely, although these days very few people are in traditional psychoanalysis 4 or 5 times a week. Managed care will not cover such treatment, and few people can afford it on their own.

As the therapist, I believe strongly that good treatment can be done when seeing people once a week. Therapists often underestimate the work that patients do between sessions, and letting the patient live with the material for the intervening week can be productive.

As the patient, I don't want the therapist pressuring me to come more often. I may read that as a sign that he or she thinks I'm unable to function on my own. If I decide that I want more sessions, I'll say so.

RELATED READING

Appelbaum, S. A. (1992). Evils in the practice of psychotherapy. *Bulletin of the Menninger Clinic* 56(2):141–149.
Gedo, P. M., and Kohler, B. J. (1992). Session frequency, regressive intensity, and the psychoanalytic process. *Psychoanalytic Psychology* 9(2):245–249.
Greenberg, S. (1986). Analysis once a week. *American Journal of Psychoanalysis* 46(4):327–335.

🔊🔊🔊🔊

Question 16: How long was the session? Did it ever run over?

Therapists have a standard session length, usually 45 or 50 minutes (group sessions are usually 90 minutes). Most of the interviewees said the session time was one of these. A few people mentioned an unusual arrangement.

> After 15 years, we switched to hour-long sessions, and I pay for a session and a third. I wanted more time.
>
> [Male, 53, Professional]

Therapists differ on how well they keep the limit. Some are very strict about the session time, and patients often are angry about that.

> It never ran over. Maybe once or twice. My therapist was the queen of the boundary line.
>
> [Female, 47, Nonprofessional]

> It was 45 minutes to the second. It never started a second before and never ran a second over.
>
> [Female, 57, Professional]

It was 50 minutes. A couple of times we ran over, but not often and it wasn't encouraged.

[Male, 52, Nonprofessional]

She ended on time and she would never start a minute early.

[Female, 62, Professional]

It started and ended on the button. It was consistent with my whole experience with her of being deprived.

[Male, 44, Professional]

It might have run over a little, but they always keep their eye on the clock.

[Female, 42, Nonprofessional]

Some patients liked the strict limits, seeing them as implying something positive about the therapist.

It rarely ran over. She was very professional, if that's the right word. This was the time we had to do it in. She was very busy, and I respected her time. She respected my time, and she was never late so that I never had to wait for her.

[Female, 40, Nonprofessional]

A number of people said the session might run a little long if they were in the middle of something.

She was flexible. Oftentimes she would say, "We're running a little bit over but it's okay because I want to wrap this up."

[Female, 44, Nonprofessional]

Occasionally it would run over, if I was really into something, or if he was in the middle of making an interpretation.

[Male, 42, Professional]

It would run over maybe a couple of minutes if something really emotional was happening.

[Female, 48, Nonprofessional]

If I was really upset about something he'd give me another few minutes to calm down, with full consciousness that the session was really over.

[Female, 52, Nonprofessional]

Once in a while it would run over, if it was the middle of some kind of deep work. She pretty much kept to the time.

[Female, 45, Professional]

If we were talking about something sensitive, he would finish the topic.

[Male, 48, Nonprofessional]

Some people liked the meaning of the extra time.

There wasn't a clock visible. I would refer to my watch but I was her last appointment of the day, so there was a looseness about the time. It made me feel a little special.

[Female, 45, Professional]

It was supposed to be 50 minutes, but she very often went over, because she was generous. That felt good.

[Female, 50, Nonprofessional]

It was 45 or 50 minutes, but if something came up she would spend the extra time. I appreciated that.

[Female, 50, Professional]

Occasionally it would run over, because we had really gotten into something and she wasn't going to stop. She was very respectful; she wasn't going to just pull the plug.

[Female, 46, Nonprofessional]

Some people found the uncertainty about the limits disturbing, even when they liked the extra time.

It was 45 or 50 minutes—it wasn't always clear, and I don't remember what the agreed-upon hour was. She didn't have a standard set way to end the session, and very often I found that I would be looking at my watch or looking at the clock that I could see and waiting for her to indicate that we had to finish, and she wouldn't give me that, so I would say, "Well, don't we have to stop now?" She would say, "Yes." That made me uncomfortable because I expected that it was her responsibility to say when we were to finish. We spent some time talking about this, and she said she was aware of this as being a general problem, and she was actually working with her supervisor on it.

[Male, 48, Nonprofessional]

Occasionally, the length of the session got shorter.

> When we switched from free EAP sessions to a regular fee, the sessions got shorter, just 45 minutes, which I thought might have been commensurate with some kind of break she was giving me on the fee.
>
> [Male, 42, Nonprofessional]

> It started at 50 minutes. Toward the end she changed her schedule and shortened it to 45 minutes.
>
> [Female, 42, Nonprofessional]

Some therapists started sessions late, and patients often found this disturbing.

> I think it was 45 minutes, but often it would start late, and it would piss me off, and that became one of our biggest problems. It didn't run over, except when he was really late, when he would offer me the extra time, but because I was a therapist I was on such a tight schedule that I couldn't stay and I got shortchanged a lot.
>
> [Female, 48, Professional]

NUMERICAL DISTRIBUTION

Professionals: Twelve people said 45 minutes; 6 said 50 minutes; 2 said a full hour. Eleven said it would occasionally run over, if they were in the middle of something; 9 said it never ran over.

Nonprofessionals: Seven people said the session was 45 minutes; 29 said 50 minutes; 3 said it was a full hour; 1 said a group session was 90 minutes. Six people said it often ran over; 17 said it occasionally ran over; 17 said it never ran over.

COMMENTS

Whatever the standard session length, alterations in the allotted time have conscious and unconscious implications about the therapist's adherence to structure and rules. Without being rigid or hurtful, the therapist can keep the time fairly consistent and help the patient contain the material.

As the therapist, I try always to start and end on time. I keep the 10-minute buffer between sessions because ending on the stroke of time is not possible, and because I need the break.

As the patient, I may resent having to stop in the middle of something, but I would prefer that to being unclear about the structure of the hour. I might enjoy the extra time and even see it as a generous gift, but I might feel guilty about taking advantage. I might also wonder about the therapist's ability to keep confidences and obey the other rules.

RELATED READING

Bierenbaum, H., Nichols, M. P., and Schwartz, A. J. (1976). Effects of varying session length and frequency in brief emotive psychotherapy. *Journal of Consulting and Clinical Psychology* 44(5):790–798.

Hammer, E. (1990). Modifications of session length. In *Reaching the Affect: Style in the Psychodynamic Therapies*. Northvale, NJ: Jason Aronson.

Turner, P. R., Valtierra, M., Talken, T. R., et al. (1996). Effect of session length on treatment outcome for college students in brief therapy. *Journal of Counseling Psychology* 43(2):228–232.

Waugaman, R. M. (1992). Analytic time. *Journal of the American Academy of Psychoanalysis* 20(1):29–47.

🔊🔊🔊🔊

Question 17: Did the therapist seem to take a break between sessions, or did your session start as another person left?

The traditional therapeutic hour of 45 or 50 minutes allows for a brief break between patients, but not all therapists take one. In the *Shrink Rap* sample, 26 did and 23 didn't, with another 11 saying they sometimes did and sometimes didn't. What are patient reactions to these behaviors?

Several patients mentioned that they liked having the therapist take a break between sessions.

> For the most part, there was no one coming in as I left. I don't want to bump into anyone in the therapist's office, even strangers.
>
> [Female, 40, Nonprofessional]

> He always took a break. I never felt like I was walking in on an assembly line.
>
> [Male, 46, Nonprofessional]

I very rarely had the feeling that someone was talking in the next room, which I would not have liked. She spaced people out so that never happened. One period of time there was someone right before me.

[Female, 51, Professional]

Some patients have a negative reaction to the absence of a break between sessions.

She didn't seem to take much of a break. I think I saw people leaving as I was entering. Sometimes it seemed a little awkward—the management of people, the traffic. And of course the session would start late as a result, if the prior session ran over.

[Male, 48, Nonprofessional]

I never had feelings of rivalry with other patients, but there was always something perfunctory about the whole relationship. This session's over—Next!

[Male, 44, Professional]

Sometimes a guy came in as I left. It was kind of weird to see and be seen.

[Female, 26, Nonprofessional]

In one situation I was her first patient. Sometimes when I left there was someone in the waiting room but I couldn't tell if that was for her or the other therapist. Sometimes it seemed that she went from one to the next. I sometimes wondered how she could go so quickly from person to person. I would think that you would want some time to clear your head.

[Female, 50, Professional]

Sometimes I wondered if he would be there for me, because this other person had just walked out of the office. Where's his mind?

[Female, 50, Nonprofessional]

As I was leaving she would be greeting the next person, and I can remember thinking, *She's so warm and friendly with these people*, and wondering if I had a special relationship with her, after she greeted these people who were very different from me.

[Female, 39, Professional]

Some people didn't mind there being no break between sessions.

She seemed very much there when I was with her. Every now and then she would take a break to use the bathroom or make a phone call, and she always gave me 5 minutes more at the end.

[Female, 45, Nonprofessional]

Often it started immediately after someone left. It didn't bother me.

[Female, 50, Nonprofessional]

Professionals were more understanding of the therapist who did not take a break between appointments.

He did not take a break. I can sometimes go without a break myself and I assumed he could too.

[Female, 57, Professional]

My session started as another person left. I identified with him as a hard-working therapist, and sometimes I was envious of him because he seemed to have a busier practice than I did. I know that I don't always take a break, and everyone is so different that the next person is a break from the person before.

[Female, 58, Professional]

Not taking a break between appointments can lead to scheduling problems, and even professionals can be angry about that.

My therapist didn't take a break. Generally it was okay, but there were times when I was working and I felt a lot of pressure to get back to the office on time. He was always willing to go late if we started late, but on my part I didn't always have the time. There were a couple of years when it was an issue, his starting late and my anxiety about whether I would get all my minutes back.

[Male, 50, Professional]

I don't think he had a break scheduled, but he sometimes needed one. He had his office in his house, and sometimes he would run upstairs to use the bathroom, but I think he did it on my time. Phone calls too. It happened many, many times.

[Female, 48, Professional]

He didn't take a break, but he would run out before my session to use the bathroom. It bothered me that he would sometimes start late.

[Female, 50, Professional]

An office with separate doors can make it easier to keep patients from encountering each other, even without a break between sessions.

> The therapist had a way of ushering me in one door and ushering the former patient out another so we wouldn't see one another.
>
> [Male, 42, Nonprofessional]

NUMERICAL DISTRIBUTION

Professionals: Twelve people said they thought the therapist did not take a break between patients; 6 said the therapist did take a break; 2 said they could not tell because they were the first or last session.

Nonprofessionals: Twenty-five people said the therapist took a break; 11 said there was no break; 4 said they couldn't tell.

COMMENTS

A much higher percentage of the professionals said that the therapist did not take a break, and, as reflected in the answers, many had feelings about that. Therapists can't assume that any behavior of theirs is irrelevant or meaningless to patients.

As the therapist, I have never understood how a therapist can see patient after patient without a break between appointments. Making notes, using the bathroom, or returning phone calls become impossible, and the therapist inevitably does some of these things anyway and winds up starting and finishing sessions late. The responses to this question suggest that this is an area in which patients have feelings about the issue that they don't always tell the therapist.

As the patient, I don't want to see the therapist rushing between patients to use the bathroom. I also don't want to be starting the session late because the therapist has gotten jammed up, which then makes me late for whatever I have to do. I want to know that the therapist is taking good care of himself as well as of me; otherwise I may wonder how well he's capable of taking care of either of us.

RELATED READING

Greenson, R. (1974). The decline and fall of the fifty-minute hour. *Journal of the American Psychoanalytic Association* 22:785–791.

Langs, R. (1982) *Psychotherapy: A Basic Text.* New York: Jason Aronson.

🔳🔳🔳🔳

Question 18: How did the therapist set the fee?

Patients know that fees can range from low to high. How did therapists tell patients about the fee?

In many cases, the therapist simply announces what the fee will be.

> He told me what the fee was.
>
> [Female, 57, Professional]

> She announced what her fee was.
>
> [Male, 48, Nonprofessional]

> He had his fee and that was it.
>
> [Female, 59, Professional]

> My impression was that there was one fee and that was it.
>
> [Male, 48, Nonprofessional]

> She told me what she charged.
>
> [Female, 52, Professional]

Often the therapist has a sliding scale, and will negotiate the fee with the patient.

> One of the reasons I went to her was that my income was quite low, and I found out that the fee would be set according to my ability to pay. So when I first started to see her the fee was set appropriately.
>
> [Female, 48, Nonprofessional]

> She told me her fee, and I told her it was a little high, and she said if I was willing to see her earlier in the day she would lower it some, so I did.
>
> [Female, 51, Professional]

> We talked about my income and she gave me a break. I was only working part-time and she gave me a low fee. She also charged me less because I came twice a week.
>
> [Female, 42, Nonprofessional]

> There was discussion of what kind of insurance I had, what my co-payment was, and what I thought I could afford.
>
> [Female, 39, Professional]

She set the fee based on what we could afford. I sensed that it was lower than her normal fee.

[Female, 44, Nonprofessional]

He told me what he typically charged and then we discussed what I could afford, and he came down to the lowest he felt he could come down to.

[Male, 30, Professional]

We discussed it. It was a different fee if I came in the evening than in the afternoon. For twice a week, the second session would be less.

[Female, 50, Professional]

We set it together. He wanted to know what I could pay and I told him and he said that was fine.

[Male, 42, Professional]

Sometimes the patient will decline the offer of a fee adjustment.

She said it was a certain amount, but that there was a sliding scale if that was a problem. I said it wasn't and I would pay the full fee.

[Female, 41, Nonprofessional]

I had the sense that I could have negotiated the fee at the beginning, if I had said that I was a starving student or something.

[Female, 39, Nonprofessional]

Sometimes the therapist will adjust the usual fee to the circumstances of the patient.

It wasn't a high fee originally because I think she was still in school. She announced the fee.

[Female, 45, Professional]

In the first place the fee was kind to me because I didn't have a lot of money.

[Male, 52, Nonprofessional]

Because I was in school he started me at a fairly low fee. He said that he had a sliding scale, but he was also considering my husband's salary. I felt it was fair.

[Female, 50, Professional]

And sometimes the therapist lets the patient indicate what the fee should be.

> I told her what I could afford and she agreed to it.
> [Female, 55, Professional]

If the patient goes through an agency, they usually set the fee.

> It was set by the clinic on a sliding scale. It was very fair.
> [Female, 48, Nonprofessional]

> The fee was set initially by the referral service and confirmed by him.
> [Male, 53, Professional]

> The center set the fee, and she was the only one who would see me at that fee, even though it felt high to me.
> [Female, 28, Nonprofessional]

In recent days, the fee is sometimes set by the HMO.

> Her regular fee was higher by $10 than my insurance covered, and she accepted the lower fee.
> [Male, 49, Nonprofessional]

> It was set by the insurance company.
> [Female, 41, Nonprofessional]

> It was an HMO and was completely covered.
> [Male, 50, Nonprofessional]

NUMERICAL DISTRIBUTION

Professionals: Ten said the therapist announced what the fee was; 8 said the fee was discussed or negotiated; and 2 said it was set by the clinic or referral service.

Nonprofessionals: Twenty-three said the therapist announced what the fee was; 11 said it was negotiated; 3 said it was set by the clinic or HMO; and 3 said there was no fee.

COMMENTS

The same proportion of the two groups answered this question the same way. In most cases the fee was simply announced and the patient accepted.

Many therapists do announce the fee, and others invite discussion and negotiation by mentioning a sliding scale. I prefer to say directly that my fee is X and, if the patient objects or has difficulty with it, to discuss other possibilities.

As a patient, I don't want to resent the fee; I want to feel I'm getting what I need without sacrificing too much of my income, without having to suffer for it. I would prefer the opportunity for negotiation if the announced fee seems too high, but the therapist who announces she has a sliding scale from X to Y and asks me what I can afford puts too much responsibility on me.

RELATED READING

Citron-Baggett, S., and Kempler, B. (1991). Fee setting: dynamic issues for therapists in independent practice. *Psychotherapy in Private Practice* 9(1):45–60.

Herrell, J. M. (1993). The psychotherapeutic value of fees: What do practitioners believe? *Journal of Mental Health Administration* 20(3): 270–277.

Herron, W. G. (1995). Visible and invisible psychotherapy fees. *Psychotherapy in Private Practice* 14(2):7–17.

Shields, J. D. (1996). Hostage of the fee: meanings of money, countertransference, and the beginning therapist. *Psychoanalytic Psychotherapy* 10(3):233–250.

⊠⊠⊠⊠

Question 19: How often did you pay the bill? Who set it up that way?

Different therapists have different policies for when payment is due. Some prefer the patient to pay monthly; some prefer payment at each session; some have other arrangements depending on the patient's schedule.

Traditionally, the patient was given a bill at the end of the month. Many therapists still do it this way.

> We paid once a month. She would give us a bill.
>
> [Female, 44, Nonprofessional]

I paid once a month. She would hand me a bill. If my last session was moved to the next month, she would mail the bill.

[Female, 47, Nonprofessional]

I paid once a month. That was what she was comfortable with.

[Male, 48, Nonprofessional]

Once in a while the arrangement changes.

I started by paying every week, and then went to once a month.

[Male, 49, Nonprofessional]

I started out paying every week, which was my idea, but she hated it and we switched to monthly. It was more bookkeeping than she liked.

[Female, 51, Professional]

Many therapists ask for payment at each session.

I paid every week. I think it was her idea, but it would have been my preference.

[Female, 50, Professional]

I paid weekly. That was what she requested.

[Female, 40, Nonprofessional]

I paid every week, at her request.

[Female, 45, Professional]

Sometimes this arrangement is the patient's idea.

I paid for each session, because I went every other week.

[Male, 30, Professional]

I always pay at the end of each session. That's what I'm used to, and it was fine with him.

[Female, 48, Nonprofessional]

This policy may have a negative meaning to the patient.

If I had to pay every time that would bother me, because it would mean we don't trust each other.

[Female, 50, Professional]

Some therapists offer the patient a choice.

> I was going 3 times a week and I paid in the third session each week. He offered the choice of the end of each week or the end of the month, and I said that paying each week would feel less expensive.
> [Female, 57, Professional]

> I paid monthly. It was just part of the culture. It was never even discussed.
> [Male, 50, Professional]

> I paid at the end of the month. I decided to do that because it was more convenient for me once a month.
> [Male, 42, Professional]

Occasionally the patient arrives at an unusual arrangement.

> I paid every 2 weeks, which was something that developed organically; nobody ever said to do it that way.
> [Male, 44, Professional]

> I paid her at the end of the month. In the beginning, because part of the problem I was having was with money, I even paid her ahead of time to insure that I didn't fuck up and not have the money at the end of the month.
> [Female, 48, Nonprofessional]

Sometimes the policy is unclear.

> He didn't explain to me at the beginning, and ended up telling me that I was paying way too late, and that angered me too.
> [Female, 48, Professional]

NUMERICAL DISTRIBUTION

Professionals: Twelve said they paid monthly; 7 said weekly; 1 said every two weeks. Overall, 14 said it was the therapist's request; 6 said it was their own decision.

Nonprofessionals: Twenty-one said they paid monthly; 17 paid weekly; 2 had no fee. Overall, 28 said it was the therapist's request; 10 said it was their own decision.

COMMENTS

The two groups were again similar in responses to this question. There is a fairly even division between monthly and weekly payment. I'm surprised that the patient so often gets to decide which it will be.

I don't think it much matters whether the patient pays weekly, monthly, or some other variation, as long as the rule is clear and the patient is consistent. Weekly payment seems easier to me because I don't have to keep track of a balance, and because monthly bills are additional work.

As a patient, I prefer to pay weekly because I don't build up a large debt at the end of each month, when I may or may not have the money.

RELATED READING

Bishop, D. R., and Eppolito, J. M. (1992). The clinical management of client dynamics and fees for psychotherapy: implications for research and practice. *Psychotherapy* 29(4):545–553.

Herron, W. G. (1994). Dealing with fees in psychotherapy. In *Innovations in Clinical Practice: A Source Book,* vol. 13, ed. L. Vande Creek, S. Knapp, and T. L. Jackson, pp. 223–235. Sarasota, FL: Professional Resource Press.

Klebanow, S., and Lowenkopf, E. L., eds. (1991). *Money and Mind.* New York: Plenum.

Knapp, S., and VandeCreek, L. (1993). Legal and ethical issues in billing patients and collecting fees. *Psychotherapy* 30(1):25–31.

🐚🐚🐚🐚

Question 20: Did your therapist ever raise the fee?

Many therapists raise the fee in the course of a long treatment, and patients often have strong feelings about the meaning of such a change.

Many therapists raise the fee regularly, as a cost-of-living increase.

> Once or twice I left and came back, and when I came back I always came back to a higher fee by five or ten dollars.
>
> [Female, 45, Nonprofessional]

> It went up a couple of times. It got a little more significant as it got higher, and it was hard for me. There was a time when I was seeing

her twice a week and it got impossibly expensive. I mentioned that it was tough but that I respected her.

[Female, 50, Nonprofessional]

Every year he raised it at least $5, and that pissed me off because I thought, *When will it end?* He would always say that it was a cost-of-living increase. It was hard when we lost our insurance. There were things that happened that he didn't seem to take into consideration.

[Female, 48, Professional]

Over the years it would go up from time to time. I never had a problem with that.

[Male, 49, Nonprofessional]

He did a couple of times. It was just inflation. It seemed fair. Initially I had a negative reaction, and we discussed it.

[Male, 48, Nonprofessional]

Some therapists wait for the patient to agree to a raise before putting it into effect.

There were numerous occasions over 25 years. It was always negotiated. I had to accept it, although he was firm. It was a combination, that I may be ready to pay this and I may have the money now, but also he stayed out of the area of my money, and said that I knew best what I could afford.

[Male, 53, Professional]

Each year he would ask me if he could have a fee increase, and what it would be, and I told him what I could afford, and we would either increase the fee or not. The first year of analysis when I didn't have much money he charged me very little.

[Male, 42, Professional]

In a few unusual situations, the patient asked for the increase.

I requested that she raise the fee. I asked her why she was charging that fee, because it was too low, and I asked her to raise it out of concern for her and her managing her practice.

[Female, 47, Nonprofessional]

At one time I asked her how come she wasn't raising my fee, because it was the same fee for 2½ years. She said that it was something she was having trouble with herself. I think it came up when she wanted to raise it like 10 cents. I felt that her not charging me enough meant that she wasn't taking it seriously and wasn't really working.

[Male, 52, Nonprofessional]

Sometimes patients accept the increase.

Her rate was going up just like mine does every year. It's a business and I understand that.

[Female, 42, Nonprofessional]

I always hated it but I understood it.

[Female, 45, Professional]

When I changed from twice a week to once a week, she raised it, and that seemed fair. She raised it again when my income went up.

[Female, 42, Nonprofessional]

The fee was set according to my income, so during the time I saw her, as my income went up, the fee was raised. Each time I resented it a little bit, but not enough to challenge it. I was very committed to the process, it was very important to me, so I never challenged how much she was worth to my life.

[Female, 48, Nonprofessional]

It went up but not much. She would give me notice in advance of about a month. I always said okay. I knew I was low when I started, so whatever she said was okay.

[Female, 45, Nonprofessional]

Occasionally the fee raise has a positive meaning to the patient.

When I started making more money, after I paid off what I owed him, he raised it, and 2 months later raised it again, and got me up to his going rate. He didn't do that until I could afford it, and I felt so proud that I was paying his full fee. I was deeply grateful.

[Female, 52, Nonprofessional]

Some people said that the absence of a fee increase had a special meaning.

He raised the fee for other people, but not for me.

[Female, 45, Nonprofessional]

> As her fees went up, she didn't raise mine as much. You had some seniority in her system. If you'd been there long enough, you got a special deal.
>
> [Female, 50, Nonprofessional]

Often patients are angry about fee raises.

> His fee became an issue, because at that time I was having a lot of trouble with money. I was a single parent and it was costing me $8,000 a year just for babysitting. Part of what I was depressed about was that I never had enough money to take care of myself. When he kept raising his fee, I remember being very angry. He was a very good dresser and very into his appearance, and I remember getting preoccupied with how much his socks cost.
>
> [Female, 58, Professional]

> I frequently felt unhappy about it, if it meant that I couldn't see him as much as I wanted to, or if it created a financial constraint for me. There were times when I was spending all of my money on therapy, and in retrospect I question whether that was in my best interest. It plays into my being more liberal and easy about my own patients. I'm not offended that people want to be in therapy and also want to be able to go out on dates.
>
> [Male, 50, Professional]

A fee raise can sometimes lead to the patient quitting therapy.

> One time it was $15, which seemed out of line. I was very angry about it and quit soon afterward.
>
> [Female, 44, Nonprofessional]

> I told her I couldn't afford it. She heard me, but there was no negotiation about it. She was going on vacation and when she came back I terminated.
>
> [Female, 45, Professional]

> It went up a couple of times. She moved to a nicer office so it seemed reasonable. I was getting a break to start with so it was just moving up to the normal rate. It helped me get out.
>
> [Male, 52, Nonprofessional]

Therapists are sometimes unwilling to discuss the merits of the increase.

She raised it once. I was angry. She said she thought she had been eminently fair, and that other people did not complain.

[Female, 55, Professional]

Fee raises can sometimes lead to awkward situations.

She raised it a couple of times in the course of treatment. I went back recently for a single session, and apparently her fee had increased, and she didn't tell me about it. I handed her a check and she sent me a supplementary bill. I would not have done it that way.

[Female, 62, Professional]

NUMERICAL DISTRIBUTION

Professionals: Eleven said the fee had been raised; 9 said it had not.
Nonprofessionals: Seventeen said the fee had been raised; 22 said it had not. One person said there had been no fee.

COMMENTS

This is a complicated question: Is it fair to raise the fee when the contract was made to meet at a specific fee? Some therapists announce in the first session that fee increases can be expected after a certain time, and this seems like a good thing to do.

As the therapist, I have recently started asking permission for any fee increase, rather than simply announcing it, as a way of making the increase feel as fair as possible. I don't want the patient to resent an increase, but I don't want to resent carrying at a low fee someone who can afford the increase.

As a patient, I'm never going to like paying more for the same product, but I realize that whenever I go to the store all the prices have gone up. All I ask is that the realities of my financial situation be recognized and that I be part of the decision process.

RELATED READING

Herron, W. G. (1996). Revisiting fee policies. *Psychological Reports* 78(3, pt. 1): 881–882.

Lien, C. (1993). The ethics of the sliding fee scale. *Journal of Mental Health Counseling* 15(3):334–341.

Power, L. C., and Pilgrim, D. (1990). The fee in psychotherapy: practitioners' accounts. *Counselling Psychology Quarterly* 3(2):153–170.

Yoken, C., and Berman, J. S. (1984). Does paying a fee for psychotherapy alter the effectiveness of treatment? *Journal of Consulting and Clinical Psychology* 52(2):254–260.

🅡🅡🅡🅡

Question 21: Did your therapist ever lower the fee?

Many therapists will lower the fee when a patient's circumstances might otherwise make it impossible to continue treatment.

> There was a period of time that I was out of work and she lowered the fee, and although I went every week, I paid her only for every other week. This was after years of treatment.
>
> [Female, 47, Nonprofessional]

> I was in a bad spot financially and emotionally, and I offered to reduce my frequency of sessions. He asked whether that would be putting myself into too much distress and jeopardy, which I felt was the case and told him so. He said, "Then why don't we consider lowering the fee?" It was extremely touching to me.
>
> [Male, 53, Professional]

> When my insurance ran out, and it was a short period when I was going more than once a week, I told her frankly it was too much and she reduced it.
>
> [Female, 45, Nonprofessional]

> She did, because my income went down. I lost my job. I felt that it increased my obligation to make the payments.
>
> [Female, 48, Nonprofessional]

> At one point when I was financially having a hard time—I was in school—she lowered the fee for about 8 months. I felt really taken care of. It felt really understanding. And it was hard for me to take, so it was also therapeutic.
>
> [Female, 45, Professional]

> She lowered it when I went back to school.
>
> [Male, 49, Nonprofessional]

Patients don't always appreciate the offer of a lower fee.

> I think it was an attempt to placate me because I was so pissed off.
> [Female, 48, Professional]

Some therapists will lower the fee at the beginning of treatment if the situation seems to warrant it.

> He started me at a low fee and didn't raise it until I could afford it.
> [Female, 52, Nonprofessional]

> We started at a fee lower than his usual fee. I appreciated his coming down, but I felt like it was still pretty high. I think I resented that I could only go every other week because I couldn't afford it.
> [Male, 30, Professional]

> At the start of therapy, she gave me a lower fee than her regular fee. I was grateful that she did, because it would have been very hard for me to afford her otherwise.
> [Male, 45, Nonprofessional]

Often, if the patient adds a session to the weekly schedule the fee is lowered.

> For a while I was seeing him for less than his usual fee to facilitate my going twice a week. There have been moments when I felt that I could give in more to my aggressive impulses if I was a full-fee patient. It also set up a lot of anxiety at times about telling him that I took my wife out to dinner.
> [Male, 50, Professional]

> When I was seeing her twice a week, the second session was a lower fee.
> [Female, 45, Professional]

> The second session each week was a lower fee.
> [Female, 50, Professional]

Occasionally the possibility of a lower fee is discussed but never implemented.

> Some discussion came up about the possibility of my continuing with her when I could no longer go through the HMO, and we talked about the fee then, but that never happened.
> [Male, 50, Nonprofessional]

There was a stage where the insurance company was giving us a hard time, and she said if necessary we would but we never needed to.
[Male, 49, Nonprofessional]

Sometimes the absence of a fee raise is experienced as a lower fee.

She let me slide at the old fee for 6 months before she raised it.
[Female, 50, Nonprofessional]

Some people were skeptical about the idea of the fee being lowered.

Are you kidding?
[Female, 62, Professional]

NUMERICAL DISTRIBUTION

Professionals: Seven said the therapist had either lowered the fee due to circumstances or started treatment at a lower fee than usual; 13 said this had not happened.

Nonprofessionals: Eleven said the fee had been lowered either at the start of therapy or during treatment; 28 said it had not. One person said there was no fee.

COMMENTS

Given the cynicism of some respondents about therapist greed, a surprisingly large portion (about one-third) of both groups said that the fee had been lowered either at the start of therapy or during the course of treatment.

If the financial situation of the patient changes radically, a fee adjustment may be necessary for the patient to continue treatment. As the therapist, I have an ethical commitment not to abandon patients over money and fees, so a lower fee may become necessary, if only temporarily.

As the patient, I want to be sure that, having become involved in and to some degree dependent on therapy, I won't get cut off if the money isn't there for some reason beyond my control. If the therapy leads me to change careers, or return to school, and my income drops as a result, I don't want to be penalized for that by losing the treatment.

RELATED READING

Cerney, M. S. (1990). Reduced fee or free psychotherapy: uncovering the hidden issues. *Psychotherapy Patient* 7(1–2):53–65.

Connolly, G. (1993). The price of growing up. *Psychoanalytic Psychotherapy* 7(1):85–95.

Erle, J. B. (1993). On the setting of analytic fees. *Psychoanalytic Quarterly* 62(1):106–108.

Levy, M. A., Arnold, R. M., Fine, M. J., et al. (1993). Professional courtesy: current practices and attitudes. *New England Journal of Medicine* 329(22):1627–1631.

🔊🔊🔊🔊

Question 22: Did you ever owe the therapist money?

At times, circumstances in the patient's life will make it impossible for him to pay the therapist's bill, and a balance will accumulate. Therapists handle this situation in different ways.

Many therapists will allow the patient to owe them a certain amount, and work out some arrangement to pay the balance.

> He allowed me to owe him the money, and kept a running total. When I was able to earn more money we worked out a payment schedule.
>
> [Male, 42, Professional]

> I think there was a period where I just couldn't pay for a little while, an accumulation of 2 or 3 months, and he was fine with that and very understanding. I paid it off soon.
>
> [Female, 46, Nonprofessional]

> It was no problem. I paid whenever I had it.
>
> [Female, 39, Professional]

> He was able to carry me. I hated owing him money, but he didn't have any problem with it.
>
> [Female, 50, Nonprofessional]

> She let me build up a large bill, because we knew that I was coming into an inheritance, at which point I paid it off.
>
> [Female, 62, Professional]

> If I ever did, it was only for a short time, a month or two. And it was always critically important to me that I pay up.
>
> [Female, 48, Nonprofessional]

For many patients, dealing with money is an important part of the treatment. Sometimes this is a positive experience.

> Early in therapy I ran up a big bill, and she realized it was counterproductive to the therapy. She gave me a deadline, which was a catastrophic happening in the therapy and a turning point for me. I actually had to take out a loan to pay my therapist.
>
> [Female, 51, Professional]

Sometimes money is at the center of a very negative experience.

> I had an emergency appendectomy and I almost died. I couldn't go to therapy for 3 weeks. I had to pay for those sessions, but I couldn't work either and didn't have money to pay him. I told him that I was able to pay him half of what I owed, and within a 6-week period I would add an extra amount to the regular fee and pay every cent that I owed him. That wasn't acceptable to him, and he asked me three times in that session when he was getting his money. I reminded him that he had known me for 13 years and I had never failed to pay him. I said, "It sounds as if you don't trust me." And then he said, "Hold on to the couch, I have something to tell you: I do trust you. But I need to know when I'm getting my money." I couldn't understand that.
>
> [Female, 57, Professional]

Occasionally the offer to carry the bill is declined.

> She offered me that option but I said it wouldn't help me.
>
> [Male, 49, Nonprofessional]

> She allowed for that, but I never took her up on it, because I was so trained by then in keeping the boundaries, that I didn't know what to do with the leniency.
>
> [Female, 47, Nonprofessional]

Occasionally a bill carries over beyond the end of treatment.

> The last session I was supposed to go to I missed, and it was a good 6 months before I paid it. He called me and reminded me.
>
> [Female, 41, Nonprofessional]

In a very rare situation, the debt was erased.

> I got into money trouble and owed him some money, and I don't know what happened but he forgave all debts from all patients. Maybe it was a write-off or something, and we started anew.
>
> [Female, 52, Nonprofessional]

NUMERICAL DISTRIBUTION

Professionals: Five said they had at some point owed the therapist a balance; 15 had not.

Nonprofessionals: Seven said they had owed the therapist money; 33 had not.

COMMENTS

More professionals said they had owed the therapist a balance, and this might reflect therapists giving greater latitude with a professional patient.

As the therapist, I try to allow some leeway in hard times for the patient to accumulate a balance, so that treatment is not interrupted. Too large a balance, however, becomes a burden to both the patient and the therapist.

As the patient, I need to know that circumstances beyond my control aren't going to deprive me of the treatment I have come to need. I also want to know that my therapist trusts me enough to allow me some latitude when necessary.

RELATED READING

Herron, W. G., and Welt, S. R. (1991). *Money Matters: The Fee in Psychotherapy and Psychoanalysis.* New York: Guilford.
Klebanow, S., and Lowenkopf, E. L. (1991). *Money and Mind.* New York: Plenum Press.

⋈⋈⋈⋈

Question 23: Did you use insurance?

Many patients use insurance to help pay for treatment. These days, managed care carefully controls how this works.

A standard arrangement is to have the patient pay the therapist the full fee and get reimbursed by the insurance company.

> I paid her the entire amount and got reimbursed.
>
> [Male, 42, Nonprofessional]

Sometimes patients wait to file claims.

> Every 6 months I would have her fill out a bill and I'd get back some money.
>
> [Female, 45, Nonprofessional]

> After 3 or 4 months, at one point after a year, I would fill out the forms, or he would give me a receipt for that period. I would pay and let 3 or 4 months go by. It was never a big deal.
>
> [Female, 48, Nonprofessional]

Sometimes the patient pays only a portion of the fee and the therapist gets the balance from the insurance company.

> I paid the co-payment and she got reimbursed by the insurance company.
>
> [Male, 49, Nonprofessional]

> He would accept the co-payment and wait for the balance from the insurance company.
>
> [Female, 41, Nonprofessional]

> I paid the co-payment and he was reimbursed by the insurance company.
>
> [Female, 45, Nonprofessional]

> He billed through the insurance company, and once they paid their part I would pay the co-payment.
>
> [Male, 43, Nonprofessional]

Rarely, the insurance company pays the entire fee.

My insurance company got billed through the time I was going and they paid the therapist directly.

[Female, 48, Nonprofessional]

It was completely paid for by the HMO.

[Male, 50, Nonprofessional]

Often insurance covers only a small portion of the cost.

My insurance paid $1,000 a year, and therapy was costing me $270 a week, so it ran out after about 4 weeks.

[Female, 57, Professional]

It didn't cover much but I used it.

[Female, 50, Professional]

A few patients decline to file insurance claims, even when coverage is available.

I don't believe in using insurance for therapy.

[Female, 45, Professional]

For a while I did with a couples counselor, but eventually I stopped submitting that, because I was uncomfortable with those bills being part of my permanent health record.

[Male, 48, Nonprofessional]

I would only get back $8 a session, so sometimes I wouldn't even send it in.

[Female, 59, Professional]

NUMERICAL DISTRIBUTION

Professionals: Fourteen said they had used insurance; 6 had not.
Nonprofessionals: Twenty-nine said they used insurance; 11 had not.

COMMENTS

As a therapist, I hate dealing with insurance on every level, from having to assign a diagnosis, to filling out forms, to revealing personal details, to justifying more sessions. Insurance carriers are more and more intrusive and invasive. I much prefer dealing with a patient who pays for therapy himself, and try to keep my fees on a level where this is possible.

As a patient, I may prefer to use insurance when I can, since it lowers the cost to me, but I will be concerned if the insurance company asks for personal information or tries to tell the therapist how to work.

RELATED READING

Angel, V. T. (1994). The influence and impact of health care systems and the relationship to the psychoanalytic process: discussion. *International Forum of Psychoanalysis* 3(1):17–19.

Canter, A. (1991). A cost effective psychotherapy. *Psychotherapy in Private Practice* 8(4):13–17.

Cummings, N. A. (1995). Unconscious fiscal convenience. *Psychotherapy in Private Practice* 14(2):23–28.

Giles, T. B. (1991). Managed mental health care and effective psychotherapy: a step in the right direction? *Journal of Behavior Therapy and Experimental Psychiatry* 22(2):83–86.

Tuckfelt, S., Fink, J., and Warren, M. (1997). *The Psychotherapists' Guide to Managed Care in the 21st Century*. Northvale, NJ: Jason Aronson.

℞℞℞℞

Question 24: Did the insurance company ever ask for details of the treatment, or try to limit the number of sessions?

Insurance policies usually come with limits, either on the amount of reimbursement or on the number of sessions allowed each year.

> There was a limit of 50 sessions.
>
> [Female, 51, Professional]

> They don't limit the number of sessions, they limit the amount of reimbursement.
>
> [Female, 39, Nonprofessional]

Some insurance carriers require that additional sessions be justified.

> She said that she had to convince them to continue treatment, because I had gone beyond the few sessions normally allotted. She

figured out a way to do it, but I don't know exactly what she said. I wasn't concerned because we discussed how she was doing it, and it was more or less the truth.

[Male, 50, Nonprofessional]

They limited the number of sessions. She kept requesting additional sessions and they finally refused, and I didn't want her to go further.

[Female, 62, Professional]

I remember us talking about it once, that they were trying to limit the number of sessions, and she was really upset.

[Female, 48, Nonprofessional]

This is sometimes a problem.

I built up this balance with my therapist and we were trying to get coverage from my insurance, and they asked for all kinds of details about my treatment, and then they said they wouldn't cover it because it wasn't precertified. Then he had to fill out a form with "measurable objectives," and they certified me for several sessions and then for one more.

[Female, 42, Nonprofessional]

We went through several battles with the various insurance companies, and the last one just refused to reimburse me.

[Male, 49, Nonprofessional]

Insurance carriers will sometimes ask for details of the case, a treatment plan or an assessment of risk. Patients and therapists may have concerns about what is revealed, and to whom.

She showed me the response before she sent it. I had no concern because it was very well couched.

[Female, 50, Professional]

She would fill out the form and be as oblique as possible. We weren't worried about it because she showed it to us before she sent it in.

[Female, 44, Nonprofessional]

I was very concerned about what he might reveal, and he supported my concern, and we jointly refused to divulge any details and negotiated for years with the insurance company. I don't think they got any more than a diagnosis out of us. They threatened to limit the number of sessions. This was all a long time ago. They hadn't yet developed the belief that they could control everything.

[Male, 53, Professional]

They requested a lot of information. I was concerned, but she told me what she was going to say and got my okay. I feel it's very dangerous for this information to be floating around.

[Male, 49, Nonprofessional]

Some patients were not worried about what was revealed to the insurance company.

Not at first, but later on he had to report some amount of information, and he talked with me before doing that to discuss exactly what he would be saying and would I be comfortable with it.

[Female, 46, Nonprofessional]

At the beginning they asked for details. And then they okayed it. I didn't care about what they were told. I figured they didn't know me, I didn't know them, it was somebody sitting at a desk pushing paper.

[Female, 40, Nonprofessional]

She had to submit a treatment plan. She never showed it to me and I never asked to see it. I had no concern about what was revealed.

[Female, 62, Professional]

NUMERICAL DISTRIBUTION

Professionals: Of the 14 who used insurance, 3 said the insurance company asked for details of the treatment; 11 said they did not. Four people said the number of sessions was limited; 10 said it was not.

Nonprofessionals: Of the 29 who used insurance, 8 said the insurance company asked for details; 21 said they did not. Eight people said the number of sessions was limited; 21 said it was not.

COMMENTS

The situation of managed care—HMOs and PPOs and such—has made the use of insurance for therapy much more complicated for patient and therapist. As the therapist, I may be told how many sessions I am allotted for a particular patient; I may be asked to explain in great detail what the patient has revealed about the problems we are addressing; I may be told what I can charge for my services; I may have to spend extra time in paperwork and phone contact with the insurance carrier. None of this is anything I want to do.

As the patient, I may be worried about what my therapist is revealing, and to whom. What will result if my therapist exaggerates my condition to justify further treatment? I may wonder where this information will wind up, who may have access to it, and its future effect on my career. I may also wonder how my therapist feels about working with me if I am aware that she is accepting a fee much lower than her regular fee.

RELATED READING

Barron, J. W., and Sands, H., eds. (1996). *The Impact of Managed Care on Psychodynamic Treatment.* Madison, CT: International Universities Press.

Browning, C. H., and Browning, B. J. (1996). *How to Partner with Managed Care.* New York: Wiley.

Cummings, N. A., Pallak, M. S., and Cummings, J. L., eds. (1996). *Surviving the Demise of Solo Practice.* Madison, CT: Psychosocial Press.

Karon, B. P. (1992). Problems of psychotherapy under managed care. *Psychotherapy in Private Practice* 11(2):55–63.

Lazarus, A., ed. (1996). *Controversies in Managed Mental Health Care.* Washington, DC: American Psychiatric Press.

᠅᠅᠅᠅

Question 25: What was the rule about cancellations and missed sessions?

Every therapist has a cancellation policy. Is the patient responsible for all sessions? If not, how much notice must be given to avoid having to pay for a missed session? Are makeup sessions offered? Whatever policy the therapist has, patients have reactions and feelings about it.

Some patients never learn what the rule is.

> I don't know because I never missed or canceled and neither did he. And we never discussed it.
>
> [Male, 30, Professional]

> I don't think it was ever stated.
>
> [Female, 48, Nonprofessional]

> I don't know—it never came up.
>
> [Female, 56, Professional]

> I don't remember. He was very loose, and it never came up.
>
> [Female, 48, Nonprofessional]

The following example shows what can happen when the rule is not clear.

> She apparently had a policy and didn't tell me. I lived an hour away, and when the weather was bad in the wintertime I didn't want to drive that distance. I assumed her cancellation policy was 24 hours' notice, and it was actually a week. So at one point I canceled and she charged me, and I was upset by that. She retracted the charge and clarified the policy. It bothered me that she had implemented a policy without telling me what it was.
>
> [Female, 62, Professional]

The traditional rule in psychoanalysis has been that the patient pays for all sessions. Patients may accept this policy but they don't always like it.

> You paid for them. Obviously I hated it, but I didn't think it was exactly unfair.
>
> [Female, 55, Professional]

> I was responsible for every session. When I chose him as my therapist, I knew how rigid he was, and I made a decision to play by his rules. I don't think it was fair.
>
> [Female, 57, Professional]

> Whether you missed or canceled you still paid for it. A little bit unfair, but I figured he was due what he was due.
>
> [Male, 46, Nonprofessional]

> I paid for all sessions. I was sort of annoyed because I work it a little differently in my own practice, and I have a different vacation policy.
>
> [Female, 59, Professional]

She was really rigid about it. If you missed a session you paid for it, even if it was an emergency. It didn't feel fair. The first time it happened and I misunderstood, she let that one go, but she explained that she kept her rates moderate and she needed to guarantee a certain income.

[Female, 45, Professional]

Here is another opinion about this rationale.

He actually said that his philosophy was that if the patient cancels for a valid reason, and the therapist bills because he wants to have a steady income, he's making the therapist's problems the patient's responsibility, and the patient shouldn't be made responsible for the therapist's income.

[Male, 42, Professional]

Another common practice is to require 24-hour notice of a cancellation.

Twenty-four hours' notice and one didn't have to pay. Less than 24 hours' notice and one did have to pay. Reasonably fair. One could easily imagine emergency situations. There was one session where I couldn't give 24 hours' notice, and I paid. I didn't discuss it. I think I just accepted that those were the rules, and I wanted to live with the rules agreed to.

[Male, 48, Nonprofessional]

Sometimes the rule is combined with a required makeup session.

I was responsible for missed sessions. She told me at the beginning that I was, so I made a point not to miss. I could reschedule if I gave 48 hours' notice, and I would have to reschedule sometime that week. That didn't seem fair because I'm a freelancer and sometimes I have to be out of town for the whole week. Also, I might have a week where I'm not working and don't have the money that week. I asked her about coming every other week but she didn't go for it.

[Female, 28, Nonprofessional]

That pissed me off too. He was very rigid about it. He gave what he called a "floating makeup," which meant if you had to cancel, but you did it with enough notice, he charged you for it but you could have another session. That's a fine idea, but when my husband was hospitalized I wasn't able to find another time, and he charged me anyway.

[Female, 48, Professional]

You got one missed session. The rule was you had to cancel with 24 hours' notice, and he wanted you to reschedule.

[Female, 41, Nonprofessional]

You had to give notice, 2 or 3 days, maybe a week, otherwise you were billed for the session. If you gave notice, you had to reschedule. It didn't seem fair, especially when I knew 2 months in advance that I was going for surgery. I was furious, but because I had a very strong level of trust, we managed to move that issue into a therapeutic experience. There was part of me that never bought into it, and was very angry.

[Female, 47, Nonprofessional]

If I gave her notice I would have to make the session up in the same week. If I went away on vacation or for a business trip, I also had to make it up. It didn't seem fair. It seemed a burden, but it felt like part of the burden of what I needed to do in being there—not a financial responsibility, but that I had to do that job.

[Female, 50, Nonprofessional]

If we canceled we were responsible for payment unless she could find another time for us during that same week. Yes, it seemed fair. But we had to pay when we were going on vacation, which didn't seem fair.

[Female, 44, Nonprofessional]

You had to call her in advance and you had to reschedule it. If you couldn't reschedule, you were charged. I didn't have a problem with it. It's kind of standard, isn't it?

[Female, 50, Professional]

Some therapists had a very flexible policy about cancellations.

She was very flexible about that—I was surprised. I once canceled a session that day and she didn't charge me because I was working on a big, long, involved project that she knew about.

[Female, 51, Professional]

Occasionally the policy gets complicated.

I had a specific time once a week. I was entitled to two weeks' vacation, whenever I wanted, not necessarily during her vacation. Otherwise I paid for it. If I was sick we'd do a telephone session. Otherwise she'd offer me a makeup time. I had a problem with it, and I would have had more of a problem if my insurance company hadn't been paying 70 percent. I guess it is fair. I don't know.

[Female, 40, Nonprofessional]

Some therapists made allowances for emergency situations.

It was displayed in the waiting room that 24 hours' notice was required, although I did have one or two emergencies when I canceled at the last moment and I wasn't charged for the sessions.

[Female, 46, Nonprofessional]

Once I was walking there and I got run over by a car. She didn't charge me—I had the police call her.

[Female, 45, Professional]

I was responsible for them, and he charged for them. There may have been an occasion where something exceptional happened and he made an exception. I didn't like it, but I could understand it.

[Female, 46, Nonprofessional]

And some made no such allowances.

I remember missing a session due to a huge blizzard, and it led to an argument because she expected me to pay. I ended up paying. I was aware that it was standard practice but I didn't like it and it didn't seem fair.

[Male, 44, Professional]

Sometimes a strict cancellation policy can lead to a patient quitting treatment.

I saw a therapist for 4 or 5 sessions, and we did not hit it off. At the time I was traveling a lot, and I had told her that. I said she had to factor that in somehow. She said that her philosophy was that if she couldn't fill the slot she would have to charge me for the session. I said that wouldn't work. I said I could give her lots of notice, and she said let's try it. The first time I had to travel I gave her 8 days' notice, and at the end of the month when I went to pay the bill, she had charged me for the session, so I chose not to go back to her.

[Female, 41, Nonprofessional]

Sometimes the policy changes over the course of a long treatment.

> When I first started with him, it was the season ticket at the opera: you were responsible for all sessions, with the exception that if you were going on vacation you weren't charged. This used to be a huge issue between us, because I never felt comfortable maintaining so rigid a stance with my own patients. It wasn't that I felt angry that he was charging me, but that I felt inadequate that I couldn't be like him. Over the years he became more liberal. What I liked about him, what enabled me to tolerate it, was that he never took the position that it was somehow for my own good to pay for a missed session. He said that it was his need, and if you wanted to work with him you had to live with it.
>
> [Male, 50, Professional]

> At first it was 24 hours' notice to avoid payment, and then he became more unusual and switched to 48 hours. On one level it was negotiated, meaning that he asked if I could agree to that. If I had put up a disagreement with a reasonable argument, I think that he would have made an accommodation.
>
> [Male, 53, Professional]

Patients may have strong feelings when the therapist fails to keep his own rule.

> I had to cancel a session with a couples counselor that my wife and I see, and he was actually very apologetic about insisting on payment, but I felt that it was as important for us as for him to follow the rules that we had agreed to. He was actually looking for a way to weasel around it and find a way to break his own rule, and I said I'd rather not do that.
>
> [Male, 48, Nonprofessional]

Patients may accept the therapist tightening the cancellation policy.

> The rule was 24 hours' notice. I went through a period where I was canceling frequently, always for a valid reason, and she finally told me she was going to start charging me regardless of how much notice I gave her. That was very smart of her, because I was messing around with my therapy at the time.
>
> [Female, 50, Professional]

NUMERICAL DISTRIBUTION

Professionals: Eight said the rule was that they were responsible for all sessions; 3 more said they had to pay but were offered a makeup hour at no additional cost if it could be scheduled the same week; 9 said there was no charge if they canceled in advance, varying from 24 hours to 1 week.

Nonprofessionals: Nine said that they were responsible for all sessions; 25 said they had to give at least 24 hours' notice; 3 said they had to give a week's notice; 1 person said she could cancel any time before the session. Two people said the rule was never stated and never came up.

COMMENTS

More of the professionals found themselves in the situation of being responsible for all sessions. Perhaps the therapists were more stringent with professional patients.

As the therapist, my problem is to balance the needs of the patient and my own needs in a way that takes care of both without either resenting the other. A deadline for cancellations, whatever the time period, seems to me the best way to do this.

As the patient, I don't want to feel responsible for the therapist's income. That's her problem. I want some recognition that circumstances sometimes prevent my being at my session, even if I want to, and I don't want to be penalized for living in the real world.

RELATED READING

Blackmon, W. D. (1993). Are psychoanalytic billing practices ethical? *American Journal of Psychotherapy* 47(4):613–620.

Fay, A. (1995). Ethical implications of charging for missed sessions. *Psychological Reports* 77(3, pt. 2):1251–1259.

———— (1996). Charging for missed sessions: Ethical problem or straw person? *Psychological Reports* 78(3, pt. 1):924–926.

Furlong, A. (1992). Some technical and theoretical considerations regarding the missed session. *International Journal of Psycho-Analysis* 73(4):701–718.

℞℞℞℞

Question 26: Did your therapist have any other rules?

Every therapist has rules about cancellations, but sometimes they have additional rules about patient behavior.

Sometimes these rules are also about money.

> His vacation rule wasn't fair. He would announce when he was taking his vacation, and if you didn't take your vacation at the same time you paid for the sessions scheduled during your vacation time.
>
> [Female, 58, Professional]

> She would give me the bill each month, and if I couldn't pay it by the next session, she asked that I bring it up and talk to her about it.
>
> [Female, 42, Nonprofessional]

> I used to pay him relatively late in the month, and at one point he was going to demand payment by the tenth of the month or charge a late fee. I threatened to leave therapy over it because it offended me so much, and the rule died.
>
> [Male, 50, Professional]

Some rules were about sobriety.

> Show up sober.
>
> [Male, 49, Nonprofessional]

> One time I went to a session after snorting some cocaine and he ended the session and said that he wouldn't work with me if I was using anything.
>
> [Male, 46, Nonprofessional]

Some therapists had specific rules for group therapy.

> In group, after we had been together for a while, once a month he would start the session and then we would continue without him. He discouraged relationships outside the group.
>
> [Female, 50, Professional]

> The group was allowed to talk while they were there, and to have no interaction outside the group.
>
> [Male, 43, Nonprofessional]

A few people mentioned rules about the therapy itself.

> Probably there were implied rules: no jumping around, no acting, just talking.
>
> [Male, 53, Professional]

> He had a definite rule about not eating in the session.
>
> [Female, 48, Nonprofessional]

> She required that I take it seriously, that it was a very serious commitment she was making to me and she expected me to match her in that.
>
> [Female, 45, Professional]

> She had very strong boundary rules: never walking into another room, never disclosing anything personal. As we went on, there was a slow relaxing of those rules.
>
> [Female, 47, Nonprofessional]

> She had a rule that she wouldn't tell me anything personal about herself.
>
> [Female, 39, Nonprofessional]

> The rule was to say what you think.
>
> [Female, 52, Nonprofessional]

One person commented about the idea of rules in general.

> The most characteristic thing about the therapy was the lack of rules, of what I thought were supposed to be the rules.
>
> [Male, 30, Professional]

NUMERICAL DISTRIBUTION

Professionals: Three people mentioned rules; 17 did not.
Nonprofessionals: Eight people mentioned rules; 32 did not.

COMMENTS

As the therapist, I try to keep the rules to a minimum. I have to have some rules about fees and payment, because this is my business, and these are fairly standard within the field. There are a number of implicit rules that should perhaps be more explicit: no violence, no threats, no intoxication, no sex. Too many rules makes me feel like a controlling parent.

As the patient, I want the rules to be clear and consistent. I have to decide whether they're acceptable, or discuss anything I find objectionable. I don't want the therapist to appear arbitrary or parental, and I don't want to feel controlled.

RELATED READING

Halpert, E. (1992). Structuring the psychotherapeutic situation. In *Psychotherapy: The Analytic Approach,* ed. M. J. Aronson and M. A. Scharfman, pp. 41–51. Northvale, NJ: Jason Aronson.

Hellman, I. D., Morrison, T. L., and Abramowitz, S. I. (1987). Therapist flexibility/rigidity and work stress. *Professional Psychology: Research and Practice* 18(1):21–27.

🐾🐾🐾🐾

Question 27: Did you ever discuss with the therapist what kind of therapy it was?

There are many different schools of therapy, and many different kinds of treatment. The *Shrink Rap* sample mentioned more than twenty-five different labels for their theoretical orientations. Is this a significant issue for new patients, and how many ask about and discuss with the therapist the type of therapy they're in?

Professionals seem to be more educated about what kind of therapy they are getting.

> I knew what kind of therapy it was. It was strict Freudian psychoanalysis.
>
> [Female, 57, Professional]

> Over the years I have spent an inordinate amount of time talking with my therapist about whether what he was doing with me was really analysis, with me claiming it wasn't because it didn't fulfill the formal requirements and with him taking the position that he was an analyst and therefore what he did was analysis.
>
> [Male, 50, Professional]

All the time, we were talking about what were doing.

[Male, 30, Professional]

It was obvious that it was psychoanalysis.

[Female, 48, Professional]

He had raised it in the first or second session. He had showed me a book, and indicated that he was more of an object relations kind of person, the mother–child interaction, and he said that this is the way he worked. I wasn't quite sure what he was trying to explain, but the picture on the book showed a mother holding the baby.

[Female, 59, Professional]

She said that at that time she was working in body-oriented gestalt work, that was what she was training in, and I saw her in an office there. Eventually I also trained in that method. At the time I didn't really understand her answer, and found it a little scary.

[Female, 45, Professional]

I spent some time talking about the previous therapy, and he had a look of horror on his face, and he said that he was shocked by some of the things she did. Because of that I asked him a lot of questions about his credentials and experience.

[Female, 50, Professional]

I knew what it was when I started. It's called control-mastery.

[Female, 62, Professional]

I knew it was hypnotherapy and EMDR [eye movement desensitization and reprocessing].

[Female, 56, Professional]

I knew it was Gestalt therapy.

[Female, 45, Professional]

We talked a little about it. She was connected with a particular institute. Sometimes it would get mixed in with my own work as a therapist, comments she would make. At one point we talked about why neither of us was a self psychologist.

[Female, 51, Professional]

She said she had put together her own brand of therapy, based on ego psychology and self psychology.

[Female, 52, Professional]

Nonprofessionals are sometimes experienced enough to be familiar with the different approaches.

> We touched on that a little bit, particularly since, about a little more than a year into it, she announced that she was relocating across the country and had to terminate therapy, and she was recommending a number of therapists as appropriate to work with me. Then we touched on theoretical issues, and she did talk about some of the analysts that she believed in and that she studied and so on. She thought a lot of Winnicott, and Klein, and one other. Some of this I found useful and some I found extremely unuseful.
>
> [Male, 48, Nonprofessional]

> She said it was eclectic, and I needed to know how eclectic and what the mix was. Initially I went to her because she was trained in bio-energetics, but she was also trained in Gestalt and her practice evolved and her training evolved.
>
> [Female, 47, Nonprofessional]

> I believe it was cognitive therapy.
>
> [Female, 28, Nonprofessional]

> Briefly we would talk about it. Even though I had heard she was a Freudian she really had an eclectic approach.
>
> [Female, 42, Nonprofessional]

> I was told that it was a systems family therapy approach.
>
> [Female, 44, Nonprofessional]

> Right at the beginning, I talked to her about what she did, and how she did it, and what her feelings about it were, what her theories were.
>
> [Male, 52, Nonprofessional]

Sometimes patients are not educated enough to understand the therapist's answer.

> It was several years into the therapy. I finally broke down and said to her, "So what do you actually practice? Is there a name for this?" and she did tell me. She said she was an adherent to the British school of object relations, which didn't mean much to me.
>
> [Female, 45, Nonprofessional]

I asked her what her approach was, but I wasn't sufficiently grounded in the field to understand her answers.

[Female, 39, Nonprofessional]

Fully half the nonprofessionals said they had never discussed what kind of therapy they were in.

We didn't discuss that to any extent. Occasionally I would ask if something was this or that, but he didn't seem to be into that very much. He was kind of integrated.

[Male, 48, Nonprofessional]

I don't think we did, except in very general ways, because it was working so well and I never felt like stepping back and examining the mechanics.

[Male, 49, Nonprofessional]

I believe he told me the type of work that he did, but not in any clinical description.

[Female, 48, Nonprofessional]

Sometimes the answer is a little vague.

I asked questions about that, and he said that it was to let out the anger I had inside of me, and to work with that, and to see how the others in the group brought out their problems.

[Male, 43, Nonprofessional]

He never put a name to it, but we talked about how his was different from the groups I was going to.

[Female, 52, Nonprofessional]

It was somewhat vague, although I know it was Gestalt therapy.

[Female, 46, Nonprofessional]

She was a pragmatist, and she didn't have a single theory, but had a lot of different theories and different tools and used them as needed.

[Male, 50, Nonprofessional]

When I first went in, I asked him what his approach was, and he said he was humanistic. It seems that he came from a much more personal-relationship type of thing than a clinical approach, because he was very sincere, made a lot of eye contact, and tried to be very reassuring and compassionate.

[Female, 48, Nonprofessional]

She felt her therapy was very action-oriented, and focused on your here-and-now life.

[Female, 45, Nonprofessional]

She used to use the word "Gestalt" but I think her meaning of the word was a "little bit of everything."

[Female, 50, Nonprofessional]

Sometimes patients know, even when the subject is not discussed.

It was a combination of bioenergetic and Gestalt therapy.

[Male, 46, Nonprofessional]

We never did discuss it, but I know enough about therapy to know that she seemed very Freudian.

[Female, 40, Nonprofessional]

I knew up front that it was Jungian therapy. I don't think I followed through in her therapeutic way, in the sense of writing down dreams and talking about them. I just didn't do it.

[Male, 52, Nonprofessional]

I knew it was hypnotherapy, though it turned into more traditional therapy.

[Male, 53, Nonprofessional]

Sometimes knowing what it is doesn't help.

It came up in talking about what I wanted and what he offered. He was a psychotherapist of a psychoanalytic nature, and he didn't hide that that was his orientation, and I was disappointed when I found out because that wasn't what I wanted. I guess I know enough about the field to say that wasn't what I wanted. We talked about it, and I thought, "Well, I'll just try it," but we many times came to crises. I used the analogy when I left that it was like being with a married man who kept saying he'd break off the marriage. When I said that this isn't what I want, he kept saying he'd try some other techniques, but he couldn't.

[Female, 48, Nonprofessional]

NUMERICAL DISTRIBUTION

Professionals: Twelve said they had discussed it; 8 said they knew what kind of therapy it was and didn't need to discuss it.

Nonprofessionals: Twenty said they had discussed it; 19 said they had not; 1 person said he didn't remember.

COMMENTS

All the professionals either discussed the kind of therapy they were getting or knew beforehand, but half the nonprofessionals never asked about or discussed what kind of therapy they were in, or what the theoretical rationale was for what was going on. For me this raises the concern that it makes more likely what one therapist in the *Shrink Rap* sample called "therapy by the seat of your pants."

As the therapist, I want patients to have some idea of what we're doing and why we do it this way. Otherwise I will probably get something less than full cooperation and enthusiasm.

As the patient, on the other hand, I may not care what the therapist uses as a theoretical model, or what label he puts on what he does, as long as I feel that it's working.

RELATED READING

Brunink, S. A., and Schroeder, H. E. (1979). Verbal behavior of expert psychoanalytically oriented, gestalt, and behavior therapists. *Journal of Consulting and Clinical Psychology* 47(3):567–574.

Giles, T. R., Prial, E. M., and Neims, D. M. (1993). Evaluating psychotherapies: a comparison of effectiveness. *International Journal of Mental Health* 22(2):43–65.

Lindon, J. A. (1991). Does technique require theory? *Bulletin of the Menninger Clinic* 55(1):1–21.

Rice, D. G., Gurman, A. S., and Razin, A. M. (1974). Therapist sex, style, and theoretical orientation. *Journal of Nervous and Mental Disease* 159(6):413–421.

Tremblay, J. M., Herron, W. G., and Schultz, C. L. (1986). Relation between therapeutic orientation and personality in psychotherapists. *Professional Psychology: Research and Practice* 17(2):106–110.

❧❧❧❧

Question 28: What did the therapist tell you about confidentiality?

Confidentiality is one of the basic principles of most psychotherapy. Recent changes in the way insurance coverage works, and some recent court decisions, have limited the extent of what is confidential.

Many of the professionals did discuss this issue with the therapist, especially in regard to a specific situation.

> I'm sure it was brought up at the beginning. but I don't remember discussing it at any length.
>
> [Male, 44, Professional]

> In the beginning we did because it was in an institute. I was pretty concerned about that.
>
> [Female, 55, Professional]

> When I referred a friend to her, we discussed it.
>
> [Female, 39, Professional]

> That was one of the things he said in the very first session, and then again when we were in group. He was very scrupulous about that.
>
> [Female, 50, Professional]

Many of the professionals, apparently due to their knowledge of the facts, never discussed this issue with their therapists.

> We never needed to. I knew his rules about it.
>
> [Female, 57, Professional]

> It was assumed.
>
> [Female, 51, Professional]

> It never even crossed my mind.
>
> [Female, 48, Professional]

About half the nonprofessionals who discussed the issue were told that confidentiality was total and complete.

> It was always made clear in the beginning that everything was confidential, and I was advised not to share what was going on with anybody.
>
> [Female, 48, Nonprofessional]

> I was told that everything we discussed was totally confidential, and I absolutely trusted that.
>
> [Female, 40, Nonprofessional]

But many nonprofessionals, many of whom were not so knowledgeable, never discussed the issue.

> I don't remember her specifically telling me anything.
>
> [Female, 45, Nonprofessional]

> I don't think that we ever discussed it.
>
> [Female, 48, Nonprofessional]

> I don't remember discussing it. My assumption was that what we said was totally confidential.
>
> [Male, 52, Nonprofessional]

> I guess I just assumed that, but I don't think she ever made some sort of statement to that effect.
>
> [Male, 45, Nonprofessional]

> I can't remember him talking about it. I just assumed that it was very confidential.
>
> [Male, 48, Nonprofessional]

Sometimes the issue is the question of what will be revealed to the insurance carrier.

> It was a major issue, heightened by the entanglement with the insurance company.
>
> [Male, 53, Professional]

> She raised it and we discussed it in terms of the insurance. At first I said I didn't care, but I feel now that it's very dangerous for the information to be floating around.
>
> [Male, 49, Nonprofessional]

Occasionally there are specific situations that need discussion.

> My therapist knew a lot of people that I knew, and a lot of her patients were friends of mine, so it was an important issue and we discussed it. She said she would ask my permission to mention me to other authority figures, and sometimes we would discuss in advance what

she would say, and limit it so it was very clear. Sometimes it was hard with my friends, because they would talk about their sessions with her and then it would be like a "Mom loves me best" kind of thing.

[Female, 42, Nonprofessional]

I discussed it in terms of my brother, who was also seeing her. Plus my mother was still seeing her father. I was totally unconscious of how concerned I was.

[Female, 45, Nonprofessional]

Her husband is also a therapist, and I saw him occasionally at conferences and workshops, and she got a little indignant when I asked if she had told him that I was seeing her.

[Female, 62, Professional]

He had seen my father, and he made it very clear that he wasn't going to discuss anything with regard to my father, so I assumed that would apply to me too.

[Male, 53, Nonprofessional]

A friend of mine is a therapist in her supervisory group. Sometimes I would say, "I'm not sure if I should even be telling you these things," and she was very clear that what I told her was never discussed. Also, there was a time after my divorce when I was dating a man who had been in couples counseling with his ex-wife with my therapist, and she explained why she couldn't say anything about that until I found it out from him.

[Female, 46, Nonprofessional]

I wanted to thank the woman who referred me, but she had died, and I asked him about her, and he said that confidentiality didn't stop even with death.

[Female, 52, Nonprofessional]

NUMERICAL DISTRIBUTION

Professionals: Eight said they had discussed the issue, briefly or at length; 12 said they never had, mostly because it was assumed.

Nonprofessionals: Fourteen said they had discussed the question of confidentiality; 26 said they had not. Of the 14 who had, at least 7 were told that everything was confidential.

COMMENTS

Because of the recent changes in the law and in the way insurance coverage works, patients need to be informed early in treatment, perhaps in the first session, about the limits of confidentiality. Recent laws require the therapist to report threats of violence or child abuse. Insurance companies demand personal details before approving treatment. Not all patients are aware of this current reality.

As the therapist, I want to offer complete confidentiality, and hate the changes in the law that have limited my control of this area. I am trying to teach people to be responsible for their own lives, and the law now puts the therapist in the role of watchdog, policeman, and informer. I have noticed that very few of my patients have ever asked about this issue.

As the patient, I want to know that my therapist will contain my revelations and keep them within the office. If there are limitations, I need to know about them.

RELATED READING

Joseph, D. I., and Onek, J. N. (1991). Confidentiality in psychiatry. In *Psychiatric Ethics,* 2nd ed., ed. S. Bloch and P. Chodoff, pp.313–340. Oxford: Oxford University Press.

Levine, M., Doueck, H. J., Anderson, E. M., et al. (1995). *The Impact of Mandated Reporting on the Therapeutic Process: Picking Up the Pieces.* Thousand Oaks, CA: Sage.

Shuman, D. W., and Weiner, M. F. (1987). *The Psychotherapist–Patient Privilege: A Critical Examination.* Springfield, IL: Charles C Thomas.

Somberg, D. R., Stone, G. L., and Claiborn, C. D. (1993). Informed consent: therapists' beliefs and practices. *Professional Psychology; Research and Practice* 24(2):153–159.

🔊🔊🔊🔊

Question 29: Did your therapist take notes during the session?

Some therapists take notes in the session, and some do not. In the *Shrink Rap* sample, 30 did (at least at times) and 30 did not. Patients have different reactions to this behavior.

Some therapists, especially analysts, take notes regularly.

He didn't initially when I was sitting up, the first year, but he did when I was on the couch.

[Male, 42, Professional]

The first few years there were notebooks full.

[Female, 45, Nonprofessional]

For some people, the therapist who takes notes is part of what they expect from therapy.

I remember being very observant, and I could tell some of what he was writing. For example, if there was a long silence, he would put three dots down. Somehow I had a feeling that this was how it was done.

[Male, 53, Nonprofessional]

Some therapists write down only selected material, particularly dreams.

Sometimes, especially when there was a dream; he kept a notebook.

[Female, 59, Professional]

The first time I told her a dream, she whipped out a notebook, but that was the only time.

[Male, 44, Professional]

Especially in the beginning, when he was getting the background and family history, he took some notes. When I was on the couch he always took down every dream. He would write things from time to time. In the beginning when I was sitting up I would wonder why he was writing something down, but most of the time it was something he needed to remember. With dreams, he told me from the beginning that he would take every word down.

[Female, 50, Professional]

Occasionally, if there was something she wanted to ruminate about, she would write that down. It was fine with me.

[Female, 51, Professional]

Sometimes she did, though not very much. If I was talking about a dream, or if I would have an important memory, or what she called a "nugget," she would write that down. Or if I had a transference reaction to her. It was okay.

[Female, 42, Nonprofessional]

A couple of times she said, "You know, I really want to remember that specifically, so we can pick it up next time."

[Female, 39, Professional]

Some patients liked the therapist to take notes, and it had a positive meaning for them.

I liked that he took everything I said very seriously.

[Female, 62, Professional]

It wasn't constantly—it was intermittent. I liked it, because it made me feel that he was there and paying attention. And it seemed to help him keep track of things. He might in a subsequent session bring up something that happened before. Obviously one can do that without taking notes, but it might facilitate it.

[Female, 46, Nonprofessional]

He did very rarely, only for dreams. At first I was put off by it, and I asked about it, and then I realized that I was flattered that my dreams were important enough that he would write them down.

[Male, 53, Professional]

I liked it because I felt that she would remember more from session to session.

[Female, 45, Nonprofessional]

He had said when I was in supervision that he took great joy in taking notes and evaluating them, so that he could figure out a game plan for the future. So when he took notes with me I thought he would be using them for my benefit.

[Female, 57, Professional]

I assumed that it was helpful to take notes while you're hearing the story. There were a large number of characters to keep track of.

[Male, 51, Nonprofessional]

I'm never certain how they remember all that stuff, so it made me feel that she had things to refer to if she needed to.

[Female, 42, Nonprofessional]

Sometimes the meaning changes.

Especially in the beginning, when I first started to see her, she took a lot of notes. But over the years, she no longer did that. It confirmed that this was important and she needed to write to write it all down. Later on, I realized that what she was probably doing was taking extensive notes because she was under supervision, and it was very important that her notes be accurate when she discussed it with a supervisor, but I didn't realize that for a while.

[Female, 48, Nonprofessional]

Several people said they had a very negative reaction to note-taking in the session.

He was writing all the time and it really pissed me off. It didn't seem like he was taking notes. Maybe he was.

[Male, 48, Nonprofessional]

Other people had mixed feelings about it.

She had the most amazing technique: she could write in her notebook without looking down, even to turn the page. I think she even made the notebooks herself because they had very loose rings, not a binder. I asked her once if she ever looked at the notes, because it bothered me that she did all that writing. I thought that she did, but I also thought that it was a way that she listened.

[Female, 50, Nonprofessional]

Some patients seemed a little disturbed that the therapist never took notes.

I thought she would have, at least at first, taken down some general notes, but she never did.

[Male, 45, Nonprofessional]

Some people were able to guess that the therapist, while not taking notes in the session, must have done so later on.

I always used to guess that she took notes afterward. I know that she did, because I saw her look at things sometimes. It would not have been okay if she took notes during the session because it would have been very distracting.

[Female, 40, Nonprofessional]

I was amazed at his memory, because he never took notes and he didn't take a break, and he seemed to remember everything. He must have written things down because even when I went back a year later he knew exactly when I had been there and he remembered the issues.

[Female, 41, Nonprofessional]

I remember that she did have notes on me. She wrote things down afterward. I thought it was good because she would remember where we were.

[Female, 50, Nonprofessional]

One person mentioned an unusual arrangement.

For a while he taped the sessions, and I still have those tapes. I never listen to them but I keep them.

[Female, 52, Nonprofessional]

NUMERICAL DISTRIBUTION

Professionals: Twelve said the therapist took notes, often or occasionally; 8 said not at all.

Nonprofessionals: Seventeen said the therapist took notes; 23 said no.

COMMENTS

Apparently note-taking in sessions is still common: almost half the total sample reported that the therapist did take notes at least some of the time.

As the therapist, I've never believed that it's possible to be fully present while taking notes, and I think that therapists who do that during the session may be using them to avoid the immediacy of contact with the patient. Notes afterward are a completely different story and are extremely valuable in organizing one's thinking about the patient and the treatment, as well as providing a long-term record of trends and progress.

As a patient, while I might like to see the interest of the therapist who takes notes, I don't want to be distracted by wondering why he writes down this and not that. I would much prefer that he demonstrate his attention by remembering what I tell him.

RELATED READING

Albeck, J. H., and Goldman, C. (1991). Patient–therapist codocumentation: implications of jointly authored progress notes for psychotherapy practice, research, training, supervision, and risk management. *American Journal of Psychotherapy* 45(3):317–334.
Hickling, L. P., Hickling, E. J., Simon, G. F., and Radetsky, S. (1984). The effect of note-taking on a simulated clinical interview. *Journal of Psychology* 116(2):235–240.
Presser, N. R., and Pfost, K. S. (1985). A format for individual psychotherapy session notes. *Professional Psychology: Research and Practice* 16(1):11–16.
Wolfson, A., and Sampson, H. (1976). A comparison of process notes and tape recordings: implications for therapy research. *Archives of General Psychiatry* 33(5):558–563.

ᘒᘒᘒᘒ

Question 30: Did you ever use the couch?

Psychoanalysis and psychoanalytic psychotherapy are often conducted with the patient lying on the couch, unable to look at the therapist. Theoretically this frees up the patient to attend more completely and deeply to his own thoughts and feelings, and to speak more freely to the therapist.

Some people found it useful in exactly those ways, though it often took some time to get used to it.

> I hadn't even thought of using the couch initially, but then I entered analytic training. I really wanted to but I was nervous about it. I loved the couch, because I found it very disinhibiting. I would not talk to someone face to face and say the same things that I would say on the couch.
>
> [Female, 48, Professional]

> It took a long time but I finally did. It was very hard at first, lying down and not seeing her. But it was better, because I got out of the conversational mode. For a long time, I thought I had to make conversation. It was an incredible responsibility, as if I were at a cocktail party. Part of the reason for lying down was so I wouldn't have such a burden of being social.
>
> [Female, 50, Nonprofessional]

It was relaxing, and I liked it.

[Female, 62, Professional]

At first I didn't, because I thought it made me subservient. After a while, because we were doing hypnosis, it seemed like a reasonable thing to do, and then I used it pretty much exclusively, even when we weren't doing hypnosis.

[Male, 53, Nonprofessional]

In the beginning it was quite strange, because I really am very visually aware of people, so the first few times it felt very bizarre. He suggested it, and I thought it was a good idea. I got used to it very fast.

[Female, 50, Professional]

I didn't use it a lot. I remember the first few times I did, feeling *really* uncomfortable with the idea.

[Female, 48, Nonprofessional]

I was actually surprised that she asked me to use it. I sat on the couch for about 6 months before she suggested that I lie down on it. I was somewhat embarrassed. It felt like a cartoon. I got used to it immediately.

[Male, 52, Nonprofessional]

Some patients are willing to comply with the suggestion to move to the couch, but not everyone who does likes it.

I did not like it. I felt it was kind of infantilizing. I wasn't used to it because I had gone through a whole course of therapy without it. I wasn't willing to make the adjustment.

[Female, 55, Professional]

I did for a period. I had a hard time with it—it was scary. It made me very uncomfortable.

[Female, 52, Nonprofessional]

It kept me more withdrawn. It created more of a schizoid thing for me. It brought a lot of regression, but I also lost a lot of words.

[Female, 59, Professional]

At first it was very uncomfortable, because of the caricature of the psychiatrist and the mental patient. It felt like a very unnatural position at first.

[Female, 39, Professional]

Professionals may feel that using the couch is part of their training, but even then may have mixed feelings about it.

> He suggested it, and I wanted to use it as part of my training. He thought it would help me get into certain feelings and a certain state of mind that was more conducive to analysis. It occasionally did, but I don't think it made a significant difference, but occasionally it made some difference.
>
> [Male, 42, Professional]

> It's always been my decision. It was hard for me. I had a lot of fantasies that I couldn't hear him, that he couldn't hear me. I began using the couch with some regularity when I started at the institute. But my supervisor, who I saw right after my therapy hour, was so sadistic that I needed to sit up and face my therapist, to get something from him to help me deal with the abuse that I was getting in supervision. And I've stayed sitting up most of the time since then.
>
> [Male, 50, Professional]

> It was Freudian analysis. I felt perfectly comfortable. I think if I had been face-to-face I would have been able to work more with our relationship.
>
> [Female, 57, Professional]

> It was his idea, and I was uncomfortable with it, but I was willing to put myself in his hands some of the time. I also had the idea that this was the real way to do it, it's legit. It really helped me to get to more memories and more feelings. At times, it was a source of fights between us. I went months at one point refusing to speak at all.
>
> [Male, 53, Professional]

Some patients simply refuse to use the couch.

> She offered the couch to me several times, but I turned it down. I didn't want to lie down. It must have been a control issue.
>
> [Female, 42, Nonprofessional]

> She invited me to try it but I wanted to stay in the chair.
>
> [Female, 45, Nonprofessional]

> I was not interested in doing anything on the couch. I had done that for many years and felt that I didn't accomplish very much.
>
> [Female, 53, Nonprofessional]

She wanted me to, and I could tell that she would have really liked it, but she saw the terror in my face. It would have made me feel a lot more vulnerable to be lying down.

[Female, 40, Nonprofessional]

He tried to get me to but I wasn't cooperative and eventually he gave up. I wanted whatever was going on to be face-to-face.

[Female, 45, Nonprofessional]

I can't lose control like that.

[Female, 50, Nonprofessional]

Sometimes people try the couch, even for a while, but then return to the chair.

I asked to use it because I was curious to see what the sessions would be like. I pushed myself past a point of discomfort, but this was all self-initiated. It was very powerful, after having sat in my chair for years. I felt extremely vulnerable. It lasted only a couple of months and then we went back to sitting up.

[Female, 47, Nonprofessional]

I began sitting up, for a year or two, then spent a couple of years on the couch, then a few more years sitting up. It seems that the couch years were times I was going twice a week. If I was lying down, I was more relaxed, but I was missing the eye contact.

[Male, 49, Nonprofessional]

One nonprofessional had some thoughts about the usefulness of the couch.

I take issue with the couch. I'm not sure it's an appropriate route to take. It's too autistic, and disconnected. And when you're autistic you have no verbal language.

[Female, 44, Nonprofessional]

NUMERICAL DISTRIBUTION

Professionals: Eight said they had used the analytic couch occasionally or regularly; 12 said they had not.

Nonprofessionals: Eight said they had used the couch; 32 said they had not.

COMMENTS

Twice the percentage of professionals reported using the couch as the nonprofessionals, which is not surprising since many do so as part of their training. The couch is the legacy of the psychoanalytic method, and analytically oriented therapists often suggest it, even when the patient is not in traditional psychoanalysis.

As the therapist, I used to suggest the couch myself, but I haven't for years. If the patient is having difficulty talking to me while facing me, I'd prefer to deal with that directly rather than try to make an end run around it, which strikes me as an avoidance or resistance on the part of the therapist.

As a patient I might be interested in seeing what effect using the couch can have, but since I believe that the relationship with the therapist is the core of the therapy, I want us to be relating as much as possible, and the couch diverts us away from that relationship.

RELATED READING

Frank, A. (1995). The couch, psychoanalytic process, and psychic change: a case study. *Psychoanalytic Inquiry* 15(3):324–337.

Jacobson, J. G. (1995). The analytic couch: facilitator or sine qua non? *Psychoanalytic Inquiry* 15(3):304–313.

McAloon, R. F. (1987). The need to feel like an analyst: a study of countertransference in the case of a patient who refused to use the couch. *Modern Psychoanalysis* 12(1):65–87.

Sadow, L. (1995). Looking, listening, and the couch. *Psychoanalytic Inquiry* 15(3):386–395.

Waugaman, R. M. (1995). The analytic couch as transference object. *Psychoanalytic Inquiry* 15(3):338–357.

ຮຮຮຮ

Question 31: Where was the clock?

Every therapist has at least one timepiece with which to keep track of the therapeutic hour. Where to put it is an individual decision. Should the patient be able to see it as well? Is it a distraction if he can? Patients have very different feelings about this too.

A few people said they could see the clock.

There was always a small clock somewhere in the room that I could see.

[Female, 48, Nonprofessional]

Some found not seeing the clock acceptable.

In my first therapy, I remember being bothered that I couldn't see the clock, but I don't remember feeling that way with this one.

[Female, 50, Professional]

She had a little clock on her desk so that she could see it, but I couldn't. I remember thinking about the fact that I couldn't see it, but it didn't bother me.

[Female, 42, Nonprofessional]

Some actively preferred being able to see the clock.

It was helpful that I could see it, because I could help to regulate my own time.

[Male, 53, Professional]

I could see the clock. I remember thinking that it was a way for her not to have to tell me that we were running out of time. I liked it because then I could keep track of myself. I've always found it intrusive when we're on a roll and suddenly the therapist says we're running out of time. I'd rather have a sense of that myself.

[Female, 46, Nonprofessional]

It was facing me. I could see the clock. I liked that because I always knew how much time I had left.

[Female, 50, Nonprofessional]

I could see the clock and I watched it all the time, because I'm a control freak.

[Female, 48, Professional]

One person found the clock he could see symbolic of something in the therapist.

There were two clocks. The clock I could see was on a nonfunctioning mantelpiece, and one of the issues I had was that it was one of these artistic decorative clocks where the time was not clearly readable. It was a little bit ambiguous, and I pointed that out to her, and it was interesting because she had some issues about clearly terminating the hour.

[Male, 48, Nonprofessional]

Some people who could see the clock would have preferred not to.

It was on her desk, and we could both see it. I would have preferred not to, because I kept looking at it to see how much time we had left. When it came near the end of the hour, I would find myself saying, "Well, that's it."

[Female, 48, Nonprofessional]

Most people said they could not see the clock, and were divided between those who liked that arrangement and those who did not.

Some people were glad not to know the time, or found it helpful.

It was to the side; I could see it if I turned to my right. Once we got into the session, the time didn't matter to me. Most of the time I found the session over with a lot sooner than I had hoped. Not seeing the clock probably helped because I was unencumbered by thinking I had to rush to get a lot in in a short period of time.

[Male, 45, Nonprofessional]

I couldn't see it. I didn't want to be focusing on how much time we had left—that would have driven me crazy.

[Male, 46, Nonprofessional]

It used to be facing both of us; later on, she moved it. I preferred not seeing it because when the clock was visible I was aware of pacing myself in terms of how much I would allow myself to open up, depending on how much time was left, and was fearful that I couldn't close myself up adequately, because I had an early morning appointment and I had to go to work.

[Female, 47, Nonprofessional]

Some found it disturbing not to know the time.

It was behind me where I couldn't see it, and it was a little disconcerting.

[Female, 52, Professional]

It was over my shoulder. It was annoying at first, because I sometimes felt cut off, but after a while I got a sense of winding down.

[Female, 48, Nonprofessional]

I couldn't see it, and I wanted to, but I didn't tell her.

[Female, 45, Professional]

She had a clock in front of her that I couldn't see. It bothered me, but I could look at my watch.

[Female, 50, Nonprofessional]

She could see the clock, and I couldn't. For the first 5 years of therapy, I kept track of the time anyway, being overly responsible.

[Female, 45, Professional]

At least one person found disturbing the therapist's need to be aware of the time, and to control the session.

I always look for that. It was to my left and behind me, so she was always watching it. I would have preferred that there be no clock.

[Female, 42, Nonprofessional]

At some point, I realized that the clock was on the table facing her. Perhaps it felt like another aspect of deprivation, that she could see it and I couldn't, or if I looked around to check the time it was a cause for comment.

[Male, 44, Professional]

NUMERICAL DISTRIBUTION

Professionals: Seven said they could see the clock; 10 said they could not; 3 said they could see it when sitting up but not from the couch.

Nonprofessionals: Thirteen said they could see the clock; 25 said they could not; 2 said there was no clock.

COMMENTS

One of the therapist's jobs is to keep track of the session and maintain the structure and boundaries of the hour, so a clock is necessary. Some patients consciously complain about the "rigidity" of the therapist, but letting sessions run significantly over the allotted time can be profoundly disturbing, because it raises questions about the therapist's boundaries and his commitment to his own rules (see also Question 16).

As the therapist, I usually keep the clock where I can see it and the patient cannot, since most people find it distracting. Occasionally a patient will ask to turn the clock so we both can see it, and I will do that.

As the patient, I don't want to see the clock. It's too distracting, and may keep me from bringing things up if I don't think there's enough time. I know the therapist has to watch the time, but I don't want to see her eyes swinging toward the clock very often, which would suggest to me that she's more concerned with the time than with what I'm saying.

RELATED READING

Ingram, D. H. (1979). Time and timekeeping in psychoanalysis and psychotherapy. *American Journal of Psychoanalysis* 39(4):319–328.
Wiggins, K. M. (1983). The patient's relation to time during the final minutes of a psychotherapy session. *American Journal of Psychotherapy* 37(1):62–68.

⊠⊠⊠⊠

Question 32: Did your therapist smoke? Did you?

These days this question is less of an issue than in previous generations. Few therapists smoke. (Out of 60 therapists in the *Shrink Rap* sample, only 1 person smoked in his office.) But patients often do smoke, and the question arises of whether they will be permitted to smoke in the therapist's office.

Only 3 people said that the therapist allowed them to smoke in the office.

> I did, and I'm astounded that he let me smoke. I was, until I was 25, a really addicted smoker, maybe three packs a day, and would smoke four or five during a session. He didn't object to my smoking.
>
> [Male, 53, Professional]

> I did for many years. I would berate myself for smoking, and he never joined with me in that. He said I was taking care of other things and I'd take care of that in time.
>
> [Female, 52, Nonprofessional]

One therapist who had allowed smoking changed his mind.

> When he decided to stop letting people smoke in his office I told him he was being a hypocrite.
>
> [Female, 50, Nonprofessional]

Only 2 people said that the therapist smoked during the sessions.

> She did in the beginning of therapy—it was weird. I can't believe it now. I didn't like it because my mother smoked and I always hated it. I was fairly amazed that I was so tolerant of it. It was an indicator of how much I wanted the therapy to be good and to have a positive experience that I tolerated and even ignored it.
>
> [Female, 45, Professional]

> He did, but I had no reaction, because I smoked too.
>
> [Female, 50, Nonprofessional]

One person pointed out why her therapist didn't allow it.

> Not only did she not smoke, she had a lot of allergies, so there was an air purifier in the room going all the time.
>
> [Female, 45, Nonprofessional]

NUMERICAL DISTRIBUTION

Professionals: Did the therapist smoke? One yes; 19 no. Did the patient smoke? One yes; 19 no.

Nonprofessionals: Did the therapist smoke? One yes; 39 no. Did the patient smoke? Two yes; 38 no.

COMMENTS

In practical terms, this is not much of an issue nowadays. Fewer therapists and fewer patients smoke, or expect to do so in the the therapist's office. In theoretical terms, though, it's still an interesting question.

As the therapist, I don't think it's unreasonable to ask patients not to smoke for 45 or 50 minutes, and most patients never question that rule. I don't want smoke in my carpets or my upholstery or my clothes or my lungs.

If I am a patient who smokes, while I might find it hard not to, I appreciate the therapist taking good care of herself by not allowing it. If I don't smoke myself, I certainly don't want a therapist who does, not only because I have to inhale, too, but also because it raises questions about how well she takes care of herself.

RELATED READING

Kozlowski, L. T., Pillitteri, J. L., Sweeney, C. T., et al. (1996). Asking questions about urges or cravings for cigarettes. *Psychology of Addictive Behaviors* 10(4):248–260.

Munetz, M. R., and Davies, M. A. (1987). Smoking by patients. *Hospital and Community Psychiatry* 38(4):413–414.

Patton, D., Barnes, G. E., and Murray, R. P. (1993). Personality characteristics of smokers and ex-smokers. *Personality and Individual Differences* 15(6):653–664.

Sterling, R. C., Gottheil, E., Weinstein, S. P., et al. (1994). The effect of a no-smoking policy on recruitment and retention in outpatient cocaine treatment. *Journal of Addictive Diseases* 13(4):161–168.

∞∞∞∞

Question 33: Did the therapist eat or drink anything in the session? Did you?

This is another behavior that may seem innocuous on the surface, yet patients may have strong feelings about it.

Many patients, professionals and nonprofessionals, said they brought beverages (and occasionally food) into the session.

I sometimes had tea.

[Female, 50, Nonprofessional]

I had some juice sometimes because I'm diabetic.

[Male, 46, Nonprofessional]

I couple of times I brought something to drink, like juice.

[Female, 41, Nonprofessional]

The last few years I saw him on my lunch hour, and would bring my lunch with me. I always made sure it wasn't a messy lunch. It never bothered him.

[Female, 50, Nonprofessional]

Occasionally I brought food if I was rushing in between things. The therapist made no comment.

[Male, 48, Nonprofessional]

When the patient brings food or drink into the office, the therapist sometimes has a reaction.

It was the first session in the morning and she would have a thermos of Earl Grey tea, and we would both have a cup of that. I really liked that. At one point, she said that maybe my therapy would improve if I stopped drinking tea, but I didn't want to give it up.

[Female, 42, Nonprofessional]

I sometimes would bring in coffee, but it wasn't something she was happy about. She didn't say anything but I felt an awareness not to spill it. It made her a little nervous so I stopped doing it.

[Female, 45, Nonprofessional]

I remember one time I also brought a muffin, and I had been bitching about being overweight, and she pointed that out.

[Male, 49, Nonprofessional]

Once I brought something, and she said that she preferred that I didn't. She said that she found it distracting. We negotiated for water, water was okay.

[Female, 47, Nonprofessional]

The therapist may have a beverage.

Rarely she had coffee.

[Female, 50, Professional]

She might have had some coffee.

[Female, 55, Professional]

Sometimes she would drink water.

[Female, 39, Nonprofessional]

> He had tea from time to time, or water.
>
> [Female, 50, Professional]

> Every now and then she would sip from a cup of what I assumed to be tea or water.
>
> [Female, 45, Nonprofessional]

This is sometimes part of the "morning ritual."

> He would accommodate me by having very early appointments, and a few times he would bring something in.
>
> [Female, 52, Nonprofessional]

> When I added a second session, we met very early in the morning, and she may have had coffee in that session.
>
> [Male, 48, Nonprofessional]

Therapists occasionally eat in the session.

> Once or twice he asked my permission to eat a sandwich.
>
> [Male, 30, Professional]

When therapists eat or drink in the office, this may be acceptable to the patient.

> There would be a cup of tea or coffee. It was fine. It conveyed a sense of warmth and conviviality.
>
> [Male, 44, Professional]

> Occasionally she would sip something from a cup. I thought she deserved it after talking all day. She always offered me water if I wanted it.
>
> [Female, 46, Nonprofessional]

> Sometimes he would have coffee or food. When I started therapy I was unaware that there was any controversy about that, so it just became normal.
>
> [Male, 50, Professional]

Or it may not be acceptable.

> She ate and drank, which I found disconcerting. I never told her. She asked my permission and I should have said no. I thought if she was

going to sit there being hungry and longing to eat, it's better that she eat.

[Female, 51, Professional]

That would have been a real problem. I wouldn't go to a therapist who does that. I can't believe any therapist would.

[Female, 40, Nonprofessional]

He used to eat during the session and it pissed me off.

[Male, 48, Nonprofessional]

Sometimes therapists and patients share a beverage, and it becomes a kind of connection.

We might have shared coffee.

[Female, 41, Nonprofessional]

She had tea. I did too. She gave it to me.

[Female, 56, Professional]

She would sip tea. It felt very comfortable. There was a setup in the waiting area so it was available for you to help yourself.

[Female, 45, Professional]

He would have coffee or tea. I did, too. In fact, that was a bonding thing sometimes. I would bring my own, but we both loved coffee.

[Female, 48, Nonprofessional]

Patients don't always accept the offer.

She often had a hot beverage. She always offered it to me and I always said no.

[Male, 49, Nonprofessional]

There was coffee in the waiting room, which he offered to me, and I could have had it if I wanted.

[Female, 48, Nonprofessional]

And sometimes therapists don't share.

Sometimes she drank tea. She never offered me any.

[Female, 45, Professional]

NUMERICAL DISTRIBUTION

Professionals: Did therapists eat or drink? Twelve yes; 8 no. Did patients? Six yes; 14 no.

Nonprofessionals: Did therapists eat or drink? Fifteen yes; 25 no. Did patients? Seventeen yes; 23 no.

COMMENTS

Though we might have expected therapists to be less stringent about rules with a professional patient, there was no major difference between the two groups here, except that more nonprofessionals brought beverages to the session than the professionals.

Patients bring things to drink all the time, and occasionally things to eat, and as the therapist I rarely say anything about it unless it becomes clear that these things are being used to avoid working or reduce anxiety. I never eat or drink in the therapy office.

As a patient, I would like the freedom to drink when I'm thirsty or even eat something, if I don't have any other chance to do that, without feeling like I'm being scolded by a controlling parent. I don't want the therapist eating or drinking anything because if he's thinking about that he's not paying attention to me.

RELATED READING

Kahn, S. R. (1993). Reflections upon the functions of food in a children's psychotherapy group. *Journal of Child and Adolescent Group Psychotherapy* 3(3):143–153.

℞℞℞℞

Question 34: Did the therapist answer the phone during the session?

Answering the phone during the session is another behavior that may seem reasonable or even unimportant to the therapist, but it can bring up powerful feelings in the patient.

Most therapists did not answer their phones during the session, but when they did patients had different reactions. Some patients accepted the behavior, sometimes after some work on the issue.

He would answer the phone, and speak briefly, and typically would arrange to speak with people at other times. I found it annoying, and he helped me to resolve that. At times it was helpful, in that it gave me a break. The narcissistic injury was softened by the understanding that I could get through to him, that he'd want to hear from me as well if I needed to reach him. Later on, he had a child, and that was another dimension of his life, that his kid could reach him, and we talked about it as a technique issue with patients of mine.

[Male, 53, Professional]

I think once or twice the answering machine wouldn't pick up and she answered, probably a call she was waiting for. It threw my concentration off, but I didn't resent it or anything.

[Male, 49, Nonprofessional]

He did very rarely, and he would always say that he had to get the call, and would only be on for 30 seconds. At first it threw me, but it wasn't a big deal.

[Female, 50, Professional]

Occasionally he did. He was supposed to have his phone calls screened, so it must have been something important, and he would only stay on for a second. He didn't have a machine to deal with. The secretary was supposed to deal with that. It didn't bother me because he clearly was annoyed and didn't stay on.

[Female, 48, Nonprofessional]

It happened once, and it was an obvious distress to her that the phone even rang. My reaction was to her reaction—it was positive to see affect.

[Male, 44, Professional]

She did, but only when she told me in advance that there was something going on. I was mildly annoyed, but only mildly. I figured she worked in a high-pressure clinic and there was a lot going on and that's the way it went.

[Male, 50, Nonprofessional]

She would tell me at the beginning if there was an emergency.

[Female, 50, Professional]

It happened only once or twice. She was expecting an emergency call that she had to take or else her whole evening would be screwed up, and she would go into the other room, which was her bedroom. It didn't bother me because it gave me a chance to regroup and see where I was.

[Female, 50, Nonprofessional]

She did only when the machine wasn't working. She seemed embarrassed about it.

[Female, 44, Nonprofessional]

It happened rarely. I was a little annoyed, but he didn't stay on the phone long.

[Female, 59, Professional]

And others had some negative reactions.

I felt that someone who was a strict Freudian analyst, who started and stopped at the precise moment, should not have been picking up the phone. Sometimes it rang three or four times during a single session. I told him about it and he didn't do anything about it. He didn't seem to relate to the point I was making.

[Female, 57, Professional]

He didn't get into conversations. It was just, "I can't talk right now," or, "I'll call you back." But if it happened four or five times in a session it was a big distraction. Sometimes it gave me a break I wanted. Sometimes I felt "saved by the bell" and sometimes if I was thinking about something it gave me an extra 30 seconds to think about what I wanted to say. Other times I felt like I couldn't even pick up where I left off.

[Female, 58, Professional]

It really pissed me off. I hate that. I don't do that.

[Female, 48, Professional]

I hated it. I told him and he would apologize. Sometimes he would tell me beforehand, and then it was okay.

[Female, 50, Nonprofessional]

Once I had a reaction to his answering the phone at the very end of my session and putting the phone down to finish talking to me as I was about to leave, and I told him that, as far as I was concerned, if I was still here the session was still on and I wanted to be able to say to him whatever I wanted to say without someone on the other end of the phone being able to hear my conversation. He accepted that.

[Male, 42, Professional]

Patients don't always tell the therapist how they feel about the behavior.

I thought it was inappropriate. I didn't tell her because it was only occasionally and she would always say in advance that she was waiting and she would have to get it because it was important. I still didn't like it.

[Female, 44, Nonprofessional]

It was annoying. I didn't tell her.

[Female, 53, Nonprofessional]

I wasn't crazy about it. The longer I saw her the more our relationship changed, became less formal, and the more she would answer the phone. Sometimes she'd even tell me who it was. I didn't tell her it upset me. It was breaking my rhythm in the session.

[Female, 45, Nonprofessional]

I hated that. I never told her. I wasn't good at confrontation. She always took a message, but she had an answering machine so I was never clear on why she would do it.

[Female, 42, Nonprofessional]

Patients can be understanding of the need to speak on the phone during an emergency situation.

I got the impression through the whole time I was with her that it was really an emergency in those times that she did. I remember once the phone rang and rang and rang and she finally had to answer it. Whenever she did it, it was okay, and she would get off the phone right away.

[Female, 48, Nonprofessional]

It happened maybe a couple of times. Each time she would apologize and explain that it was a call that she'd been expecting. I got the impression also that it was quite important, that it wasn't the dry cleaner.

[Male, 52, Nonprofessional]

Patients sometimes tell themselves that their angry feelings about this behavior are not justified.

> He has a separate emergency phone, and when that one rang he answered it. He was on for no more than 30 seconds. I didn't care for it but my reaction seemed totally irrational because it was his emergency line. He would do it only once every 4 months or so.
> [Female, 52, Nonprofessional]

Sometimes even when the therapist has an answering machine, the phone is still a distraction.

> When the phone rang he would always look to see that the answering machine was connected, so he sometimes got momentarily distracted by the phone, but he never actually picked it up and talked to someone.
> [Male, 51, Nonprofessional]

> Her answering machine had this horrendous ring, and it was very distracting, and I asked if she could do something about it, but she never did and I got used to it.
> [Female, 47, Nonprofessional]

> She didn't answer the phone, but she would have to answer the buzzer to the front door, which was on a kind of phone. I thought it would be annoying but it never was.
> [Female, 41, Nonprofessional]

NUMERICAL DISTRIBUTION

Professionals: Ten said it never happened; 10 said it had happened. Of those people, 3 said they got angry or annoyed; 7 said they understood and accepted it.

Nonprofessionals: Twenty-five said it never happened; 15 said it had happened. Of these, 7 said they were upset by it; 8 said they were not.

COMMENTS

Almost half of both groups reported that the therapist answered the phone during the session. Many people said they didn't like that, and a number of them said they never told the therapist that they were upset about it. Therapists who answer the phone need to re-examine why they are doing that.

As the therapist, I can find no acceptable reason for answering the phone during the session. Modern technology makes certain that messages will be received. Patients know the therapist is likely to be in a session when they call, and there are few situations that can't wait 45 minutes for the session to end. If the therapist's situation is so out of control that he can't wait for the end of the session, maybe he shouldn't be working that day.

As the patient, I can't think of a time when I wouldn't be upset with the therapist answering the phone in the middle of my session. Such behavior would convey to me that the therapist's priorities are much more important than mine, and would raise doubts about his ability to contain his own anxiety, not to mention mine.

RELATED READING

Meek, C. L. (1986). Guidelines for using an answering machine in your practice. In *Innovations in Clinical Practice: A Source Book*, vol. 5, ed. P. A. Keller and L. G. Ritt, pp. 101–106. Sarasota, FL: Professional Resource Exchange.

Weiss, S. S. (1975). The effect on the transference of "special events" occurring during psychoanalysis. *International Journal of Psycho-Analysis* 56(1):69–75.

🔊🔊🔊🔊

Question 35: Did you take any psychoactive medications during treatment?

When the patient's problems don't respond to treatment, or when the patient needs help coping while therapy proceeds, prescription medications are sometimes indicated.

The most commonly prescribed medications fall into two major categories: antidepressants and antianxiety agents. The same proportion of professionals took medications as the nonprofessionals, although the nonprofessionals were more likely to take antidepressants. Sometimes the therapist suggests it.

> I took Zoloft for about a year. She suggested it, but I was perfectly willing to try it. It helped.
>
> [Male, 49, Nonprofessional]

> I took Zoloft. She suggested it and I was very relieved when she did. It helped a lot.
>
> [Female, 44, Nonprofessional]

Sometimes the patient suggests the medication.

> I took Prozac for a year. I suggested it. It helped a lot.
>
> [Female, 41, Nonprofessional]

> I started Zoloft about a year before I stopped therapy. I suggested it, but she was open to it.
>
> [Female, 50, Professional]

Occasionally the patient will get medication on his or her own.

> At the beginning I took tranquilizers. It was only for about a year. I found the psychiatrist myself.
>
> [Female, 50, Nonprofessional]

> I started with Prozac, which was not effective, and switched to Wel-butrin, which was. I started taking them before I started therapy.
>
> [Male, 51, Nonprofessional]

> I referred myself to a psychiatrist, someone I know. I tried Prozac for 2 weeks, and thought I was going to have a heart attack. I switched to Zoloft.
>
> [Female, 39, Professional]

The professionals were more likely to take an antianxiety medication.

> Maybe occasionally I would take some Valium to help me sleep.
>
> [Male, 53, Professional]

> I requested some at one point, and she did refer me to the psychiatrist she worked with, but I never went. I did take Valium at some point for anxiety control as needed.
>
> [Male, 44, Professional]

Most psychotherapists are not permitted to prescribe medication, and therefore need to refer patients to a psychopharmacologist or psychiatrist. Patients are often relieved when the therapist does suggest medication.

> She suggested Prozac, and I reacted with relief. She referred me to a psychopharmacologist.
>
> [Female, 52, Professional]

> For about 3 or 4 years I was on a number of antidepressants. I think the therapist suggested it. I was really in bad shape for a while. The therapist had to refer me to an M.D., who was able to prescribe the medication.
>
> [Female, 48, Nonprofessional]

Some patients react negatively when the therapist suggests a medication.

> I took Paxil for 18 months, then 5 months off it, and then again for a year. She suggested the medication. I said, "Absolutely not, no way." Because I was afraid of it, I don't like taking medication. It meant that I had failed on my own. I was very, very against it. But talking to her and realizing that it was worth the risk made me change my mind. It helped tremendously.
>
> [Female, 48, Nonprofessional]

> For a long time she encouraged me to take an antidepressant, which I resisted. Eventually I did. I started out with Serzone, but I switched to Prozac. I had to pick a psychiatrist that was covered by my plan, and the only one I could find never returned my phone calls. So I got my physician to write the prescription after he talked to my therapist.
>
> [Male, 49, Nonprofessional]

Patients are not always happy with the psychiatrist, even when the medication is working.

> The staff psychiatrist prescribed it, and I had to see him. I was told that he had to prescribe it and had to monitor the people on it. I thought he was a jerk, because the first time I went in there, I was in for about 8 minutes, and I thought, "He knows absolutely nothing about me." I realized that he wasn't there to analyze me but how could he get any kind of reading in 5 or 10 minutes? After that, when I had to deal with him, I was totally frustrated by his lack of communication.
>
> [Female, 48, Nonprofessional]

I took Elavil for 6 months. I was having such difficulty sleeping she thought I needed something, and she referred me to a psychiatrist who I saw a couple of times. I was leery of it, but I was so desperate that I needed something. It was a little like cold water because he wasn't as warm and fuzzy as my therapist. He was nice enough, and saw me only once, and agreed to monitor my medication over the phone.

[Female, 42, Nonprofessional]

NUMERICAL DISTRIBUTION

Professionals: Five said they had taken medication during treatment; 15 had not. Of those who did, 2 took occasional Valium, and 3 took an SSRI (selective serotonin reuptake inhibitor) antidepressant (Prozac, Zoloft, or Paxil); all said the medication helped.

Nonprofessionals: Nine said they had taken medication; 31 had not. One person took antianxiety medication, and 8 took antidepressants; all said the medication helped.

COMMENTS

There were no significant differences here between the groups; the professionals required medication just as often as the nonprofessionals.

As the therapist, I'm aware that new medications can be very effective in treating certain symptoms, such as depression, anxiety, or obsessive-compulsive behavior. I have an association with a psychopharmacologist to whom I refer anyone I think needs medication. At the same time, I don't want this to be a substitute for investigation and understanding of the patient's psychodynamics.

As the patient, I want relief from my distress. If there is a simple and easy way to get that relief, I will want to consider it and even try it. I may be concerned about the implications of taking "medicine" and may feel like this makes me "sick," but I hope that won't stop me from getting the relief I need.

RELATED READING

Biondi, M. (1995). Beyond the brain–mind dichotomy and toward a common organizing principle of pharmacological and psychological treatments. *Psychotherapy and Psychosomatics* 64(1):1–8.

Drescher, J. (1995). Psychotherapy, medication and belief. *Issues in Psychoanalytic Psychology* 17(1):7–28.

Freimuth, M. (1996). Combining psychotherapy and psychopharmacology: with or without prescription privileges. *Psychotherapy* 33(3): 474–478.

Granet, R. B. (1993). The cotreatment of patients: when psychotherapists and pharmacotherapists collaborate. *Journal of Psychotherapy Practice and Research* 2(3):222–229.

Kriegman, D. (1996). The effectiveness of medication: the *Consumer Reports* study. *American Psychologist* 51(10):1086.

Sarwer-Foner, G. J., ed. (1993). Special section: Psychotherapy and pharmacotherapy. *American Journal of Psychotherapy* 47(3):387–423.

🔊🔊🔊🔊

Question 36: Did you ever work with dreams?

Therapists have traditionally worked with and analyzed patient dreams. There are many different ways of doing this.

> I would describe the dream, associate to the various aspects of the dream, and he would ask me more about certain elements of it.
>
> [Female, 58, Professional]

> I would recite the dream and she would give a short interpretation, an arrow up or an arrow down as an indicator of progress.
>
> [Female, 52, Professional]

> Depending on what part of the dream I was connected to in the telling, she would focus on that part and get me to take on that part.
>
> [Female, 45, Professional]

> In a very psychoanalytic way, going through every element in the dream. I liked it a lot and it was very helpful.
>
> [Female, 48, Professional]

> Occasionally I would bring in a dream and he would interpret it and we would talk about the symbolism. We also did some visualization work.
>
> [Male, 30, Professional]

> We dealt with a dream by looking at it so that all the people in the dream were me. It was interesting, but I think I should have free-associated more to the different elements.
>
> [Female, 50, Professional]

> It was a kind of who's who in the dream. It was his choice to raise transference issues, like where would he be in the dream, if at all.
>
> [Male, 53, Professional]

Sometimes the therapist would write down the dreams.

> We worked with dreams quite a lot. I would frequently bring in dreams and we would discuss them in great detail. She would write extensive notes, she would write down the whole dream, and we would talk about it. We would talk about what the elements of the dream might mean to me, and what they could be saying about what I was feeling or experiencing in my life. She might say what she thought it meant, but never led me in a particular direction. It took a while for me to understand how to use the dreams, and perhaps in the beginning she was more directive, but after a while I became experienced in using the dreams on my own. It was very useful.
>
> [Female, 48, Nonprofessional]

And sometimes the patient would be asked to keep a dream journal, or even decide on his or her own to do that.

> I kept a journal and she would read it, or I would mail stuff in with dreams. She would read them and we would discuss it.
>
> [Male, 49, Nonprofessional]

> She read my dream journal, between sessions. She told me things she noticed, that there was a lot about my mother.
>
> [Female, 48, Nonprofessional]

> She suggested that I try to take notes of my dreams, and any ones that caught my attention in particular to try to analyze them a little and see if I could come up with what they might be alluding to. We didn't do that very often, but it was something that she brought up and I tried to do a little of that. It was interesting, because before that I never thought much about my dreams, but now I was actually thinking about them and writing them down. With one dream I went into great detail as to what I thought it meant. I wrote a whole page about what I thought it meant, and brought it in and read it to her,

and we talked about it for a while. It was interesting, and I think it could have been useful if I had gotten more deeply into it. I think she was just trying to show me this as an alternative, something I could do on my own and carry with me.

[Male, 45, Nonprofessional]

I would write them down and bring them to her and we would talk about them a lot. We talked a lot about my house dreams. It was useful.

[Female, 44, Nonprofessional]

If I had a dream, she told me to write it down, and then we would talk about it. She was interested in the feelings I was having in the dream and the associations I would have.

[Female, 42, Nonprofessional]

Patients know when working with dreams is significant to the therapist.

He was very interested in dreams, and I've always had a problem remembering them, so it was a rare occurrence. He suggested writing them down, and I did that a couple of times. He felt that it was unusual that I didn't remember dreams. His attitude seemed to be that I was suppressing them.

[Male, 53, Nonprofessional]

It was a very big interest of the therapist, and she expressed that to me, and I immediately started dreaming. I think the day I went there I had a dream, a classic and repetitive dream that recurred over the years. I had other dreams as well, but I had that one dream almost every week. It changed its nature but it was basically the same dream.

[Male, 52, Nonprofessional]

He loved talking about dreams! It was interesting, but I don't know if it was useful. I would tell him the dream, and he would say, "What do you think this is about?" They were interesting, though I didn't always know what to do with them, but I enjoyed that.

[Female, 48, Nonprofessional]

Occasionally the patient seems more interested in the dreams than the therapist.

> If I had a major dream I would bring it in and we would talk about it.
>
> [Female, 48, Nonprofessional]

> Sometimes if I brought it up, if there was a dream that I considered very significant, she would ask me about it, ask me what I thought it meant, why it seemed significant to me.
>
> [Female, 45, Nonprofessional]

> I don't think she ever asked for them. I would say, "I had the wildest dream." It sounds like a cartoon of a therapist, because she would say, "What do you think that means?" And I'd almost always get it right, because I don't think you have to be a rocket scientist to interpret dreams. We didn't work with dreams that much, but it was very useful. And I still sometimes will write down a really strange dream and try to think about it.
>
> [Female, 40, Nonprofessional]

Several people said that being in therapy had educated them to think more about their dreams.

> After 3 years he was able to tease dreams out of me. It was fascinating. There was one common dream, and as I got healthier, the dream changed and it was easy to see it.
>
> [Female, 45, Nonprofessional]

> I would always find the dreams a great source of support, like somebody was telling me the right thing.
>
> [Female, 50, Nonprofessional]

Oddly enough, it can happen only once or twice.

> I think I must have once or twice. We would talk about it, but I wouldn't do any classical free association. I would interpret my own dreams.
>
> [Male, 48, Nonprofessional]

> We did once, and it was very interesting. It never came up again.
>
> [Female, 41, Nonprofessional]

A few people reported specific dreams.

> Aside from allowing me to feel and cry about the losses in my life from having parents who were damaged themselves, one wonderful thing that happened was that I had a terrific dream about my father,

who had always been a very remote figure and a scary guy to me. In the dream I was in a terrifying situation, and he appeared as an encourager, encouraging me to save myself. It was so moving to me, and I brought it into therapy, and it was a major moment, bigger than all the dreams I had had about myself. It changed the way I felt about my father, even though in real life we never had that kind of exchange. It made me realize that he would have liked to have that exchange.

[Male, 52, Nonprofessional]

I remember a dream about a small dog falling out of a window and hanging on the ledge by its fingernails. Actually, it was my mother.

[Female, 48, Nonprofessional]

I once told her about a dream where I was in the car, and the steering wheel was loose and the brakes weren't working, and she asked what I thought that meant, and I said "That I'm not in control?" And we just laughed.

[Female, 40, Nonprofessional]

Several people said they did not find dream work valuable.

I was uncomfortable doing it and was resistant to doing it so it wasn't very useful. I was incredibly insecure and had no self-esteem.

[Female, 42, Nonprofessional]

We didn't do it a lot; there was too much else to talk about.

[Female, 44, Nonprofessional]

I would report it and then we would nibble away at it and try to find connections. It was useful as an exercise rather than as progress. I never saw it as the serious part of therapy, more of a fun game.

[Male, 49, Nonprofessional]

Several people said they had had trouble remembering their dreams.

We did a little bit but not much. It would have been very helpful if I had done it more. I just didn't remember them.

[Male, 52, Nonprofessional]

I don't know if it was useful, because it wasn't very often, it wasn't consistent.

[Female, 50, Nonprofessional]

We didn't do it a lot because I don't remember them often. I don't think it was any more useful than working with day-to-day material.
[Male, 51, Nonprofessional]

We did a little, but I don't remember dreams very often. It was interesting, but I don't know if it was useful.
[Male, 50, Nonprofessional]

One person reported changing her opinion about working with dreams.

She asked me to pay attention to them. When I remembered them we would talk about what struck me about them, what struck her about them, what they might suggest. I thought it was somewhat bogus but we did do it. It started feeling useful when we actually did it.
[Female, 39, Nonprofessional]

NUMERICAL DISTRIBUTION

Professionals: Only 2 people said they did not work with dreams in treatment; 18 said they did.

Nonprofessionals: Fifteen people said they often worked with dreams; 17 said they did occasionally; 8 said they never did.

COMMENTS

More professionals than nonprofessionals seem to recognize the value of working with dreams, or at least their therapists seem to have been more into it.

Whatever dreams may be and wherever they come from, they have always seemed to me useful clues to what may be going on with the patient just below the surface of his or her conscious mind. As the therapist, I encourage patients to remember and bring in dreams, and most people are able to do this once they start paying attention. Only a few people find this work uninteresting or irrelevant.

As the patient, I love the idea that I know more than I know consciously, and may have access to that material through dreams. Dream work is usually fun, and often exciting. It adds a whole other dimension to therapy.

RELATED READING

Barrineau, P. (1996). A reexamination of the role of dreams (from a person-centered perspective): practical implications for mental health counselors. *Journal of Mental Health Counseling* 18(1):3–15.

Cartwright, R. D. (1993). Who needs their dreams? The usefulness of dreams in psychotherapy. *Journal of the American Academy of Psychoanalysis* 21(4):539–547.

Heller, M. B. (1989). Dream work in analytic psychotherapy. *British Journal of Psychotherapy* 6(2):154–159.

Keller, J. W., Brown, G., Maier, K., et al. (1995). Use of dreams in psychotherapy: a survey of clinicians in private practice. *Psychological Reports* 76(3, pt. 2):1288–1290.

🔖🔖🔖🔖

Question 37: Did you ever have a dream about your therapist?

In *Shrink Rap*, I asked if the therapist had dreams about the patient, and 52 out of 60 therapists said they had. Here the question explores the other direction: whether the patient dreams about the therapist.

Usually when the patient has a dream about the therapist, the dream is discussed.

> I had a number of dreams about her over the years, and we discussed them.
>
> [Female, 48, Nonprofessional]

> It was one of the more significant dreams. We discussed it at length.
>
> [Female, 46, Nonprofessional]

One person was surprised it didn't happen more often.

> I remember being surprised that I only had one dream about the therapist.
>
> [Male, 49, Nonprofessional]

And another waited until after terminating.

> I have dreamt about him since I stopped, but not while I was in therapy.
>
> [Female, 48, Nonprofessional]

Even when the patient dreams about the therapist, the dream is not always discussed.

> I had some dreams about her, but I don't know that I brought them up in therapy except to mention that I had such a dream.
>
> [Female, 45, Professional]

> It's hard for me to do that, because it's very hard for me to talk to him about my feelings for him.
>
> [Female, 50, Nonprofessional]

NUMERICAL DISTRIBUTION

Professionals: Eleven people said they remembered dreaming about the therapist, and 10 of them discussed the dreams while 1 person did not; 9 said they had not had such dreams.

Nonprofessionals: Seventeen people had dreams about the therapist, and 12 discussed the dreams while 5 did not; 23 did not have such dreams.

COMMENTS

Slightly more than half the professionals said they had dreamt about their therapists, and slightly less than half the nonprofessionals did.

It usually takes a while for the therapist to become important enough to appear in a dream, although I have occasionally had patients report such dreams in the second week of treatment. As the therapist, I am especially interested in hearing these dreams, because they give me such direct feedback about what I'm doing right and doing wrong. Of course, I may also appear in dreams in disguised form, but the dreams in which I make an appearance as myself are often turning points in the therapy.

As a patient, a dream about the therapist can be reassuring, if positive, or disturbing if not. I think of these dreams as monitoring the therapist and place a lot of trust in the implicit evaluations they make.

RELATED READING

Lippmann, P. (1996). On dreams and interpersonal psychoanalysis. *Psychoanalytic Dialogues* 6(6):831–846.

Lipschutz, L. S., Blum, H. P., Yazmajian, R. V., et al. (1993). Resistance, transference, and dreams. In *Psychoanalytic Articles on Dreams,* ed. T. M. Alston, R. M. Whitman, H. Deserno, et al., pp. 477–581. Madison, CT: International Universities Press.

Myers, W. A., and Solomon, M. (1989). Dream frequency in psychoanalysis and psychoanalytic psychotherapy. *Journal of the American Psychoanalytic Association* 37(3):715–725.

Rohde, A. B., Geller, J. D., and Farber, B. A. (1992). Dreams about the therapist: mood, interaction, and themes. *Psychotherapy* 29(4):536–544.

🐎🐎🐎🐎

Question 38: Did you ever ask the therapist to look at something you had written, painted, or made?

Sometimes the patient will bring in some artistic creation, and ask the therapist to look at it.

Usually this takes the form of a piece of writing.

> I gave him some poetry. He commented about the quality of it; he liked it. They were poems about issues we had been talking about a lot, so I didn't need for him to say much about the content. I was just showing it to him as a different slant on the topic.
>
> [Female, 58, Professional]

> I brought in some short stories that I wrote, and more recently my professional articles. There are times when I've told him that he'd better react a certain way, and we negotiate whether he's willing to read it under those conditions. In regard to the article, he responded very positively. He's been very actively supportive of my writing and presenting.
>
> [Male, 50, Professional]

> It was a letter I wrote to my father, and I also read her a letter from my uncle and my response to him. She was very supportive.
>
> [Female, 41, Nonprofessional]

> She would read my dream journal and we would discuss it.
>
> [Male, 49, Nonprofessional]

He read my dissertation, and not many people do that. He considered it a work of love. He sensed my interest in the work and my attachment to it. It was a very touching experience for me.

[Male, 53, Professional]

I asked him to look at a syllabus I wrote for a course on abstinence and gratification. He was very positive in his comments. I also asked him to look at a collection of things my friends had written for my fortieth birthday. He didn't do it in any depth, but I didn't expect that.

[Female, 48, Professional]

I asked him to look at some papers I had written, and my final analytic case that I presented. His feedback was very helpful.

[Male, 42, Professional]

Occasionally the patient wants the therapist to look at (or experience) some other kind of creation.

I brought in some of my pottery.

[Female, 50, Professional]

I would show her a lot of my photographs. She reacted very supportively, and she was very complimentary.

[Male, 45, Nonprofessional]

I played the violin for him. He was very supportive and encouraging.

[Male, 30, Professional]

I made a pouch, and I showed it to her because one of my problems was that I couldn't finish anything, and I was pretty proud of it. She was very happy.

[Female, 48, Nonprofessional]

I did a drawing in the session.

[Female, 45, Professional]

Several people said that they had brought in photographs, often of the family.

I did bring pictures of my family, and she was interested.

[Female, 62, Professional]

I showed him some photographs from my trip.

[Female, 52, Nonprofessional]

Once in a while this kind of exchange takes place outside the office.

I had a show of my work at a gallery and I asked him to come to the show and he came and said something really important. He said, "Yep, it's all here."

[Male, 46, Nonprofessional]

Most people indicated that they got positive or supportive feedback.

I gave her some of my poems. She was very interested and said she liked them a lot.

[Male, 50, Nonprofessional]

I brought her some letters I had written. She read them and commented on them.

[Male, 52, Nonprofessional]

She often looked at things that I wrote. She always thought that they were great.

[Female, 51, Professional]

I read her some of my angry journal entries. She listened and said, "That certainly says a lot about how you feel."

[Female, 50, Nonprofessional]

I was having a lot of trouble writing, so I asked her to look at something I had written. She was pretty objective about it—looking at my handwriting and saying it looked like I was having trouble.

[Female, 42, Nonprofessional]

But a few said there was little or no reaction.

I did a couple of times. She was willing to do it but she didn't say much of anything. She asked me how it felt for me to do it.

[Female, 45, Professional]

I had kept a notebook in college of poems and writings, and I showed that to her. She said that it was interesting; it gave her some information.

[Female, 44, Nonprofessional]

> I brought in an article I had written. It was right at the end of therapy so I didn't get any feedback.
>
> [Female, 51, Professional]

> It was a memorial statement, a eulogy, I had written for my mother. He just listened.
>
> [Female, 41, Nonprofessional]

A few patients said they had wanted to or considered bringing in something for the therapist to look at but decided against doing so.

> I didn't do it because I knew that he wouldn't.
>
> [Female, 57, Professional]

> I was doing all this writing; you would think I would have. There are a lot of things you just don't think of because they don't seem part of the system.
>
> [Female, 50, Nonprofessional]

Occasionally the therapist seems hesitant to participate.

> I'm an artist and I make my living with my hands and I thought it was important that she see what I do and she was very reluctant to do that and we had to discuss it for a long time.
>
> [Female, 44, Nonprofessional]

One person discussed some of the complexities of asking the therapist to look at a long piece of writing.

> I asked her to read a novel that I had written and published, and we spent a fair amount of time talking about the novel. That turned out to be a much more complicated question than I had anticipated. It's a very long novel, and there was the issue of the time she would spend reading it, and also, because she was in graduate school at the same time, she found it difficult to read it on a timely basis. She hadn't finished it even at the time we terminated. On the other hand, I wasn't really sure it was fair for me to ask a therapist to read a 600- or 700-page book for free, in effect.
>
> [Male, 48, Nonprofessional]

NUMERICAL DISTRIBUTION

Professionals: Ten people did bring in something they had created; 10 did not. Three people brought in family photographs.

Nonprofessionals: Nineteen brought in something they had created; 21 did not.

COMMENTS

Patients often want the therapist to read what they have written, as another way of seeing into the psyche. As the therapist, I'm always willing to look at what patients bring: writing, painting, whatever they want me to see. I always learn something new and sometimes the patient does too.

As the patient, I'd always like feedback about what I'm doing creatively or professionally from someone who knows me as well as my therapist does.

RELATED READING

Aldridge, D. (1994). Single-case research designs for the creative art therapist. *Arts in Psychotherapy* 21(5):333–342.

Mazza, N. (1993). Poetry therapy: toward a research agenda for the 1990s. *Arts in Psychotherapy* 20(1):51–59.

Rabinor, J. R. (1991). The process of recovery from an eating disorder: the use of journal writing in the initial phase of treatment. *Psychotherapy in Private Practice* 9(1):93–106.

Torem, M. S. (1993). Therapeutic writing as a form of ego-state therapy. *American Journal of Clinical Hypnosis* 35(4):267–276.

🏵🏵🏵🏵

Question 39: Did the therapist ever recommend a particular book?

Therapists are often aware of books about issues that the patient may be dealing with, and sometimes the therapist will recommend such a book.

> A couple of books. One was called *The Hidden Injuries of Class* and I read it and enjoyed it. The others were the Alice Miller books, *Prisoners of Childhood* and the others. I thought they were terrific. I bought copies of both of those and gave them to many people.
>
> [Male, 52, Nonprofessional]

I did read it. It was about alcoholism, its history and treatments. It was helpful.

[Male, 49, Nonprofessional]

He recommended several. *The Psychiatric Interview* was one. I read parts of it. He also mentioned the Bowlby books on attachment and separation. Parts of them were very useful. He gave me a paper to read once that was very helpful.

[Female, 52, Nonprofessional]

Patients, however, don't always take the recommendation.

It was called *He, She, and We.* I didn't read it, because I thought it was bullshit, the same old stuff I'd been hearing for too many years.

[Male, 52, Nonprofessional]

I read a little. The whole time I was thinking, "What did she want me to read this for?" I just said forget it.

[Female, 50, Professional]

She recommended *The Drama of the Gifted Child.* I bought it but I didn't read it. I started it but it didn't seem to resonate with me.

[Male, 49, Nonprofessional]

Sometimes patients find the books useful: informative, enlightening, thought-provoking.

It was helpful because I was able to see parallels in my own life.

[Female, 48, Nonprofessional]

The first book she lent me was *The Drama of the Gifted Child* and that blew me away, that there was this book that was written about me and everyone I knew. It was an eye-opener.

[Female, 45, Professional]

Sometimes patients read the book more for information about the therapist than for its content.

I read it more out of curiosity, to find out why she thought it would help me.

[Female, 46, Nonprofessional]

When the patient is a professional, the therapist may recommend books in the field.

> He recommended something by Spotnitz, and a book called something like *Telling Your Own Story*. I read pieces of that, and another book by Spotnitz. I was very taken by the one about telling your own story. It was the first glimpse of what my therapist's theory was, where he was coming from.
>
> [Male, 53, Professional]

> A few times he gave me articles; he was the editor of an analytic journal. There were times he would give me things as a colleague, more than as a patient.
>
> [Female, 50, Professional]

> I did read them. One was *The Shaman's Body*, by Arnold Mandel, a Jungian who's gotten into Eastern and shamanic practices and integrated them.
>
> [Male, 30, Professional]

> She mentioned Winnicott and Searles as people to read. I was familiar with them.
>
> [Male, 44, Professional]

Sometimes the patient has a very negative reaction to the written material.

> When she lent me a psychoanalytic paper by one of the four therapists she was recommending, I found it very disturbing. It was very, very heavy psychoanalytic jargon, and everybody seemed to be a case history proving the theoretical position, and I really didn't want to be thought of in those terms, as a case history proving somebody's theory.
>
> [Male, 48, Nonprofessional]

> It was one of those self-help books. I didn't like it at all, because it was so poorly written. I was amazed that she liked it, and it made me question her judgment.
>
> [Female, 42, Nonprofessional]

Books can be a way of connecting between patient and therapist.

> We talked a lot about books. We even at times shared books. She would lend me a book, or we actually bought a few books together.
>
> [Female, 51, Professional]

> We would talk about books, but she never recommended a book to me. I would recommend books to her.
>
> [Female, 42, Nonprofessional]

Even when the therapist has written books, the patient doesn't always want to read them.

> She's written a lot of books and I've never even thought about reading them.
>
> [Female, 56, Professional]

NUMERICAL DISTRIBUTION

Professionals: Nine said the therapist had recommended a book; 11 said the therapist did not. Of those who did, all 9 read at least some of the book.

Nonprofessionals: Fourteen said the therapist had recommended a book; 26 said the therapist had not. Of those who did, 10 read the book and 4 did not.

COMMENTS

In the past, patients were often advised not to read anything related to therapy or psychology, a position that grew out of a concern that this would only feed resistance. Therapists don't appear to worry so much about this anymore, and often recommend books that relate to patient issues.

As the therapist, I often recommend books that I think will help a patient understand an issue or a concept. The Alice Miller books, especially *The Drama of the Gifted Child* (also known as *Prisoners of Childhood*) are particularly helpful, although patients often say they are hard to read, partly because of the material and partly because of a clumsy translation.

As the patient, I'm glad when the therapist suggests a book. It's something I can do between sessions to continue what we're doing in the office. I'm in favor of anything that speeds up the process. Of course, if I hate the book, or don't see the way my therapist thinks it applies to me, that can be disturbing.

RELATED READING

Gould, R. A., Clum, G. A., and Shapiro, D. (1993). The use of bibliotherapy in the treatment of panic: a preliminary investigation.
Behavior Therapy 24(2):241–252.

Pardeck, J. T. (1994). Using literature to help adolescents cope with
problems. *Adolescence* 29(4):421–427.

Rileigh, K. K. (1993). Good reads in psychology: recommended books
beyond the required textbook. *Teaching of Psychology* 20(3):183–185.

Warner, R. E. (1991). Bibliotherapy: a comparison of the prescriptive
practices of Canadian and American psychologists. *Canadian Psychology* 32(3):529–530.

🔊🔊🔊🔊

Question 40: Did you ever discuss the relationship with the thera-pist?

In many therapies, especially psychoanalytic orientations, the relation-ship with the therapist is central to the work, and becomes an essen-tial aspect of the treatment.

> She used that a lot in the therapy. For example, if I pulled my chair toward her, she would ask what that might mean. Or how I would avoid things. She used what was going on in the room a great deal.
> [Female, 45, Nonprofessional]

> I would talk about my feelings about her, the nature of the relationship I was asking of her, how confident I felt in her. Whenever she did anything that disturbed me I would tell her. After having been in a lot of therapies, I feel pretty comfortable telling therapists when I don't like what they've done, or when something they've done makes me anxious or uncomfortable, and I'm aware of my familiarity with the theory that the relationship is really the heart of the therapy.
> [Male, 48, Nonprofessional]

> If I had certain feelings about him I would tell him, and occasionally he would infer that something I was saying was also related to him.
> [Male, 42, Professional]

We did talk about her rule against self-disclosure, and we did talk about my feeling that I needed to be loved by everybody and whether I was acting in such a way as to make her love me, and how I thought she felt about me.

[Female, 39, Nonprofessional]

We discussed it all the time. For example, I told him many times how terrible the message on his machine was, the extreme rigidity of it, and after a while he did change it a little bit. He kept trying to get at sexual feelings I might be having toward him, and asked me repeatedly why I wore a jacket on the couch. I said I always wore a jacket, except when it was a very warm day and then I didn't wear one. He seemed to feel that I thought that if I took my jacket off I would be totally alluring and he would be unable to resist me. I told him that was not the case but I don't think he believed me.

[Female, 57, Professional]

One of my beliefs is that much of the change in therapy happens at the boundaries of the relationship.

[Male, 30, Professional]

Some people said that examining the relationship with the therapist didn't seem an important part of the treatment.

Compared to everything else that we were doing it seemed very minor. I talked about relationships all the time, but my relationship with her didn't seem like a big topic.

[Female, 50, Nonprofessional]

Some people said that for different reasons they avoided that part of the relationship and the therapy.

I don't remember doing that. I always thought of it as a very formal relationship, and the relationship itself wasn't an issue beyond that.

[Female, 48, Nonprofessional]

We did very little, but part of that was my problem. I had trouble saying things to her. There was a block between us.

[Female, 50, Professional]

It was really hard for me to do that, especially at the beginning.

[Female, 50, Nonprofessional]

It felt dangerous to talk about the intensity of the relationship with her.

[Male, 44, Professional]

Some people thought the therapist was avoiding it.

I remember thinking at times that she was being the mother that I had needed, and I said that to her. She smiled, but I felt that it was a little embarrassing to her, and she shifted the conversation to focusing on my having a better relationship with my own mother.

[Female, 46, Nonprofessional]

A couple of times I would bring up her rigidity, and she would get into my anger at her as some sort of a generic thing.

[Female, 62, Professional]

I found myself discussing the relationship with her usually at times when I was about to end the therapy, in terms of somehow being too comfortable with her. She didn't seem challenging enough.

[Female, 45, Nonprofessional]

I kept telling him that he wasn't giving me what I wanted. I told him that I felt that it had gone beyond the point of no return, and he kept saying, "But you could use that feeling and try to work on this," and I said that some relationships are not worth doing that. He really just kept at it. He never accepted my dissatisfaction.

[Female, 48, Nonprofessional]

Many people said they discussed their feelings about the therapist.

When I was concerned that he was thinking something bad, good, about me or what I was saying, then we would talk about that.

[Female, 46, Nonprofessional]

There were times when I was feeling very angry, maybe about paying for missed sessions. There were a couple of times when I felt he didn't understand me and I felt very betrayed. Other times I felt very positive.

[Female, 59, Professional]

Once I talked to her about the fact that she knew so much about me and I knew nothing about her, and that bothered me because it's so unequal.

[Female, 40, Nonprofessional]

We talked about the friends who also saw her who would talk about their special relationship with her, and then I came to understand that every patient had a special relationship with her, and I could hear other people talk about her and not be bothered.

[Female, 42, Nonprofessional]

I had a conflict because, on one hand, after working with him for years I felt like a friend and a special person in his life, and yet I always felt he was awkward with me outside of the treatment setting, a spaced-out aloofness. We talked about that.

[Male, 46, Nonprofessional]

Sometimes the structure of the relationship after termination is discussed.

Wanting a relationship with her and contact after therapy ended was discussed a lot at different points in therapy.

[Female, 47, Nonprofessional]

In discussions about the relationship, some of the therapist's feelings may also be revealed.

Toward the end of treatment, I started to see a man with whom I was very much in love, and the therapist acknowledged that he was happy for me, but it was difficult for him to see me so glowingly in love with someone else.

[Female, 45, Nonprofessional]

At a certain point there was a flirtatious energy, and we discussed that a little bit.

[Female, 48, Nonprofessional]

Some people, especially the professionals who know how important the relationship with the therapist is, were disappointed with that aspect of the treatment.

I didn't discuss the relationship as much as I should have, and I don't think he encouraged it very much. He would say at times, "What do you think this has to do with me?" but he mostly waited for me to bring it up. I think I was avoiding it, and he wasn't helping me not avoid it.

[Female, 58, Professional]

In my previous therapies it was constantly discussed, constantly, and this time it was only once. I came in feeling that I had nothing to talk about.

[Female, 39, Professional]

We didn't discuss the relationship until the last session. It was very intriguing to me that we did talk about it because a lot of things came up that I was really conscious of, about what had been happening between us. It was really fascinating. The last few times I went I was thinking about not making another appointment. In the last session I said, "I don't really need to be here, but I like coming here," and she suggested not making another appointment and asked me how I felt about it. I thought I was okay with it, and she said, "You know, you might be angry at me, you might feel abandoned," which really surprised me but I realized why she was saying it and how it could happen. I got teary-eyed for a few moments. And then she talked about the trust I had in her, and why I might feel angry or abandoned. I never realized consciously how much I trusted her, that everything she ever asked me to do, or suggested that I try, I did, no matter how painful or horrific it seemed. I never equated that with my trust in her. I wish we had done more of that, because I had read about it and I knew about it, but I never related it to my own experience until that last session.

[Female, 48, Nonprofessional]

NUMERICAL DISTRIBUTION

Professionals: Seventeen people said the relationship with the therapist was discussed often or all the time; only 3 said it was rarely or never discussed.

Nonprofessionals: Three people said the relationship was often discussed; 15 said it was sometimes; 11 said rarely; and 11 said it was never discussed.

COMMENTS

Anyone who has read my previous book will know that I believe that the relationship with the therapist is the heart of therapy, so these responses are disturbing. While professionals seem to realize the importance of such discussion, fully half the nonprofessionals said that they had discussed that relationship only a little or not at all.

As the therapist, I'm always listening for explicit or encoded references to me or to the therapy, and try to pursue whatever leaning they may have. Most patients will follow me into this area, although a few patients regard this as a distraction and may get angry if I keep doing it.

As a patient, I watch carefully to see how the therapist deals with this aspect of the therapy. I want the therapist always to keep the focus on what is happening between us. Any discomfort, hesitation, or reluctance in addressing feelings, issues, or conflicts between us is a very bad sign.

RELATED READING

Gelso, C. J., and Carter, J. A. (1994). Components of the psychotherapy relationship: their interaction and unfolding during treatment. *Journal of Counseling Psychology* 41(3):296–306.

Held, B. S. (1995). *Back to Reality: A Critique of Postmodern Theory in Psychotherapy*. New York: Norton.

Pantone, P. J. (1993). Transference: solutions to integrate the past with the present. *Contemporary Psychotherapy Review* 8:44–67.

Winslade, J., Crocket, K., and Monk, G. (1997). The therapeutic relationship. In *Narrative Therapy in Practice: The Archaeology of Hope,* ed. G. Monk, J. Winslade, K. Crocket, and D. Epston, pp. 53–81. San Francisco: Jossey-Bass.

৳৳৳৳

Question 41: What difference do you think the gender of the therapist made?

Almost half of both groups reported in Question 3 that they wanted the therapist to be a specific gender. Here they were asked what difference that choice made in the treatment.

Many people who had a preference said that it was easier to trust, to feel safe.

It helped me to establish a trusting relationship.

[Female, 45, Nonprofessional]

I probably had a more easy initial rapport with her, trusted her more quickly.

[Female, 56, Professional]

It made a very big difference, because I don't like men. I don't trust men, and don't feel comfortable.

[Female, 50, Nonprofessional]

I think it made a big difference. There were some issues I was working on that had to do with my feelings about being female, and it helped there. Also, I felt more comfortable with her because I expected her to be more sympathetic.

[Female, 39, Nonprofessional]

Given my own family dynamic, I trusted her more, and that made it easier to talk about some issues. I've done work with male therapists since then, but that was where I needed to begin.

[Female, 45, Professional]

Some people said they felt more comfortable with a therapist of the same sex.

I could feel more comfortable talking to him about sexuality and sex than a woman.

[Male, 48, Nonprofessional]

Consciously, I felt that it was easier for me, that I wouldn't be seductive, I wouldn't be on the make with him. Gradually it looked like it neutralized and simplified things some, and it was easier to identify with him.

[Male, 53, Professional]

I was more comfortable with a woman, because women are on a different level than men emotionally.

[Female, 48, Nonprofessional]

The relationship was very open, and I felt comfortable talking about everything with her.

[Female, 62, Professional]

It made a tremendous difference. I felt safer with a woman, and felt that she would be able to get to certain stuff. I think that women can do a lot of unconscious seduction with male therapists that they're not aware of.

[Female, 50, Professional]

Some of those who saw therapists of the opposite gender still felt safe.

I knew that I could trust him, and that he would never make a sexual overture toward any of his patients, because he had talked about that. Even though he was a man, I felt great safety with him.

[Female, 57, Professional]

I had had a woman therapist before, and I found her on the distant side. Because most of my problems stem from my mother, I think that creates a more difficult time with female therapists and a more benign time with male therapists. He was a warm person, so he was a good male model.

[Female, 59, Professional]

Others said the therapist's gender helped them feel better understood.

After I got to know her for a few years, I realized that her situation in life was very much like mine. When I learned that, it was very helpful to know that she had experiences like mine. She could understand me better.

[Female, 42, Nonprofessional]

It helped me to open up to female energies in me that the male therapist couldn't get to.

[Female, 45, Professional]

The initial reason I went to her was trouble with a man, and she seemed very empathetic about that. I had issues about my body and how I viewed myself that a woman would be more understanding with.

[Female, 42, Nonprofessional]

My previous therapists were both men. She understood in a way a man would not have.

[Female, 62, Professional]

The process is hard enough, and I wanted someone who I knew would understand certain things without having to explain everything.

[Female, 44, Nonprofessional]

It's hard to say because all my previous therapists had such different styles: the first guy hardly said anything; the second guy wanted me to discuss everything with him before I made a move, which really made me crazy. This time it was a woman, who I could really identify with, and she was much more nurturing, and she had been through all these things that I was dealing with. I never had a male therapist with those qualities.

[Female, 39, Professional]

Both men and women said they saw the female therapist as more nurturing.

It made an incredible difference. She really did do the mothering that I had lacked as a child. I had always been attracted to authoritative people, and she was totally the opposite. I hadn't realized how much I needed that.

[Female, 46, Nonprofessional]

I was looking for a mother. I made men into fathers very easily, and I really wanted someone who was like a mother. I was working with a lot of men and also trying to have more friendships with women. I wanted a mother in the sense of something nurturing but I also wanted to be closer to women.

[Female, 50, Nonprofessional]

I have a nurturing, maternal presupposition about women.

[Male, 44, Professional]

Some people said the therapist provided a role model they could identify with.

It made an enormous difference with me because most of my friends are women and I was never close to my father, and I never had a close relationship with a man until him.

[Male, 46, Nonprofessional]

It's been incredibly meaningful to me, because despite whatever technical strengths and weaknesses he has, he's given me a man in the world to identify with.

[Male, 50, Professional]

She was a great role model, which my mother was not. She was a role model in a lot of ways, how to be a mother, how to be a professional person.

[Female, 51, Professional]

Some people were more comfortable with a therapist of the opposite sex.

> I find that talking to women for me is a lot easier than talking to men, and I think I was a lot freer and open with a woman.
>
> [Male, 45, Nonprofessional]

Some people said having a therapist of the opposite gender was very useful to them.

> I think I was much more open to her because of that. I had a much more open relationship with my mother than my father. Also it allowed me to attack the key underlying issues, namely my mother's anxieties, which were transferred to me, her fears of everything. And here was a woman who didn't have those fears. And if she did, she would tell me that this was something she was not good at, while my own mother couldn't tell me anything. All she could do was worry.
>
> [Male, 52, Nonprofessional]

> It was a good thing at that time, because I didn't have any trust for men. He was a kind person, so I felt trusting of him.
>
> [Female, 48, Nonprofessional]

> The fact that I had a very loving relationship with my father, but he died when I was young, must have played a role in our relationship. I had a level of trust.
>
> [Female, 46, Nonprofessional]

> I trusted him more easily in the beginning, because my relationships with the men in my family are better than with the women.
>
> [Female, 52, Nonprofessional]

> I was seeing a therapist because of the failure of my marriage, and I wanted a woman to talk to because I couldn't talk to my wife.
>
> [Male, 42, Nonprofessional]

> I find it easier with a man, because I feel that the woman is probably not going to like me as much as the man is going to like me. I feel more accepted with a man.
>
> [Female, 48, Nonprofessional]

A therapist of the opposite sex can be useful even when the work is more difficult.

> I think it was very important because it gave me an opportunity to deal with a lot of issues about women. It made it particularly difficult

in some areas because a lot of what I was talking about was erotic and sexual feelings and a lot of fantasies and things of that nature, and that was more difficult for me to discuss with a woman, but I think that it was also very beneficial that I was able to.

[Male, 48, Nonprofessional]

It was hard with a male. It's taken me a long time to have relationships with men that I could just be friends with. I could work out my stuff with my dad with him.

[Female, 44, Nonprofessional]

Some people said that having a therapist of the opposite gender created some roadblocks.

I think in the beginning it was difficult to be as open about certain areas. I thought that he couldn't completely understand because he was a man.

[Female, 50, Professional]

I think sex issues might have been discussed more if she had been a man, but I felt more comfortable with a woman.

[Male, 52, Nonprofessional]

It was another layer I had to work through to feel comfortable talking.

[Female, 48, Nonprofessional]

It brought up all that sex stuff, and I know you're supposed to talk about that, but I wouldn't.

[Female, 50, Nonprofessional]

A number of people said they thought the therapist's gender was not a significant factor.

I don't think it made any difference—it's the individual personality.

[Male, 43, Nonprofessional]

Her personality made more of a difference than the fact that she was a woman.

[Female, 53, Nonprofessional]

I don't think it made much difference. I didn't have certain feelings toward him that I would have had toward a woman, and I think that if I went into analysis again I would pick a woman, because it's hard for me to have an erotic transference to someone with a beard. Certain issues would emerge with a woman that didn't with a man.

[Male, 42, Professional]

I don't think the gender makes a lot of difference. It's how sympathetic the person is to your individual issues.

[Female, 48, Nonprofessional]

It was more her personality that I valued, because she was much more giving and responsive than my previous therapists, but I don't think it was her gender.

[Female, 41, Nonprofessional]

I don't think it made any difference. I felt that he heard what I was saying and understood it.

[Female, 41, Nonprofessional]

Some people's opinions changed over time.

In the beginning it was very important, but after years it became completely unimportant.

[Female, 47, Nonprofessional]

I think the initial degree of comfort was greater than it would have been with a woman, but over time it might not have made much difference.

[Male, 51, Nonprofessional]

A few people mentioned the importance of having therapy experiences with both men and women.

I was more comfortable initially with a man. I sought out my next therapist, who is female, so I could work on the issues that I wasn't ready to before then.

[Male, 30, Professional]

I was able to focus a lot on mother issues. But I never touched a lot of stuff about men. I think I should have also seen a man. I think people need to do both, or they miss a tremendous amount.

[Female, 45, Nonprofessional]

That was actually helpful. My previous therapist had been a woman, and I wanted a different experience, and his being a man helped.

[Female, 58, Professional]

NUMERICAL DISTRIBUTION

Professionals: Thirteen said the therapist was the same gender; 7 said the opposite gender. Six said that it was easier to trust; 4 said that they felt better understood; 5 said the therapist provided a role model; 2 said a female therapist was more nurturing; 3 said they didn't think it made a significant difference.

Nonprofessionals: Twenty-one said the therapist was the same gender; 19 said the opposite gender. Nine said that it was easier to trust; 4 said that they felt better understood; 8 said the therapist provided an opportunity to work on specific issues; 2 said a female therapist was more nurturing; 10 said that the gender made the therapist easier to talk to; 7 said they didn't think it made a significant difference.

COMMENTS

With most patients, there may be different transferences and other reactions to a man than to a woman. At the same time, the female therapist may be experienced as a father figure or the male therapist as a mother. As the therapist I don't automatically assume that I'm a male figure to the patient. For example, someone whose father was very distant and rejecting but whose mother was warm and nurturing may experience gentle giving and acceptance as female qualities.

As a patient, having seen both male and female therapists, I know that each evokes different responses and different issues. I'm glad to have had both experiences.

RELATED READING

Brown, L. S. (1990). What female therapists have in common. In *Women as Therapists: A Multitheoretical Casebook,* ed. D. W. Cantor, pp. 227–242. New York: Springer.

Erickson, B. M. (1993). *Helping Men Change: The Role of the Female Therapist.* Newbury Park, CA: Sage.

Farber, B. A., and Geller, J. D. (1994). Gender and representation in psychotherapy. *Psychotherapy* 31(2):318–326.

Morgan, M. E. (1992). Therapist gender and psychoanalytic couple psychotherapy. *Sexual and Marital Therapy* 7(2):141–156.

≋≋≋≋

Question 42: Did you ever have any physical contact with the therapist?

Physical contact between therapist and patient is a controversial issue in the field. Many writers on the topic suggest that it can be a prelude to sexual contact, and is therefore dangerous. Others say that helping patients differentiate between sexual and affectionate contact can be valuable.

Many people reported occasional handshakes with the therapist.

> There was an occasional handshake at the beginning of treatment or before a vacation.
>
> [Male, 42, Professional]

> I think we shook hands when we met and at our last session.
>
> [Male, 48, Nonprofessional]

> Maybe years into the therapy there was a handshake before a vacation.
>
> [Female, 50, Professional]

Some people said that the therapist was available for hugs.

> There were Christmas hugs.
>
> [Female, 52, Professional]

> There was a group hug at the end of every group.
>
> [Male, 43, Nonprofessional]

> I usually hugged him at the end of the session. That came out of the old marathon days.
>
> [Male, 50, Professional]

When a patient is upset, a touch from the therapist can be soothing.

> When my father died he hugged me, and when I stopped seeing him.
>
> [Female, 50, Nonprofessional]

> When I was in deep distress he would hold me, and it felt very good.
>
> [Male, 46, Nonprofessional]

There was one time in group when he put his hand on my head when I was really upset about something. I think we hugged a couple of times on really special occasions.

[Male, 53, Professional]

If I seemed really distressed, she would touch my arm as I was leaving and tell me to take care. A few times on parting we hugged.

[Male, 49, Nonprofessional]

She might put her feet on top of mine to ground me, or put a hand on my shoulder. More of a neutral kind of thing.

[Female, 45, Professional]

A few people reported some unusual kinds of contact.

We wrestled once, and did some pillow fighting once. It blew the lid off what I thought was acceptable, what people would do. In this litigious society, he wasn't as worried as I would be. It was a lot of fun.

[Male, 30, Professional]

Some people seemed to sense that the therapist was avoiding any physical contact.

I don't even remember a handshake.

[Female, 28, Nonprofessional]

There were times I wanted to give him a hug after the session, when I felt a lot of things had been brought up, and it was more of a comfort hug, but I never felt that I could, because of the distance, so I would just leave. I'm not sure we even shook hands.

[Female, 41, Nonprofessional]

We started doing some bioenergetic work, but she stopped doing that because she was working with a lot of trauma survivors and decided that this way of working was really inappropriate a lot of the time.

[Female, 45, Professional]

I don't even remember hugging her when I left. I think the absence of physical contact is so weird. A pat on the hand—something.

[Female, 50, Nonprofessional]

Sometimes the therapist avoids physical contact, and sometimes the patient does, too.

> She hugged me maybe once, and that was because I wouldn't let her—I was really hands-off. I was afraid of being engulfed.
> [Female, 50, Professional]

Physical contact, especially when unexpected, can be disturbing.

> I remember her helping me on with my coat when my back problem was acting up. That was unsettling because it was so unusual.
> [Male, 44, Professional]

NUMERICAL DISTRIBUTION

Professionals: Six people said they had hugged the therapist; 4 said handshakes; 2 mentioned other kinds of physical contact; 8 people said there had been no physical contact of any kind.

Nonprofessionals: (Some people gave more than one response.) 17 said they had hugged the therapist; 5 mentioned handshakes; 2 mentioned a touch on the arm or shoulder; 19 said there had been no physical contact.

COMMENTS

The professional group reported more physical contact than the non-professionals, and this may reflect the therapists' greater comfort with sophisticated patients who are less likely to misinterpret or to sue.

Physical contact is a charged issue in these days of malpractice suits and allegations of sexual misconduct, but an ability to distinguish between sex and affection is an important asset in the world of adult relationships. As the therapist, my guidelines are pretty clear: patients get hugs only when they initiate and ask for them.

As the patient, I want to know that my therapist is comfortable with touch and affection and is himself (or herself) able to distinguish these from sex.

RELATED READING

Barak, Y., and Rabinowitz, G. (1995). Gestalt elements in D. W. Winnicott's psychoanalytic technique. *Gestalt Journal* 18(2):87–91.

Corey, G., Corey, M. S., and Callanan, P. (1993). A special case: non-erotic physical contact with clients. In *Issues and Ethics in the Helping Professions,* 4th ed. Pacific Grove, CA: Brooks/Cole.

Field, T. M. (1993). The therapeutic effects of touch. In *The Undaunted Psychologist: Adventures in Research,* ed. G. G. Brannigan and M. R. Merrens, pp. 3–11. Philadelphia, PA: Temple University Press.

Hedges, L. E. (1994). Appendix: Informed consent regarding limited physical contact. In *Working the Organizing Experience: Transforming Psychotic, Schizoid, and Autistic States,* pp. 252–261. Northvale, NJ: Jason Aronson.

🈀🈀🈀🈀

Question 43: Did you like your therapist?

Patients want to like the therapist and many feel this is necessary if they are to reveal themselves and explore their issues.

Most people said they liked their therapist.

> Very much, he was very likable.
>
> [Female, 59, Professional]

> I liked him as a person.
>
> [Male, 42, Professional]

> I thought she was great.
>
> [Male, 52, Nonprofessional]

> Yes, tremendously.
>
> [Male, 30, Professional]

Sometimes this takes a while.

> I grew to like her.
>
> [Male, 48, Nonprofessional]

For some people, their feelings went beyond liking the therapist.

> I loved her—she's a wonderful woman.
>
> [Female, 42, Nonprofessional]

> I loved her. She was wonderful.
>
> [Female, 46, Nonprofessional]

I thought she walked on water.

[Female, 40, Nonprofessional]

The patient may like the therapist and yet not be satisfied with the therapy.

I liked her as a person. She wasn't the greatest therapist, but as a person she was very nice.

[Female, 50, Professional]

She was a very generous-spirited person, and I really liked her. Toward the end of treatment I still liked her but I might have lost some respect for her, because we used to converse about some things that were going on with her, like choosing an apartment, or decorating, or what she was going to do with her career and her practice. It would usually happen at the end of the session, and she would open up, and I discovered that she was an extremely indecisive person. It took her forever to make a decision. It weakened her power for me. I was giving her advice about things that I was more expert on.

[Female, 50, Nonprofessional]

Whether the patient does or does not like the therapist, the therapist's professional distance can evoke feelings in the patient.

I didn't like her formality, her aloofness.

[Female, 62, Professional]

I don't know if it was in reaction to feeling that he didn't like me.

[Female, 48, Nonprofessional]

She was nice, but she was not an easy person to communicate with outside of just talking about my feelings.

[Male, 42, Nonprofessional]

I liked him a lot but I always felt there was something keeping us from being friends.

[Male, 46, Nonprofessional]

NUMERICAL DISTRIBUTION

Professionals: Seventeen people said they had liked the therapist; 3 said they had not.

Nonprofessionals: Thirty-eight people said they liked the therapist; 2 did not.

COMMENTS

As the therapist, I want the patient to like me, because that tends to indicate a level of trust and openness that makes the work easier. I can live with it for a while if the patient doesn't like me, but if that doesn't change reasonably soon I have to wonder what's going on. Patients who don't like me will probably leave after a few sessions.

As a patient, I want to like my therapist, because I can't imagine trusting someone or working so intimately with someone I don't like. I have seen therapists I didn't like much, and even accomplished some things, but in each case the therapy ended badly in a way that validated my reservations about the therapist.

RELATED READING

Callaghan, G. M., Naugle, A. E., and Follette, W. C. (1996). Useful construction of the client–therapist relationship. *Psychotherapy* 33(3): 381–390.

Hatcher, R. L., and Barends, A. W. (1996). Patients' view of the alliance in psychotherapy: exploratory factor analysis of three alliance measures. *Journal of Consulting and Clinical Psychology* 64(6):1326–1336.

Kleckner, T, Frank, L., Bland, C., et al. (1992). The myth of the unfeeling strategic therapist. *Journal of Marital and Family Therapy* 18(1): 41–51.

Tryon, G. S., and Kane, A. E. (1995). Client involvement, working alliance, and type of therapy termination. *Psychotherapy Research* 5(3): 189–198.

🔊🔊🔊🔊

Question 44: Did you ever think you were in love with your therapist?

A common stereotype is that of the patient falling in love with the therapist. Most people said this had not happened. One person explained why.

188 📖 SECOND OPINIONS

> I didn't feel the kind of intimacy that would allow me to do that.
>
> [Female, 48, Nonprofessional]

A few said that they had at times had feelings of love for the therapist.

> I was crazy about him for a while.
>
> [Female, 48, Professional]

> I idolized her.
>
> [Female, 45, Professional]

Sometimes the patient is aware of what is happening.

> I worried about that at one point. It probably was around the time I had a dream about him that was explicitly homosexual. It had more the flavor of parent and child.
>
> [Male, 53, Professional]

> It felt like I thought I was in love with him, but I also knew that he was my therapist and I was just thinking that I was in love with him. I wasn't thinking about it too seriously.
>
> [Female, 48, Nonprofessional]

> There was a period where I knew what was going on but he was in my dreams. There was definitely that transferential thing happening, but because I was a little more sophisticated I didn't identify it as being in love.
>
> [Female, 50, Professional]

> I thought that I loved him in a way, but it was so unreal.
>
> [Female, 52, Nonprofessional]

A few people mentioned a fantasy of continued connection with the therapist after treatment ended.

> I felt that she had become a very good friend.
>
> [Male, 45, Nonprofessional]

> I really wanted to be friends with her after I wasn't her patient any more.
>
> [Female, 42, Nonprofessional]

NUMERICAL DISTRIBUTION

Professionals: Four people had had feelings of being in love with the therapist; 16 had not.

Nonprofessionals: Two people said they had been in love with the therapist; 38 had not.

COMMENTS

In spite of the stereotype, most people did not fall in love with their therapists. I don't think it's happened to me as a therapist more than three or four times in 20 years, at least that I was aware of. I don't think falling in love with the therapist is conducive to self-disclosure or self-examination, so no matter what Freud may have thought I don't believe it's useful to encourage this in a patient. On the other hand, if the patient does have such feelings, I want just to accept them and not make the person feel foolish or vulnerable.

As the patient, I might not feel entirely comfortable with this kind of feeling, wondering what it might lead to and whether the therapist could contain it without overreacting.

RELATED READING

Elise, D. (1991). When sexual and romantic feelings permeate the therapeutic relationship. In *Gays, Lesbians, and Their Therapists: Studies in Psychotherapy,* ed. C. Silverstein, pp. 52–67. New York: Norton.

Gabbard, G. O. (1994). On love and lust in erotic transference. *Journal of the American Psychoanalytic Association* 42(2):385–403.

Hill, D. (1994). The special place of the erotic transference in psychoanalysis. *Psychoanalytic Inquiry* 14(4):483–498.

Kernberg, O. F. (1994). Love in the analytic setting. *Journal of the American Psychoanalytic Association* 42(4):1137–1157.

🐚🐚🐚🐚

Question 45: Did you ever have sexual feelings or fantasies about your therapist?

Again, here is a common stereotype of the analytic situation, in which the patient has erotic or sexual feelings for the therapist. Most people said this had not happened.

A few people acknowledged such feelings.

> In my dreams sometimes I did, even though he was not normally someone I would find attractive.
>
> [Female, 50, Professional]

> There have been times when I've had uncomfortable or disquieting fantasies with some some sexual content.
>
> [Male, 50, Professional]

> I did have one dream about him that was explicitly homosexual.
>
> [Male, 53, Professional]

Several people seemed to be almost experimenting, to see if they could have such feelings.

> I would say yes, but it was minor. Actually she served as a pretty good model of what I found attractive in women, in that she was competent but not hostile.
>
> [Male, 52, Nonprofessional]

> I think I may have had a mild sexual fantasy about her, just to see what that was like.
>
> [Male, 48, Nonprofessional]

> I did only mildly, not intensely.
>
> [Male, 42, Nonprofessional]

Some people found the feelings disturbing or difficult to handle.

> I had them, and then I banished them from my mind.
>
> [Male, 44, Professional]

> I did have some, but I wouldn't discuss those with him.
>
> [Female, 50, Nonprofessional]

> I had a few, but not in a real way. It would feel sick or strange, as if I had those feelings about my brother.
>
> [Female, 52, Nonprofessional]

NUMERICAL DISTRIBUTION

Professionals: Only 5 people said they had had sexual feelings or fantasies; 15 denied having any.

Nonprofessionals: Eight people acknowledged some sexual feelings or fantasies; 32 denied having any.

COMMENTS

Again, only a quarter of the combined group acknowledged having sexual feelings toward the therapist. Perhaps other people in the sample also had such feelings but were unable to admit it to me. As the therapist, I'd like to hear about such feelings, because they may be revealing of something important, but I know that it might be hard for someone to disclose this kind of material.

As a patient, I might have such feelings from time to time. If I enjoyed those thoughts I might even reveal them to the therapist. If they were disturbing they would be very difficult to talk about.

RELATED READING

Altman, M. L. (1995). Vicissitudes of the eroticized transference: the impact of aggression. *Psychoanalytic Review* 82(1):65–79.

Bridges, N. A. (1995). Managing erotic and loving feelings in therapeutic relationships: a model course. *Journal of Psychotherapy Practice and Research* 4(4):329–339.

Lester, E. P. (1985). The female analyst and the erotized transference. *International Journal of Psycho-Analysis* 66(3):283–293.

Silverman, H. W. (1988). Aspects of the erotic transference. In *Love: Psychoanalytic Perspectives,* ed. J. F. Lasky and H. W. Silverman, pp. 173–191. New York: New York University Press.

🔊🔊🔊🔊

Question 46: How much did the therapist talk?

The silent analyst is a common stereotype. Most therapists are willing to speak when they have something to say.

Several people in traditional psychoanalysis described a therapist who was quiet much of the time.

> In the first 2 sessions in the week, almost nothing, and then in the last session, he would make some great interpretation. I would point this out to him, that this was the end of the week and perhaps he

would say something. On occasion he would say something in the other sessions.

[Female, 57, Professional]

When he had something to say it was well thought out. He would very seldom react to anything I said. If I said something really outlandish he would raise his eyebrows, and that was as much as he would give.

[Female, 41, Nonprofessional]

He didn't talk a whole lot, but especially when I was on the couch he would comment, and at the end of the session would talk for 4 or 5 minutes about his feelings about what I had said.

[Female, 50, Professional]

Others found the therapist more willing to talk when they wanted that.

She talked a bit, and she would answer questions, which I liked, because in the past I didn't find that psychologists would respond, they'd just listen. I felt that I needed some answers about what to do when I'm having a panic attack, and she would give suggestions about what to do.

[Female, 28, Nonprofessional]

He talked. He was a good listener, but I wouldn't call him a silent therapist. I never thought, "Oh, why doesn't he say something?"

[Female, 59, Professional]

She talked freely. It was very much all right with me. I don't like silent, nondirective therapists.

[Male, 48, Nonprofessional]

She left the driving to me on that. If I wanted to sit there and talk for the whole 50 minutes, that was fine. If I solicited a response, I would get one.

[Male, 49, Nonprofessional]

She was quite interactive, and talked a fair amount.

[Female, 52, Professional]

She talked more than I expected. I expected someone completely silent.

[Female, 50, Nonprofessional]

She was very active in the session. She's not a blank slate.

[Female, 45, Professional]

Some people said how much the therapist talked depended on how much they themselves had to say.

There were times when she knew I didn't have much to say, and she would kind of take over, and there were the nights when I had a lot to say and she wouldn't say much, so it depended on how much I had to say.

[Male, 45, Nonprofessional]

She could be quiet and listen for a long time, and I could talk for weeks.

[Female, 62, Professional]

It depended on what I was dealing with. Sometimes I wouldn't say a word and she would be pretty quiet. If I didn't open up, she would start the conversation by asking questions. There were other times when I couldn't shut up and she didn't need to say anything. Other times where it was just conversational, talking about life in general.

[Female, 42, Nonprofessional]

Several people were pleased when the therapist said a lot.

He spoke a lot, because it was hypnosis. I used him to some extent as an advisor, which meant that he would answer questions. He was older, so I was ready to take his advice more readily.

[Male, 53, Nonprofessional]

A number of people said they were frustrated by therapist silence.

I had many wishes that he be more active than he was. He would just analyze them. My need for him to be a real person with me was very great, and that was not his style.

[Female, 58, Professional]

She said less than me, not as much as I wanted. I would have appreciated more guidance.

[Female, 44, Nonprofessional]

I've always had the impression that she said nothing for 7 years, but I realize now that she talked more than I gave her credit for.

[Male, 44, Professional]

> He said very little. I would have liked him to tell me what to do, how to do it, when and where. He didn't not talk when he should have, but he didn't talk a lot.
>
> [Female, 52, Nonprofessional]

> There were times that I wanted more from her. I had come into therapy to deal with the issue of my husband who doesn't talk, so words were very important to me.
>
> [Female, 62, Professional]

> I wished she would have said a little more, but she probably shouldn't have. Had she talked more, I might not have liked it. I have the fantasy about therapy that she knows the answer, and she's waiting for me to find it, and why won't she just tell me?
>
> [Female, 39, Nonprofessional]

> I always wanted more.
>
> [Female, 46, Nonprofessional]

Some of these people tried to get more response from the therapist. This was sometimes successful.

> I actually asked him to give me more feedback than he was giving me, and he did. Sometimes he had brilliant insights, and I told him when he did.
>
> [Female, 48, Nonprofessional]

> If I told him I wanted more input from him he would give it to me.
>
> [Male, 42, Professional]

Other patients were unable to get more from the therapist.

> I wanted her to talk more. I told her and she didn't say anything.
>
> [Female, 50, Professional]

> I told him that he had to talk more, and it was a constant problem. He would always try in the immediate session to do what I wanted, but I always felt he was placating me. I didn't think he was really getting what I was saying. So it never held.
>
> [Female, 48, Professional]

A few people said they accepted therapist silence because they believed that was the way it was done.

I see someone now who talks more, but I never knew then it could be done differently. It's like a parent—you accept however it is and you don't know for a long time that there are other ways of doing it.
[Female, 45, Nonprofessional]

Other people found that the therapist talked more than they wanted.

Sometimes he talked a lot. Sometimes that was okay, and sometimes I had to tell him I didn't want to hear anymore about his tennis game. At times he talked when I didn't want him to, and it was hard for me to tell him that. I pushed myself to be more revealing of my feelings at a given moment about his talking.
[Male, 50, Professional]

Sometimes she said too much. She made a lot of references to other patients, not names but stories about them, and I didn't care about them. I thought, *Why are you telling me this?* It also made me wonder what she was telling other patients about me.
[Female, 39, Professional]

He talked about himself in the context of what was being discussed in the group, and sometimes I resented it. Sometimes I wanted him to shut up.
[Female, 48, Nonprofessional]

NUMERICAL DISTRIBUTION

Professionals: This one is hard to quantify. Almost everyone said the therapist's talking varied, sometimes a little and sometimes a lot, depending on what was going on in the session. Four people said the therapist did not talk as much as they wanted.

Nonprofessionals: Again, people usually said it varied, but overall 12 said the therapist talked only a little; 22 said a moderate amount; 6 said a lot. Twenty-nine said the therapist talked as much as they wanted; 9 said the therapist said too little; 2 said the therapist said too much.

COMMENTS

Part of our psychoanalytic legacy is the image of the silent analyst. A few practitioners still work that way, but it's clear from the responses that patients today want a therapist who responds to them, who interacts and reacts, and says what he or she thinks.

As a therapist who believes that the relationship is the therapy, I am very interactive and talk a lot. Of course, I still have to be aware and sensitive and not talk too much or too revealingly. Occasionally someone will say that even as much as I do talk is not enough, and even more rarely someone will tell me to be quiet.

As the patient, I want a therapist who talks to me, who participates in the dialogue, who tells me what hypotheses he is considering or what associations he's having to what I'm saying. Otherwise, the therapist appears frightened and tentative, afraid to risk his thoughts with me, which would be an impossible situation to tolerate for very long.

RELATED READING

Anthony, E. J. (1991). The dilemma of therapeutic leadership: the leader who does not lead. In *Psychoanalytic Group Theory and Therapy: Essays in Honor of Saul Scheidlinger,* ed. S. Tuttman, pp. 71–86. Madison, CT: International Universities Press.

Ehrenberg, D. B. (1996). On the analyst's emotional availability and vulnerability. *Psychoanalysis and Psychology* 32(2):275–286.

Lindon, J. (1994). Gratification and provision in psychoanalysis: Should we get rid of "the rule of abstinence"? *Psychoanalytic Dialogues* 4(4):549–582.

Schwaber, E. A. (1996). Toward a definition of the term and concept of interaction: its reflection in analytic listening. *Psychoanalytic Inquiry* 16(1):5–24.

⬯⬯⬯⬯

Question 47: Did your therapist make interpretations?

The traditional image of psychotherapy is that the therapist interprets the patient's material, connecting the past to the present and the therapist to other significant figures in the patient's life history.

Most therapists did make interpretations.

> If I told a story and showed some puzzlement, she would come in and make some connections.
>
> [Male, 49, Nonprofessional]

She would usually ask me if this reminded me of anybody in my childhood, and it was usually obvious, but if it wasn't she would say, "But what about so-and-so?"

[Female, 39, Nonprofessional]

He would often interpret things back to my childhood and family. It was very useful.

[Female, 41, Nonprofessional]

She did a little bit—some things that I'd been thinking, or something from the past that I'd said—and bring it together with something else.

[Female, 28, Nonprofessional]

They were very useful. I thought that was the point of therapy.

[Male, 52, Nonprofessional]

A few people indicated that they would have liked more such interventions.

It was helpful when she did, because I thought she was very insightful, but she didn't do it a lot.

[Female, 48, Nonprofessional]

She did sometimes, but not enough. I wanted more.

[Female, 47, Nonprofessional]

Some therapists made interpretation a collaborative process.

If I agreed, I would say so, and if I disagreed I would say so. It developed over a period of time in my mind as a dialogue. Over time, I realized that my input was valid too, and it was a dialogue. They were useful, unless I thought that something was being said that was totally off-base, but that was rarely the case.

[Female, 48, Nonprofessional]

It was a give-and-take. It wasn't just a presenting of "Here's what this means."

[Female, 46, Nonprofessional]

He allowed me to make those connections. He never offered very much in that way. Sometimes in review at the end of the session we would talk about those connections and he would confirm what I had found.

[Male, 46, Nonprofessional]

> Occasionally she did. More often she would throw it back to me and ask me to interpret it, to say what it meant to me.
>
> [Female, 46, Nonprofessional]

A few therapists did not make interpretations because of the kind of therapy they were doing, such as hypnosis or behavior therapy. But for some other therapists, it was simply not their style.

> As I came to understand the way he worked, I saw that it was explicitly avoided. Interpretations can be insulting. It was rarely, "You do this because of that," it was more, "What impact does that have? Can you think of another way to do it? Do you want a suggestion?"
>
> [Male, 53, Professional]

> She's not an analyst. There were conclusions that she would come to about what was going on.
>
> [Female, 45, Professional]

Most people said they found the interpretations useful, at least some of the time.

> They were very down-to-earth and pragmatic, useful.
>
> [Female, 62, Professional]

Sometimes the meaning was not immediately clear.

> I didn't always agree, and I didn't always understand.
>
> [Female, 45, Professional]

Some people said that the usefulness of the interpretations varied.

> Sometimes they were helpful, but other times when they were totally out of whack they weren't. Those made me feel that he was human, that he could be wrong.
>
> [Female, 57, Professional]

Some people said that interpretations were not very useful.

> They were very general, so they weren't very helpful, and she didn't pursue them or force me to consider them.
>
> [Female, 50, Nonprofessional]

A few people found the interpretations difficult to hear.

It was sometimes infuriating, but I guess it was helpful.

[Female, 52, Nonprofessional]

At the time they were difficult, but I can see now that they were useful.

[Female, 42, Nonprofessional]

I didn't always want to think about it.

[Female, 26, Nonprofessional]

If I was ready to hear it, it was helpful. If I wasn't ready then I'd get mad.

[Female, 42, Nonprofessional]

NUMERICAL DISTRIBUTION

Professionals: Only two people said interpretations were not made or made only rarely; 18 said they were made fairly often. Of these, everyone said they were sometimes useful, and often very useful.

Nonprofessionals: Twenty-four people said interpretations were made often or regularly; 9 said they were made occasionally; 7 said they were not made at all. Of the 33 who had interpretations made, only 2 said they were not useful.

COMMENTS

Interpretation is the meat of the work, the way the therapist conveys to the patient insight, understanding, connection, or experience. In most traditional therapies, interpretation is what the therapist has to offer. In the group of nonprofessionals, more than a quarter said that there were few if any interpretations made, and this is a little disturbing. What was done instead?

As the therapist, I make interpretations when I see something that I don't think the patient sees. Patients either validate what I offer or turn it away; in either case they will think about it. Most patients seem to find interpretations useful, especially as conceptual frameworks for organizing their self-knowledge.

As a patient, I welcome the thoughts of the therapist about what things mean, what connects this with that, how the past might still be affecting the present. Sometimes these explanations will seem off the mark, or won't make sense, or will feel just plain wrong, but I still want to hear them.

RELATED READING

Fordham, M. (1991). The supposed limits of interpretation. *Journal of Analytical Psychology* 36(2):165–175.

Joyce, A. S., and Piper, W. E. (1993). The immediate impact of transference interpretation in short-term individual psychotherapy. *American Journal of Psychotherapy* 47(4):508–526.

Levin, F. M. (1980). Metaphor, affect, and arousal: how interpretations might work. *Annual of Psychoanalysis* 8:231–245.

Pearson, M. (1995). Problems with transference interpretations in short-term dynamic therapy. *British Journal of Psychotherapy* 12(1):37–48.

Skolnikoff, A. Z. (1992). The evolution of the concept of interpretation. In *The Technique and Practice of Psychoanalysis,* vol. 2, ed. A. Sugarman, R. A. Nemiroff, and D. P. Greenson, pp. 117–134. Madison, CT: International Universities Press.

Spillius, E. B. (1994). On formulating clinical fact to a patient. *International Journal of Psycho-Analysis* 75(5–6):1121–1132.

◎◎◎◎

Question 48: Were you ever aware of deciding not to talk about something that was on your mind?

The cardinal rule in analytic therapy is to say whatever comes to mind, but this can be difficult at times. Most people admitted that they had sometimes edited themselves.

Sometimes feelings of embarrassment or shame are the reason.

> Some things I found shameful and embarrassing, and I wasn't ready to bring them up. Some I eventually talked about and some I didn't.
> [Male, 48, Nonprofessional]

> There were some things that made me feel so small and embarrassed that it took me a long time to talk to him about them. And for a long time I didn't talk to him about how I didn't make eye contact with him or how anxious I was when I did make eye contact.
> [Male, 50, Professional]

> I didn't say it because I was ashamed. I had broken up with someone and was very embarrassed that the person was still on my mind, about still being obsessed. The obsession gradually went away, but I discussed it only vaguely.
> [Female, 59, Professional]

I was afraid to bring it up. I was bulimic and had never told anyone. It took me more than 3 years to tell her. I had tremendous humiliation and shame about it.

[Female, 45, Professional]

Lack of trust in the therapist can prevent disclosure.

I lied to him for a long time about something major, which told me that I didn't trust him. It was that I had been seeing a married man. I finally told him.

[Female, 48, Nonprofessional]

Sometimes the therapist contributes to the break. The patient becomes aware of the therapist's reaction.

I didn't say it because she saw my husband and me in couples therapy, and she took him on also as an individual patient. And when I wanted to talk about problems with my husband, she took them personally as therapy failures with him.

[Female, 45, Nonprofessional]

The only time I can remember something like that, I get very bad menstrual cramps, and the one time I mentioned that she said that was because of separation problems with my mother. I thought there were plenty of physical reasons, and so I quit talking to her about that.

[Female, 42, Nonprofessional]

Sometimes the patient just doesn't like being pressured.

A couple of times because he suggested that I do otherwise and I didn't follow his suggestions.

[Male, 53, Professional]

I found it hard when she would ask me how I felt about something; she would try to probe me and get me to go deeper, but I would have trouble.

[Male, 49, Nonprofessional]

Concern about the confidentiality of what is revealed, about the boundaries of the relationship, can interfere with free expression.

She knew the people involved and I didn't trust that boundaries could be kept. It felt too incestuous.

[Female, 45, Professional]

> It was probably an issue of trust and confidentiality, given that it was in an institute.
>
> [Female, 55, Professional]

Some people said that at times the material felt too difficult or upsetting to discuss.

> I didn't want to deal with it. It was going to be too difficult. I didn't want to bring all that up.
>
> [Female, 42, Nonprofessional]

> There were some things that had happened to me in my life that were really very painful, and it took me a long time to tell her about them, and then another long time to say I wanted to talk about it. I knew that I wasn't talking about it but I didn't feel that I could.
>
> [Female, 39, Nonprofessional]

Awareness of the impending end of the session can inhibit some people.

> I didn't have time left. That was part of the reason I moved to the couch. I would see how much time was left, and if I didn't think it was enough time I wouldn't bring it up. Or if I didn't want to cry afterwards. I was always doing that strategizing.
>
> [Female, 50, Nonprofessional]

Certain kinds of feelings can seem dangerous.

> I had some feelings of anger, and I didn't want to go to that level in therapy.
>
> [Male, 42, Nonprofessional]

Thoughts and feelings about the therapist can seem especially difficult.

> I was aware early on in therapy that I had negative feelings about her that I didn't talk about.
>
> [Female, 51, Professional]

> I was reacting to him as if he were a person and not a therapist, and I was thinking that maybe I don't want him to know that I feel like that.
>
> [Female, 48, Nonprofessional]

I concealed things that had to do with criticisms about her, because it would get too close to me.

[Female, 62, Professional]

I'm too uncomfortable to talk about feelings about the therapist.

[Female, 50, Nonprofessional]

I never said anything about my feelings about how he dressed, for instance. I avoided it because I was suspicious of what my anger was really about, and I was a little embarrassed about it.

[Female, 58, Professional]

It felt catastrophic to talk about the intensity of the relationship with her. I did get to it eventually, but it was cyclical, feeling again too intense and too dangerous.

[Male, 44, Professional]

There was one instance. She had revealed something to me about herself that I thought she shouldn't have, and it bothered me. On the one hand, I wanted to talk to her about it, and on the other hand I didn't want to talk to her about it because I feared somehow if I told her that it bothered me to know this about her it would somehow jeopardize our relationship.

[Female, 45, Nonprofessional]

Although the therapist might see the relevance, sometimes thoughts or feelings can interfere with the patient's plan for the session.

I did that more so in group, because I wanted to save it for individual first.

[Female, 47, Nonprofessional]

I wanted to use the session for something else.

[Male, 30, Professional]

It mostly happened in couples session, and things would come up in my own head that I felt would not be so appropriate to bring up at that point.

[Female, 44, Nonprofessional]

Sometimes the patient feels that a specific behavior needs to be concealed.

It had to do with drinking. I was drinking heavily when I started, though I didn't think I was, and then I stopped drinking in the course of therapy for about 6 years. Then I started again, and I remember consciously and deliberately not talking about it. Eventually I did.

[Male, 49, Nonprofessional]

A few people mentioned that when they overcame their resistance they felt better.

I found it very difficult to talk about the explicit details of sex. My feeling was that an awful lot of analysis tends to be voyeuristic. Once I did and it was really instructive.

[Female, 45, Nonprofessional]

Many people said they consciously tried not to hold back from saying what was on their minds.

I saw him as someone I could tell anything to.

[Female, 52, Nonprofessional]

My feeling was I'm here once a week, this is costing a lot of money, and goddamn it, I'm working hard and I'm not going to sit here and bullshit anybody.

[Female, 40, Nonprofessional]

I was as honest as anyone can be with a therapist.

[Male, 48, Nonprofessional]

It was expensive for me and I wasn't going to waste any time.

[Female, 44, Nonprofessional]

A couple of times I started to edit myself, and then I thought, "How is he going to be able to help without knowing what's going on?"

[Female, 41, Nonprofessional]

I was aware of not wanting to talk about certain things, but I would force myself, because I was paying for it.

[Female, 51, Professional]

In fact my attitude is that you're a fool if you have something on your mind and you don't share it with the therapist. You're wasting your money.

[Male, 46, Nonprofessional]

NUMERICAL DISTRIBUTION

Professionals: Sixteen people acknowledged consciously withholding material; only 4 said they did not. Of those who did, 6 said it was due to shame or embarrassment; 4 said it was due to lack of trust; 2 said it was a fear of being judged; 2 said they withheld criticisms of the therapist. Of the 16 people who withheld material, 10 got to it later on; 6 never did discuss that material.

Nonprofessionals: Twenty-four people said they had consciously withheld material; 16 said they had not. Of those who did, 6 said it was due to shame or embarrassment; 6 said it was feelings about the therapist, positive or negative; 5 said because the material was too painful; 2 said it was lack of trust; 2 said the material didn't fit with what they were discussing; 1 said because of a fear of being judged; 1 said because the material didn't seem important; 1 said because they were aware the session was almost over. Of the 24 who withheld material, only 12 brought it up later.

COMMENTS

In the past, patients were told the Basic Rule: say whatever comes to your mind. But no patient really does, and it strikes me as unrealistic and slightly ridiculous to expect that anyone will all the time. The idea that the patient is allowed no secrets from the therapist is infantilizing and condescending. Patients usually say more than enough to work with, and pressure to say more is unnecessary.

As the therapist, I assume that people are withholding something most of the time. Maybe they'll get to it later, maybe they won't. That's up to them. My job is to work with whatever they do give me, and there's almost always plenty to keep me busy.

As a patient, I want to know that the therapist respects my boundaries and my timetable. The therapist who pressures me to say more, or who sits silently refusing to talk until I say everything, is not on my side and the therapy will probably get stuck soon.

RELATED READING

Astor, M. H. (1994). Therapeutic neurosis: the need to resist the healing process in psychotherapy. *Journal of Contemporary Psychotherapy* 24(1):39–50.

Bisese, V. S. (1990). Therapist specific communication styles and patient resisitance: an analogue study. *Counseling Psychology Quarterly* 3(2):171–182.

Coltart, N. (1991). The silent patient. *Psychoanalytic Dialogues* 1(4):439–453.

Osherson, S., and Krugman, S. (1990). Men, shame, and psychotherapy. *Psychotherapy* 27(3):327–339.

ᴥᴥᴥᴥ

Question 49: Did you think your therapist was smart? Was the therapist smarter than you?

Most patients want the therapist to be smart, to not be easily fooled by their tactics and resistances. Sometimes they do see the therapist that way.

> I thought she was brilliant.
>
> [Female, 40, Nonprofessional]

> I remember being impressed with her memory. If I said something in January, she would tie it in with something I'd said the previous January.
>
> [Male, 49, Nonprofessional]

> I thought he was beyond smart. I think I knew a little bit more about the world than he did, but in that room he amazed me with his mental powers.
>
> [Male, 46, Nonprofessional]

> She was brilliant.
>
> [Female, 45, Professional]

Some patients saw the therapist as more knowledgeable in specific ways.

> I didn't think she was brilliant, but she knew things that I didn't know at all.
>
> [Male, 52, Nonprofessional]

> He's more emotionally intelligent than me.
>
> [Male, 30, Professional]

She knew how to operate on something other than an intellectual level.

[Female, 46, Nonprofessional]

She was more knowledgeable in certain areas that I needed knowledge in.

[Female, 39, Professional]

In terms of people and behavior, definitely smarter than me.

[Female, 41, Nonprofessional]

I thought she was life smart—wiser than me but not smarter.

[Female, 42, Nonprofessional]

A few people did not think the therapist was particularly intelligent.

He was kind of dense.

[Female, 48, Professional]

This is not necessarily a problem.

I thought she was kind of dumb, but she was very helpful to me.

[Female, 62, Professional]

Even when the patient sees the therapist as smart it does not automatically mean there is no problem. This can take the form of not feeling understood.

I often thought that while he was bright, he was not bright enough. I feel like he didn't get me, who I am.

[Female, 48, Nonprofessional]

She was smart, but she didn't quite get me.

[Female, 50, Professional]

One patient balanced things out this way.

I thought I was smarter, but that she was prettier, so we each had our own edge.

[Female, 45, Nonprofessional]

NUMERICAL DISTRIBUTION

Professionals: Only 2 people said they thought the therapist was not smart; 18 said their therapists were smart, of whom 11 said the therapist was as smart or smarter than they were; 4 said not as smart; 3 didn't know who was smarter.

Nonprofessionals: Thirty-five people said the therapist was smart; 5 said the therapist was not smart. Of the 35, 15 said the therapist was smarter than they were; 11 said they were smarter than the therapist; 9 said it was about the same.

COMMENTS

I think you have to be very smart to be a good therapist. You need a good memory and a quick mind. You need to know a lot about therapy and about human dynamics, and also about a lot of different fields, professions, and subcultures in which patients may be involved.

As the therapist, I know I'm pretty smart, and I like having a smart patient who gets what I'm saying and what I'm pointing out.

As a patient, I want my therapist to be really smart. I certainly don't want to think that I'm smarter than he is, and I might even find it reassuring to think that he's smarter than me.

RELATED READING

Baudry, F. D. (1989). A silent partner to our practice: the analyst's character and attitudes. In *Essential Papers on Character Neurosis and Treatment*, ed. R. F. Lax, pp. 397–408. New York: New York University Press.

Ferrini, R. (1996). The qualities of the analyst. *American Journal of Psychoanalysis* 56(2):161–165.

Gilbert, P., Hughes, W., and Dryden, W. (1990). The therapist as a crucial variable in psychotherapy. In *On Becoming a Psychotherapist,* ed. W. Dryden and L. Spurling, pp. 3–13. London: Tavistock/Routledge.

Mayer, E. L. (1996). Changes in science and changing ideas about knowledge and authority in psychoanalysis. *Psychoanalytic Quarterly* 65(1):158–200.

🔊🔊🔊🔊

Question 50: Were you ever aware of testing your therapist?

In a sense, every patient tests the therapist: What does he or she do with this? How does he react? Is she judgmental or accepting? Does he get scared, anxious, uncomfortable in some way? How much of me can she stand? Sometimes, however, the tests are consciously designed.
Many of the professionals acknowledged testing their therapists.

> I would up the ante in terms of how difficult things were to see if she could tolerate it.
>
> [Female, 45, Professional]

> I tested him a lot. There was a period when I was silent for weeks. Once I told him I didn't have the money to pay him, and what was he going to do about that?
>
> [Male, 53, Professional]

> I did it by telling her something that I thought might be outlandish to her, and seeing what she did with it.
>
> [Female, 39, Professional]

> I did that by trying to get her to come in and rescue me, so that I wouldn't have to put anything out there. Or being really resistant and seeing what she'd do about it.
>
> [Female, 45, Professional]

> I tested a lot. Was he going to remember something? Not only a fact about me, but things I had told him I needed from him, like talking more. And if I did the same thing, was he going to repeat the same mistake? And he always flunked.
>
> [Female, 48, Professional]

> I did it by being late.
>
> [Female, 55, Professional]

> I did it intellectually, to see how much he knew. I would bring up certain theories or ways of addressing certain material, or what his rationale was for working with me the way he was working.
>
> [Male, 42, Professional]

Some of the nonprofessionals also acknowledged testing the therapist.

> I might have tested her around the alcohol thing. That was a huge issue for me and I might have played some games around that.
> [Male, 49, Nonprofessional]

> It was all around these boundary issues, like changing an appointment.
> [Female, 47, Nonprofessional]

> I did in the beginning, in terms of how much of my rage and my anger and my viciousness can he or would he tolerate.
> [Male, 46, Nonprofessional]

> Occasionally I'd ask her personal questions that I knew she wasn't going to answer.
> [Female, 44, Nonprofessional]

> I would say something and see what she did. I evaluated everything she said, whether it sounded stupid or right.
> [Female, 39, Nonprofessional]

> I know a little bit about psychology and its historical development and I would talk about that, and see if she knew. Or philosophers or ideas. She would say that she wished my IQ were 20 percent lower.
> [Male, 49, Nonprofessional]

> There was this issue of whether she was my therapist or my cousin's therapist. That was a question I asked my therapist, in fact it was something she picked up on. I needed to ask her if she was mine, and I felt very much that she was.
> [Female, 45, Nonprofessional]

Sometimes the therapist passes the test.

> I was very provocative to see what she would do with it. And I would put stuff out to see if she would catch it. There was stuff I was doing that I really didn't want to and I was hoping she would catch me. By and large she did.
> [Female, 50, Professional]

> I think I was testing her reaction to my writing and seeing if she was comfortable with it, because of the erotic content. She passed, but I

think it was difficult for her, and she admitted that she was thinking about and dealing with things that she hadn't before, and becoming interested in subject matter that she hadn't been interested in before.

[Male, 48, Nonprofessional]

I remember reading about someone who was silent and watched the therapist's knuckles turn white, and I tried that and it didn't work.

[Male, 44, Professional]

I tested her on some feminist issues. She passed.

[Female, 52, Professional]

And sometimes the therapist fails.

I was aware toward the end that if I brought up that I was unhappy with the therapy, we'd get into our usual syndrome. I didn't do it consciously but I think I was hoping that this time he'd have a different reaction.

[Female, 48, Nonprofessional]

I tested her a little bit in terms of the fee. She didn't know that my parents were helping me pay for it. I wanted to see if it was at all important to her to keep me as a client, so I did test her on that, and she failed.

[Female, 28, Nonprofessional]

Most people said they had no need to test the therapist.

I trusted her and didn't need to test her.

[Female, 42, Nonprofessional]

That's not the way I operate.

[Female, 57, Professional]

I tested my parents enough, I didn't have to test her.

[Female, 26, Nonprofessional]

Sometimes the therapist suggests that the patient is testing, though the patient may be unaware of doing so.

As I subjectively looked at it, no, I didn't. If you looked at it from outside, you might say I did. There were times when I was actively aggressively belligerent to him. I don't know if he experienced that as testing.

[Male, 50, Professional]

He pointed out when he thought I was testing him, but I wasn't conscious of it. At one point I said I didn't want to keep coming for a while, and he thought I was running away from issues.

[Male, 30, Professional]

NUMERICAL DISTRIBUTION

Professionals: Ten said they had consciously tested the therapist; 10 said they had not. Of these, 2 said they might have been testing unconsciously.

Nonprofessionals: Twelve said they had consciously tested the therapist; 28 said they had not.

COMMENTS

Curiously, a greater percentage of the professionals (50 percent) said they tested the therapist than did the nonprofessionals (30 percent). This suggests to me greater trust in the therapists by the nonprofessionals. Maybe professionals know better.

As the therapist, I expect people to watch carefully how I handle what they say and do. It doesn't really matter whether a test is consciously designed, I still have to pass it. I hope if I don't pass that the patient will tell me rather than quit treatment, and we can look at the whole situation.

As a patient, I'm always in some way watching the therapist, evaluating her behavior and comfort level, rating the importance of any failure or error. If I've been there long enough, and have built up enough trust, I'll reveal my reactions, but if a serious error happens early I may simply decide to stop coming.

RELATED READING

Anderson, M. (1992). The need of the patient to be emotionally known: the search to understand a counter-transference dilemma. *British Journal of Psychotherapy* 8(3):247–252.

Powell, D. H. (1995). Lessons learned from therapeutic failure. *Journal of Psychotherapy Integration* 5(2):175–181.

Taurke, E. A., Flegenheimer, W., McCullough, L., et al. (1990). Change in patient affect/defense ratio from early to late sessions in brief psychotherapy. *Journal of Clinical Psychology* 46(5):567–668.

Winston, B., Samstag, L., Winston, A., and Muran, J. C. (1994). Patient defense/therapist interventions. *Psychotherapy* 31(3):478–491.

🔖🔖🔖🔖

Question 51: Did you ever give your therapist a gift?

When a therapy is successful, patients often feel they want to give something back to the therapist. Sometimes these feelings are expressed verbally and sometimes the patient will give the therapist a present.

> When I left I gave her a silk scarf, and a little wind chime. She said it was totally unnecessary and very lovely.
>
> [Female, 39, Nonprofessional]

> I chipped in with the group for a birthday present for him. It was so much part of the group thing that it wasn't an issue.
>
> [Male, 50, Professional]

> I gave him an appointment book. He seemed very pleased.
>
> [Male, 51, Nonprofessional]

> I gave him a book or two. He reacted very nicely, asked me if I wanted him to open it at the time.
>
> [Female, 50, Professional]

> I gave her an expensive pen and pencil set when I was leaving. I got a very favorable reaction.
>
> [Female, 45, Nonprofessional]

> I gave her a book lamp. She thanked me.
>
> [Female, 52, Professional]

> It was an Indian miniature painting of two figures talking to each other. I think he was touched by it and surprised that I had done it. It was at the end of my seeing him.
>
> [Female, 46, Nonprofessional]

I gave her a piece of pottery that I had made for Christmas. She was very nice and didn't analyze it.

[Female, 50, Professional]

I gave her a copy of my novel to keep. I also gave her a magazine in which a story of mine appeared. I may have done that more than once. She reacted graciously, with interest and appreciation.

[Male, 48, Nonprofessional]

Patients may try hard to find something the therapist will like.

She always wrapped a blanket around herself in the morning, so I gave her a shawl when I stopped treatment for a while. She was very touched. She really liked it.

[Female, 42, Nonprofessional]

I gave her a lovely wooden spoon, which she thought was very symbolic of womanhood, and with feeding. She was very appreciative, especially since she found it so symbolic.

[Female, 50, Nonprofessional]

Even the patient who gives a gift may have ambivalent feelings about it.

I gave her a Christmas present. The woman who referred me had given her a present the year before, and she accepted it, so I thought that I should do that too. And then I realized that I really didn't want to do that. She accepted it but didn't say much about it.

[Female, 45, Professional]

I gave him a psychology book that a friend had written, and he said thank you. I knew that patients gave him gifts, because I'd see a box of candy or something and he'd say that a patient gave it to him. I never felt comfortable with it.

[Female, 52, Nonprofessional]

Occasionally the therapist gives a mixed message about gifts.

She said she didn't accept gifts, but she did accept it.

[Female, 44, Nonprofessional]

Sometimes the patient wants to feed the therapist.

Someone sent me grapefruit from Florida, and I brought her some. Or I stopped off at a bakery on the way to therapy to get a pastry and brought her one. She was always very gracious and said thank you. In the case of the grapefruit, she told me the week after that they were the most delicious things she had ever eaten.

[Female, 45, Nonprofessional]

I brought him food. He liked it so much he wanted more.

[Female, 41, Nonprofessional]

One Christmas I gave him some of this special dish I make.

[Female, 41, Nonprofessional]

Many people said they had never had the impulse to give a present, but a few patients had thought of it and resisted the impulse.

Many times I thought of giving him a gift, but I always changed my mind because I knew he would never accept it, and would analyze it to death and take the joy out of it.

[Female, 57, Professional]

It wouldn't have felt appropriate.

[Female, 50, Nonprofessional]

Rarely the therapist will give the patient a gift.

My therapist gave me a gift when my kids were born. I was very touched that he gave me something when each of my kids was born, especially because that was not his usual style.

[Female, 50, Professional]

NUMERICAL DISTRIBUTION

Professionals: Seven said they had given the therapist a gift; 13 said they had not. Of these, 2 considered the idea but decided not to.

Nonprofessionals: Nineteen said they had given the therapist a gift; 21 said they had not.

COMMENTS

Many therapists refuse to accept gifts, especially something expensive. My concern about doing this is that it may feel extremely rejecting and even patronizing to the patient. Most patients feel that they get a lot from their therapists; sometimes they want to give something back (besides the fee).

As the therapist, I will try to accept whatever gift a patient might give. Some discussion or analysis of the impulse might be useful, but not so much that the joy of freely giving is drained away.

As the patient, I want to know that my gift is appreciated and my desire to give something back is accepted and validated.

RELATED READING

Drew, J., Stoeckle, J. D., and Billings, J. A. (1983). Tips, status, and sacrifice: gift giving in the doctor–patient relationship. *Social Science and Medicine* 17(7):399–404.

Gutheil, T. G., and Gabbard, G. O. (1993). The concept of boundaries in clinical practice: theoretical and risk-management dimensions. *American Journal of Psychiatry* 150(2):188–196.

Kritzberg, N. I. (1980). On patients' gift-giving. *Contemporary Psychoanalysis* 16(1):98–118.

Talan, K. H. (1989). Gifts in psychoanalysis: theoretical and technical issues. In *Psychoanalytic Study of the Child* 44:149–163. New Haven, CT: Yale University Press.

≋≋≋≋

Question 52: Did your therapist ever cancel a session unexpectedly?

A therapist's schedule sometimes requires canceling sessions, for vacations, conferences, and other professional and personal business. But what about the emergency that requires a last-minute cancellation by the therapist? This situation can bring up in the patient feelings of mistrust and questions about dependability.

Sometimes the patient accepts and understands.

> I remember the session was canceled unexpectedly several times, but it wasn't an issue. I always felt that my therapist was committed to me, but I permitted them to have a life of their own. If something got in the way on occasion, then that happened, and it wasn't an issue for me.
>
> [Female, 48, Nonprofessional]

He lived upstate and couldn't get into the city because of a terrible snowstorm. That happened several times. It was okay, because I couldn't get in either.

[Female, 57, Professional]

I assumed that she was a busy person and that something came up. I had to do the same to her on occasion, so I understood.

[Male, 45, Nonprofessional]

She had a life-or-death emergency with one of her patients. I was quite sympathetic.

[Female, 53, Nonprofessional]

When she was sick she would call me at 6:00 in the morning. That happened twice. She sounded terrible and I felt bad for her.

[Female, 39, Nonprofessional]

Sometimes the patient finds the therapist's absence upsetting or disturbing.

I remember once or twice I was disappointed because I really looked forward to seeing her.

[Female, 48, Nonprofessional]

He used to co-lead the marathons with his wife. There was one time where he had his wife lead the group instead of him because he had a tennis match. I was upset about that.

[Male, 50, Professional]

She became suddenly ill and was ill for quite a while and was not available for about 6 weeks, and it was very hard.

[Female, 45, Professional]

Feelings of relief sometimes arise, perhaps mixed with other feelings.

My reaction was a mixture of being relieved and feeling rebuffed.

[Female, 45, Professional]

Once there was something going on in her personal life, I think it was about her son, but I didn't want to know. I usually felt relieved that I didn't have to go.

[Female, 50, Professional]

Some patients don't want to know the reason.

> He had been to the dentist and he basically couldn't talk. We just rescheduled the session. I felt it was a little too informal that I should know this.
>
> [Female, 48, Nonprofessional]

Occasionally the therapist is unable to cancel in advance.

> Once she missed a session because she was stuck in traffic and there was no way to reach me.
>
> [Female, 44, Nonprofessional]

> She didn't show up for a session once. She was very apologetic. She was stuck in traffic and no way to get out of it.
>
> [Female, 50, Professional]

One person said she had a very strong reaction when the therapist was not there for the appointment.

> He didn't show up once, and I was sick to my stomach. He finally showed up. I think he had forgotten. For months after that I was worried about it and would ask him, "You're going to be there, aren't you?"
>
> [Female, 52, Nonprofessional]

One person said that a last-minute cancellation had led the therapist to an unusual offer.

> He said the next session was free, because if I had done it to him he would have charged me.
>
> [Male, 53, Nonprofessional]

NUMERICAL DISTRIBUTION

Professionals: Fourteen said the therapist had canceled a session unexpectedly; 6 said it had not happened.
Nonprofessionals: Sixteen said it had happened; 24 said it had not.

COMMENTS

Situations arise in which the therapist has to suddenly cancel a session, and the meaning of this event may vary from patient to patient.

Some will be relieved, some will be anxious about the therapist, some will be indifferent. Curiously, a much higher percentage of professionals reported this happening than did the nonprofessionals; perhaps the therapists were more relaxed with professional patients.

As the therapist, I try to keep this to an absolute minimum: only major illness will make me cancel a session without warning. I don't want patients to question my reliability and pull back from me.

As a patient, I'm not so disturbed by a single cancellation, but more than that and I may start to wonder whether I can rely on the therapist. I did have a therapist once who, when he was sick, had his wife call and cancel the session, and this made me wonder about his ability to keep the boundaries. Later on he demonstrated that he was unable to, and my concerns were justified.

RELATED READING

Epstein, R. S. (1994). *Keeping Boundaries: Maintaining Safety and Integrity in the Psychotherapeutic Process*. Washington, DC: American Psychiatric Press.

Gans, J. S., and Counselman, E. F. (1996). The missed session: a neglected aspect of psychodynamic psychotherapy. *Psychotherapy* 33(1):43–50.

ᕤᕤᕤᕤ

Question 53: Did the therapist ever appear tired?

Therapists work long days, often late into the evening, and sometimes it shows. Do patients notice? How does the patient react?

Sometimes patients are understanding.

> He's had some medical problems over the years.
>
> [Male, 50, Professional]

> I knew he had had some surgery.
>
> [Male, 51, Nonprofessional]

> It led me to give her an easier time because I thought she looked worn down.
>
> [Male, 44, Professional]

Therapists will often validate the perception, if the patient asks.

> Sometimes she would say she was tired, sometimes it was that she was ill, getting a cold, or getting over a cold, that kind of thing.
> [Female, 45, Nonprofessional]

> She reacted honestly. If she was tired she would say so. Then she would ask me if I was concerned.
> [Female, 50, Professional]

> When I told her she would agree, and we would go on to something else.
> [Female, 42, Nonprofessional]

> I'd ask her about it, and she'd say that she was, or wasn't feeling well.
> [Female, 45, Professional]

> I told her, and she just explained that it was a long day, or a troubling day.
> [Male, 45, Nonprofessional]

> Once he actually said, "Yes, I've been very tired lately," which I appreciated.
> [Female, 48, Professional]

> He'd say he was thinking; sometimes he would say he *was* tired.
> [Male, 52, Nonprofessional]

> I said, "Gee, you look tired," and he'd say, "Yeah, I was up very late." Once he yawned and I called him on that.
> [Female, 50, Professional]

> Once or twice she looked tired, and I said something to her and she explained it.
> [Female, 50, Professional]

Some therapists react badly to such a comment.

> She was defensive about it. She said she always appeared tired.
> [Female, 55, Professional]

> Sometimes she did look like she was falling asleep. I would tell her, and she would give me a defensive response.
> [Female, 50, Nonprofessional]

She was an older woman, in her seventies, and did appear tired sometimes. She was a little defensive about it.

[Female, 62, Professional]

We got after him at times, telling him, "It looks like you've had a hard day." If it was us going after him, he put a stop to that in a hurry because the tables had been turned, and he put us back in the right mode.

[Male, 43, Nonprofessional]

Occasionally the therapist will accept help from the patient.

Once she had a stomach ache. She was clearly ill. I told her and she said so, and I gave her an antacid, which she took, and she said it helped.

[Female, 51, Professional]

NUMERICAL DISTRIBUTION

Professionals: Fifteen people said the therapist had appeared tired; 5 said not.

Nonprofessionals: Sixteen people said the therapist had appeared tired; 24 said not.

COMMENTS

Most therapists work a long day, often starting early before patients go to their jobs and finishing late in the evening. Fatigue in the last hour or two is an occupational hazard for many therapists, at least occasionally. More professionals reported this in their therapists; perhaps they were less guarded with the professional patients.

As the therapist, I try to arrange my schedule so that I don't work too many hours in a day. Sometimes this is impossible, and I may be tired by the end of the day. I don't think it necessarily makes me less effective, unless I'm actually unable to focus. As in any other area, I try to validate any accurate perceptions if a patient notices and asks.

As a patient, I don't want to see my therapist tired, because it raises doubts about how well he or she might be listening to me and doing the job. I especially don't want to see yawning.

RELATED READING

Gerson, B., ed. (1996). *The Therapist as a Person: Life Crises, Life Choices, Life Experiences, and Their Effects on Treatment.* Hillsdale, NJ: Analytic Press.

Schwartz, H. J., and Silver, A-L. S., eds. (1990). *Illness in the Analyst: Implications for the Treatment Relationship.* Madison, CT: International Universities Press.

West, A. (1996). The risks of burnout. In *Forensic Psychotherapy: Crime, Psychotherapy and the Offender Patient,* vol. 2, ed. C. Cordess and M. Cox, pp. 229–240. London: Jessica Kingsley.

Williams, M., and Sommer, J. F. (1995). Self-care and the vulnerable therapist. In *Secondary Traumatic Stress: Self-Care Issues for Clinicans, Researchers, and Educators,* ed. B. H. Stamm, pp. 230–246. Lutherville, MD: Sidran.

⧚⧚⧚⧚

Question 54: Did the therapist ever appear bored?

While the therapist may have acceptable reasons for feeling tired, there may be no acceptable reason for boredom. Certain behaviors, such as yawns, or the therapist's lack of reaction, may make such perceptions occasionally unavoidable.

> One time he yawned. He apologized and said he had been taking some allergy medication that made him sleepy.
>
> [Female, 50, Professional]

> When she looked really neutral I wondered if she was bored, but I never asked her.
>
> [Female, 45, Professional]

> I remember her stifling yawns a few times.
>
> [Male, 44, Professional]

Many therapists simply denied the patient's perception of boredom.

> I would say that he appeared bored but he denied it, but he managed to rally round and slog through the session.
>
> [Female, 41, Nonprofessional]

I always accused him of it, and he said he wasn't.

[Female, 52, Nonprofessional]

Other therapists sidestepped the question, sometimes by focusing on the patient.

She would throw it back to me, and ask if there was something I was avoiding.

[Female, 51, Professional]

There were times that I felt that he was bored. He neither admitted nor denied—we talked about my feeling that he was feeling bored.

[Female, 46, Nonprofessional]

I remember several different responses, including one that explored the possibility that I was feeling bored as well.

[Male, 53, Professional]

He looked like he was suppressing a yawn. He said, "Can you imagine that physiologically I might have to yawn without being bored?"

[Female, 48, Nonprofessional]

There were times when he said he was not bored; there were times when he said he was thinking about something; there were times when he interpreted it as my being emotionally disconnected with what I was saying.

[Male, 50, Professional]

Occasionally a therapist would admit to being bored.

He said he *was* bored.

[Male, 46, Nonprofessional]

Some people admitted that boring the therapist was one of their fears.

I usually think it's because I'm boring, or doing something wrong.

[Male, 50, Professional]

I would bring up from time to time, when we were going over the same stuff again, that she must be bored, but I never did anything to try to make the session more interesting.

[Male, 45, Nonprofessional]

If anything it was me thinking I was boring him. I never thought it was really going on so I never brought it up.

[Male, 30, Professional]

I could worry that I was boring her, but I don't know that she ever appeared bored.

[Female, 50, Professional]

Other people said the therapist reacted in a way that was not useful.

He always tried to throw it back on some transference thing.

[Female, 48, Professional]

NUMERICAL DISTRIBUTION

Professionals: Seven said the therapist had appeared bored; 13 people said not.

Nonprofessionals: Eleven said the therapist had appeared bored; 29 said not.

COMMENTS

In *Shrink Rap* I discuss at length the therapist's reactions to a "boring" patient. Most therapists regard the feeling of boredom as a countertransferential signal indicating something about the patient. As the therapist, I'm never bored in the sense of finding someone uninteresting, but some patients do induce a feeling of exhaustion or distraction. This is best dealt with directly with the patient.

As the patient, I don't ever want to feel that I'm boring to my therapist. If I think that, I will confront it directly, and had better get a direct response.

RELATED READING

Flannery, J. (1995). Boredom in the therapist: countertransference issues. *British Journal of Psychotherapy* 11(4):536–544.

McHolland, J. D. (1987). Client–therapist boredom: What does it mean and what do we do? *Psychotherapy Patient* 3(3–4):87–96.

Tabin, J. K. (1987). Some lively thoughts on boredom. *Psychotherapy Patient* 3(3–4):147–149.

Taylor, G. J. (1984). Psychotherapy with the boring patient. *Canadian Journal of Psychiatry* 29(3):217–222.

ℝℝℝℝ

Question 55: Did you ever try to amuse or entertain your therapist?

Patients often feel that they have to entertain and amuse the therapist in order to be accepted and liked. Different therapists have different ways of responding to this kind of behavior.

Some people were aware that this was their normal way of relating to everyone.

> I did that all the time. It's just who I am. She just accepted it.
>
> [Female, 47, Nonprofessional]

> I thought that's what I should do—be charming and engaging so she would like me. She'd ask me why I was doing it, if I felt that I needed to do it.
>
> [Female, 45, Professional]

> In the beginning that was part of my pattern, not to talk about myself but to be charming. It took him years but he finally got me to talk about myself.
>
> [Female, 45, Nonprofessional]

Some people explained their behavior.

> I was trying to make sure he stayed interested.
>
> [Female, 52, Nonprofessional]

> That's what I need to do to keep someone engaged with me.
>
> [Female, 50, Professional]

> I can remember having moments of feeling that I was consciously being charming. I wanted her to like me.
>
> [Female, 45, Nonprofessional]

> It brought up an old feeling of being inadequate. I got the feeling that I was not what he wanted either.
>
> [Female, 48, Nonprofessional]

Many people said the therapist would accept such behavior for a while, and then comment about it.

> At first he'd be amused, and then suddenly communicate that I didn't have to prove anything to him, that there was a basic acceptance.
>
> [Male, 30, Professional]

> He would say that I was a very entertaining guy, a charming guy, a funny guy, with a great imagination and a way with words. Other times he would tell me to cut the shit, that he didn't want to hear any stories that day.
>
> [Male, 46, Nonprofessional]

> I would get bubbly. Sometimes she would laugh and join in, and sometimes she would ask what we were getting so funny about.
>
> [Female, 52, Professional]

> I think she'd go along with the diversion to a certain degree and then refocus the conversation on something more important.
>
> [Female, 26, Nonprofessional]

Some people said they were disappointed when they could not get the response they were looking for from the therapist.

> Early on he was more reluctant to be involved. I was disappointed that I didn't enchant him.
>
> [Male, 53, Professional]

> Sometimes he was amused and entertained; sometimes he wasn't, and I would get anxious.
>
> [Male, 50, Professional]

> I got a few laughs out of him, but not often. He didn't have a good sense of humor.
>
> [Female, 48, Professional]

> I think I was funny, and he had a good sense of humor. If I said something funny and he didn't respond I would question him about that.
>
> [Female, 50, Professional]

And others said they enjoyed and were reassured when they could elicit a reaction.

I would enjoy telling a funny story, and getting a laugh out of her, which she probably didn't want to do.

[Female, 44, Nonprofessional]

I did, just to see if I was being seen. She did see me, both my charming social self and my shadow side.

[Male, 49, Nonprofessional]

I remember trying to tell an amusing story. I was seeing if I could make him laugh, and he would chuckle.

[Female, 41, Nonprofessional]

NUMERICAL DISTRIBUTION

Professionals: Fourteen people said they had tried to amuse the therapist; 6 people said they had not.

Nonprofessionals: Twenty-three people said they had tried to amuse the therapist; 17 people said they had not.

COMMENTS

A certain degree of trying to entertain the therapist is normal, and best left alone, but some patients continue trying to amuse and get the therapist to laugh, which becomes a defense and an avoidance of doing the work. As the therapist, I want to convey to the patient that they don't have to get me to like them by bringing me amusement and entertainment.

As a patient, I'm watching to see if my therapist can join me and enjoy things with me. If that happens, it may then be easier to stop doing it than if he or she sits silently and solemnly, with what may feel like an implied judgment of what I'm doing.

RELATED READING

Luborsky, L., Diguer, L., Kasabakalian-McKay, R., et al. (1996). Laughing matters in psychotherapy: how to read their context. In *The Symptom–Context Method: Symptoms as Opportunities in Psychotherapy*, ed. L. Luborsky, pp. 279–296. Washington, DC: American Psychological Association.

Marcus, N. N. (1990). Treating those who fail to take themselves seriously: pathological aspects of humor. *American Journal of Psychotherapy* 44(3):423–432.

Richman, J. (1996). Jokes as a projective technique: the humor of psychiatric patients. *American Journal of Psychotherapy* 50(3):336–346.

Sachs, J. (1991). Psychoanalysis and the elements of play. *American Journal of Psychoanalysis* 51(1):39–53.

⬚⬚⬚⬚

Question 56: Did you ever think your therapist was trying to amuse or entertain you?

Just as patients can try to win over the therapist by being charming or entertaining, the therapist may also try this tactic with the patient.

Only about a quarter of both the professionals and nonprofessionals said they had experienced the therapist in this way, with varying results.

> He did try a few times. I don't think he was very good at it, but he did try.
>
> [Female, 48, Professional]

> I suppose on occasion that was a factor, but I don't remember ever feeling that that was the only motive.
>
> [Female, 48, Nonprofessional]

Some people saw this behavior as a strategy of the therapist.

> He would sometimes do that to get a reaction, to draw something out of us.
>
> [Male, 43, Nonprofessional]

> She did if she felt I needed it, or she wanted to get me going, if it seemed like a really slow day.
>
> [Male, 45, Nonprofessional]

> I think sometimes she was trying to respond similarly to me.
>
> [Male, 48, Nonprofessional]

Sometimes this behavior was seen as simply part of the therapist's personality.

There was a part of him that was boyish and he would want me to laugh at his joke.

[Male, 46, Nonprofessional]

I thought she was really being herself, which could be funny, but she wasn't making a special attempt.

[Male, 52, Nonprofessional]

She did, but I'm not sure it was deliberate.

[Female, 55, Professional]

Sometimes he would cut through a lot of stuff with a line from a play or something, but it was always in a therapeutic style.

[Female, 50, Professional]

Sometimes the patient can enjoy the therapist in this way.

When she talked about topics other than therapy, I found her to be very interesting and entertaining.

[Male, 49, Nonprofessional]

Sometimes the patient finds such behavior objectionable.

He would start talking about restaurants and eating, and I didn't want to talk about that.

[Female, 41, Nonprofessional]

She seemed like one of those radio shrinks, and she talked about how she'd been on television.

[Female, 44, Nonprofessional]

NUMERICAL DISTRIBUTION

Professionals: Four felt the therapist was trying to amuse or entertain them; 16 said not.

Nonprofessionals: Nine said they had felt the therapist was trying to amuse or entertain them; 31 said not.

COMMENTS

I hope that all therapists feel the freedom to be amusing and even entertaining at times without feeling as if they are compromising the importance of the work. As the therapist, I often use humor to cut through, to lighten, and to make a point.

As a patient, I don't mind if the therapist occasionally tells a joke or relates an amusing anecdote, especially when it gently makes a point that's relevant to our discussion. But more than that might lead me to feel as if the therapist weren't taking the work seriously.

RELATED READING

Lusterman, D. D. (1992). Humor as metaphor. *Psychotherapy in Private Practice* 10(1–2):167–172.

Pollio, D. E. (1995). Use of humor in crisis intervention. *Families in Society* 76(6):376–384.

Rutherford, K. (1994). Humor in psychotherapy. *Individual Psychology Journal of Adlerian Theory, Research and Practice* 50(2):207–222.

Strean, H. (1994). *The Use of Humor in Psychotherapy*. Northvale, NJ: Jason Aronson.

⧫⧫⧫⧫

Question 57: Did the therapist have a good sense of humor? Was that important to you?

Although therapy is a serious activity, a little humor can go a long way in making the work more pleasant and more playful. Most people thought their therapist had a good sense of humor, and they appreciated this quality.

> Humor is vital to me, and a therapist who couldn't share or understand that couldn't understand me.
>
> [Male, 49, Nonprofessional]

> It's important for me because, if you can laugh at yourself a little bit and the other person sees the humor in what you're saying, it makes you feel like you still have some perspective and your life isn't out of control.
>
> [Male, 42, Nonprofessional]

> The more humanity I could find in the therapist the better, and humor is such a big part of it.
>
> [Male, 46, Nonprofessional]

Some people said it was an essential quality in anyone, therapist or otherwise.

It's an important quality in a human being.
[Male, 49, Nonprofessional]

I wouldn't see someone who didn't have a good sense of humor.
[Female, 51, Professional]

I tend not to trust people who can't take a joke.
[Male, 52, Nonprofessional]

Several people said it lightened the work.

It's a leavening in the whole process.
[Female, 42, Nonprofessional]

It humanizes the therapeutic experience.
[Female, 47, Nonprofessional]

And was an important aspect of the whole process.

As a patient and as a therapist, as I loosen up my whole approach, I think it's an important part of the whole enterprise.
[Male, 50, Professional]

His sense of humor developed over the years. It grew in me too, because I was so serious for a while.
[Male, 53, Professional]

A therapist with a good sense of humor can be a good role model.

It made me feel lighter to laugh about certain things.
[Female, 48, Nonprofessional]

It allowed me to get in touch with my own, to find the light places in myself about serious issues.
[Female, 46, Nonprofessional]

Some people felt that the therapist was trying to conceal his or her sense of humor.

I think when he let it show through, he did, but he tried not to. He was the kind of therapist who doesn't want to let you know what he's thinking. On occasion I would say something funny and I would be laughing and he would sort of let me know that he thought it was amusing too.

[Female, 41, Nonprofessional]

She was very guarded with me, so that's not something she would engage in with me.

[Female, 50, Professional]

She laughed reluctantly. It seemed she didn't want to.

[Female, 44, Nonprofessional]

A few people said the therapist didn't seem to have much of a sense of humor.

I don't remember him having a sense of humor. I respond very well to being kidded out of a bad mood, laughing at me affectionately. I never was convinced that he cared about me, so I wouldn't have interpreted his kidding as affectionate.

[Female, 48, Nonprofessional]

He had no sense of humor. I think he laughed only once. It's very important to me.

[Female, 48, Professional]

Some people didn't mind if the therapist showed no sense of humor.

She didn't show it. I generally like people with a sense of humor but I don't think it would have influenced my opinion of her as a psychologist.

[Female, 28, Nonprofessional]

I like people with a sense of humor, but I don't need to know if the therapist has a good sense of humor.

[Female, 48, Nonprofessional]

It's more important that they're light, not so heavy and analytical.

[Female, 39, Professional]

And some found it disturbing.

I've had therapists who had no sense of humor, and I found that disturbing, because it meant they were not like me, and how could I possibly use them as a model if they don't have the same vision of the world as I do? There's something forbidding and off-putting about someone who doesn't think things are funny.

[Male, 52, Nonprofessional]

She never showed it. She was pretty serious. In the beginning it was important because I had a problem believing that the therapist cared about me, and it was somehow wrapped up in that.

[Female, 48, Nonprofessional]

Some people pointed out the dangers of using humor as a therapeutic technique.

It's important if used correctly, if it doesn't lead to a flip remark or dismissing what the patient is saying.

[Female, 50, Nonprofessional]

I suspect it would be a good thing, but I'd also imagine taking it as a sign of a lack of seriousness about my feelings. It depends so much on sharing a similar sense of what's humorous.

[Female, 46, Nonprofessional]

NUMERICAL DISTRIBUTION

Professionals: Fourteen said the therapist had a good sense of humor; 6 said not. Nineteen said a good sense of humor is important in a therapist; 1 said it was not so important.

Nonprofessionals: Thirty-three said the therapist had a good sense of humor; 7 said not. Thirty-six said a good sense of humor is important in a therapist; 4 said it was not important.

COMMENTS

As many people said, a good sense of humor is an important quality in any human being, and a therapist without one is something less than fully human. As the therapist, I think laughing with the patient is important, as a way of bonding and as a way of modeling. Life without humor is pretty grim, and there's no good reason for therapy to exclude it.

As a patient, I need to see a good sense of humor in my therapist, as a sign that she is smart, as a signal that she understands my point of view, and as an indicator of her sensibility.

RELATED READING

Buckman, E. S., ed. (1994). *The Handbook of Humor: Clinical Applications in Psychotherapy.* Malabar, FL: Robert E. Krieger.

Fry, W. F., and Salameh, W. A., eds. (1987). *Handbook of Humor and Psychotherapy: Advances in the Clinical Use of Humor.* Sarasota, FL: Professional Resource Exchange.

MacHovec, F. (1991). Humor in therapy. *Psychotherapy in Private Practice* 9(1):25–33.

Mann, D. (1991). Humor in psychotherapy. *Psychoanalytic Psychotherapy* 5(2):161–170.

ᘓᘓᘓᘓ

Question 58: Did your therapist ever appear angry with you?

Patients often fear making the therapist angry. Therapists are supposedly trained not to show anger, simply to analyze the patient's behavior and its provocative intentions.

Sometimes patients get the impression that the therapist is angry with them. This may in fact be true.

> I think she might have been, when I was critical.
>
> [Female, 62, Professional]

> It probably came up during the session, and she would explain her reasons for feeling angry with me. It didn't happen too often, but there were times when she let me know that something I'd said or done was inappropriate or not right.
>
> [Male, 45, Nonprofessional]

> Whenever I criticized him and he couldn't keep up intellectually, he would hit below the belt.
>
> [Female, 57, Professional]

> When I would challenge him, I could tell he was furious.
>
> [Female, 48, Professional]

One time I had made some comment about the rug in the waiting room. He was always unbelievably neat, and I made a comment that he was a little compulsive. He alphabetized his books! And he got a little defensive, saying, "But it helps me so much!" And I think he was a little angry at what I had said. He thought I was putting down his rug.

[Female, 50, Professional]

Sometimes the therapist gets angry in response to the patient's anger.

On a couple of occasions I think he felt so abused by me that he got angry in response. That was hard for me to hear. I felt so self-righteous that I was being injured that I didn't want to hear it.

[Male, 50, Professional]

If I got too vicious with him, he let me know what the impact was on him.

[Male, 46, Nonprofessional]

Sometimes the therapist is angry about the way the patient is working (or not working) on issues.

She sometimes got on my case about things I was avoiding.

[Male, 50, Nonprofessional]

I was very resistant to stepping into an issue, and she had been very patiently trying to engage me with the resistance, and she wasn't getting anywhere for weeks. She confronted me and I could feel that she was angry. It made a world of difference and helped me deal with my resistance.

[Female, 45, Professional]

He got irritated, because I'd say that I wouldn't talk about something.

[Female, 50, Nonprofessional]

Sometimes the therapist gets angry over behaviors in the therapy.

Because of a condition I have, sometimes I'll just fall asleep in the middle of a sentence. It's something physical I have no control over. It would happen there and she got really pissed off.

[Male, 52, Nonprofessional]

> I was screwing around in a major way, like delaying paying the fee.
>
> [Male, 53, Professional]

> She got annoyed when I canceled a lot of sessions.
>
> [Female, 50, Professional]

And sometimes the patient's behavior outside the office gets a reaction from the therapist.

> She didn't get angry, but she can be formidable on occasion, and she was about my drinking.
>
> [Male, 49, Nonprofessional]

Several people said the therapist seemed frustrated, annoyed, or irritated.

> Occasionally she might have been impatient with me.
>
> [Female, 42, Nonprofessional]

> Frustrated, but not angry.
>
> [Female, 50, Professional]

> On one or two occasions she got impatient with me because she felt I wasn't trying hard enough.
>
> [Male, 42, Nonprofessional]

One person remembered a discussion about anger.

> We did talk about whether I was being careful to filter things so she didn't get angry.
>
> [Female, 39, Nonprofessional]

Sometimes the therapist appears angry to the patient, but denies that perception.

> There was some kind of unnamed tension that existed right from the beginning. I always had the feeling that he was annoyed with me. I could never quite get over that. And I would ask him, "Are you mad at me?" and he'd say, "No, why do you ask that?" There was always something about his manner that seemed unfriendly.
>
> [Female, 45, Nonprofessional]

One person described how she knew the therapist was angry.

She had a physical mannerism that let me know I wasn't getting to something and she was getting impatient: her foot would begin to twitch. It took me a long time to tell her about it. She was completely unconscious of it.

[Female, 46, Nonprofessional]

Several people said the therapist got angry when they stopped therapy.

He was upset once, because I came in for my session and said I wasn't going to be in for the next month. I was going to stop for a while. He didn't get mad but I sensed that he had some reaction.

[Male, 48, Nonprofessional]

Once she appeared angry and I thought it looked acted, performed, contrived. When I terminated abruptly it was genuine.

[Male, 44, Professional]

She got angry when I finally left.

[Female, 45, Nonprofessional]

Several people mentioned specific situations where the therapist got angry at them.

Our rule in the group was that we were not allowed to date anyone from the group. One of the women had dropped out of the group, and 2 or 3 months later I met her and struck up a relationship with her. She was totally out of the group and was never coming back, so in my mind I didn't break a rule, but it angered him.

[Male, 43, Nonprofessional]

She seemed annoyed with me when she changed my hour to a time when I couldn't come because I had asked for that time a long time before, but things had changed since then.

[Female, 44, Nonprofessional]

I think probably the only time was over a misunderstanding about a canceled session, and I remember her saying that if I wasn't able to see her one week I had to come again the following week because she needed to plan her finances, and she seemed annoyed at me because she thought I believed that if I missed a session I just missed it.

[Female, 41, Nonprofessional]

NUMERICAL DISTRIBUTION

Professionals: Ten said the therapist had gotten angry; 3 said annoyed or frustrated but not actually angry; 7 said it had never happened.

Nonprofessionals: Nine said the therapist had gotten angry; 10 said the therapist had been annoyed or irritated; 21 said it had never happened.

COMMENTS

If the therapist gets angry at the patient, that is a countertransferential feeling that needs to be processed and metabolized within the therapist, not dumped on the patient. The impulse to lecture the patient, or to vent the anger, must be contained and dealt with internally, after the session if necessary. As the therapist, if I find myself feeling anger toward the patient, I have to think about how I've stepped out of the therapist position. This may reveal something important about me or something equally important about the patient, or both.

As a patient, I regard with deep mistrust and suspicion any therapist who expresses anger at me. I'm there in the therapist's office to reveal my problems and issues, and if I can't be crazy there then where can I be? If the therapist thinks what I'm doing is objectionable or even pathological, then he has to show me that calmly and rationally, not react with anger or annoyance, which only makes me wonder about his pathology, not my own.

RELATED READING

Berger, D. M. (1987). *Clinical Empathy*. Northvale, NJ: Jason Aronson.

Chessick, R. D. (1989). *The Technique and Practice of Listening in Intensive Psychotherapy*. Northvale, NJ: Jason Aronson.

Holmqvist, R., and Armelius, B. (1996). Sources of therapists' countertransference feelings. *Psychotherapy Research* 6(1):70–78.

Levine, H. B. (1996). Action, transference, and resistance: some reflections on a paradox at the heart of analytic technique. *Psychoanalytic Inquiry* 16(4):474–490.

❧❧❧❧

Question 59: Did your therapist ever appear at a loss for what to say or do?

No therapist can be completely prepared for everything. Occasionally a patient will say something to which the therapist may have no response.

> When my husband got sick, he was totally at a loss.
> [Female, 48, Professional]

> When I started telling him about my first therapy, he was stunned. One or two other times something I told him really shocked him.
> [Female, 50, Professional]

Some therapists admitted when this happened.

> Sometimes she was at a loss for something that would neatly wrap things up, and would openly admit that she couldn't do that.
> [Female, 46, Nonprofessional]

> He admitted that he didn't quite know what to say, that he was thinking. It was helpful to me, because it suggested that one could still work on things.
> [Male, 53, Professional]

> There were a few moments where we were baffled, and didn't know where to go with something.
> [Male, 50, Nonprofessional]

Some people found this admission a positive experience.

> I loved it when he did. I think he really had a difficult time with angry feelings, and the times that I was up front with him about my anger he would just sit back and allow it to happen. Maybe that was his style, and he didn't want to interfere with my expressing those feelings, but it seemed to me that he didn't know what to do.
> [Female, 58, Professional]

> It was so well used in the session. We would look at it together.
> [Male, 46, Nonprofessional]

> In the first session, I said I wanted to learn to meditate, and what about it? And he said he wasn't sure what to do with it. I appreciated his humility.
> [Male, 30, Professional]

Some people were disappointed.

I wanted something more from her, other than a nod, and I got a nod. It appeared as if she didn't know what else to say.

[Female, 47, Nonprofessional]

Some of the circumstances in my life, I was hoping she would have some response but she didn't.

[Female, 52, Professional]

He didn't seem to be able to get at the root of the problem. I was clueless and he seemed to be clueless too, even at the time we ended.

[Male, 48, Nonprofessional]

My guess is she did, but I can't think of anything specific. I remember hanging out there and wishing she could say something.

[Female, 50, Professional]

I was feeling so bad about something and there was nothing she could do.

[Female, 42, Nonprofessional]

Sometimes she wouldn't have anything new to add, so she would just repeat things that she had said before without any elaboration. I felt annoyed that I had heard it before and it didn't help me. I didn't tell her because at that point I realized that I had outgrown her.

[Female, 50, Nonprofessional]

Several people said it was hard to tell if the therapist was feeling at a loss or just thinking.

I used to say that he could get away with being at a total loss, because he said so little.

[Female, 52, Nonprofessional]

She doesn't experience those moments as a problem, so I don't know.

[Female, 45, Professional]

On occasion, he would pause and reflect and think. Maybe he was covering up well.

[Female, 41, Nonprofessional]

Sometimes she would say, "I just don't know yet."

[Female, 51, Professional]

I can't say he appeared that way, but I wonder if that might have been going on and he was covering up.

[Female, 46, Nonprofessional]

She speaks very slowly and precisely, so I wasn't sure if she was struggling to find words or if that was her style.

[Female, 62, Professional]

There were times she was quiet and I wished she had said something, so she might have been.

[Female, 45, Nonprofessional]

NUMERICAL DISTRIBUTION

Professionals: Eight said the therapist had appeared at a loss; 9 said not; 3 said there was no way to tell.

Nonprofessionals: Thirteen said the therapist had appeared at a loss; 25 said not; 2 said there was no way to tell.

COMMENTS

There will almost certainly be times in any therapy when the therapist will not know, if only for a moment, what to say to the patient. This is not necessarily an indication of anything wrong with the therapist or the treatment. As the therapist, I don't see any reason not to reveal this when it happens if the patient asks for some response. Of course, if it happens all the time then there is a problem: the therapist can't be so continually off balance and still be effective, and this would be a good time for a consultation or supervision.

As the patient, I don't mind hearing occasionally that the therapist is at a loss; it would indicate to me that she feels no need to be omniscient or more than human. Her comfort level in accepting the feeling of not knowing what to say might also be a good role model for me in accepting my own uncertainty.

RELATED READING

Abend, S. (1986). Countertransference, empathy, and the analytic ideal: the impact of life stresses on analytic capacity. *Psychoanalytic Quarterly* 55(3):563–575.

Chessick, R. D. (1993). What constitutes our understanding of a patient? *Journal of the American Academy of Psychoanalysis* 21(2):253–272.

First, E. (1993). Countertransference strain and the use of the analyst. *Psychoanalytic Inquiry* 13(4):264–273.

Satran, G. (1991). Some limits and hazards of empathy. *Contemporary Psychoanalysis* 27(4):737–748.

⚮⚮⚮⚮

Question 60: Did you ever think your therapist was trying to teach you something?

Therapists can sometimes take a didactic position, trying to teach the patient something concrete and specific. Much of the time patients experience this as positive and valuable, especially professionals still in training.

> She taught me some specific techniques. It was part of why I was there.
>
> [Female, 56, Professional]

> Occasionally she would give me some simple strategies that were very concrete and were very useful.
>
> [Female, 46, Nonprofessional]

> She was teaching me a lot about life, what it means to be human. It didn't feel preachy.
>
> [Female, 45, Professional]

> When I was in training, he would sometimes say he was doing something for a reason that he explained. I found that useful.
>
> [Female, 48, Professional]

> I always had that feeling, but not like a teacher in front of a blackboard. It felt okay.
>
> [Male, 51, Nonprofessional]

> He was trying to teach me to be more aware, more open, more trusting, more related, less detached.
>
> [Female, 59, Professional]

He was trying to teach me something about life, or share a more realistic adult perspective. It felt fine.

[Male, 42, Professional]

It felt okay because it was clearly defined.

[Female, 45, Professional]

Part of therapy is teaching, but I didn't feel it in a pedantic way.

[Female, 50, Professional]

Some people mentioned specific areas, such as interpersonal skills.

He was trying to teach me how to express my anger in a way that didn't frighten people.

[Male, 43, Nonprofessional]

She tried to help me deal with difficulties in performing and public speaking.

[Male, 44, Professional]

She thought I had trouble getting along with people, and would sometimes try to teach me things.

[Female, 62, Professional]

What the therapist believes is useful may not seem that way to the patient.

She was trying to impart to me a theoretical framework that she believed in and sometimes I found that useful and sometimes I didn't.

[Male, 48, Nonprofessional]

There were times when she got into feminist politics, and I didn't like that.

[Female, 50, Professional]

Sometimes it felt all right and sometimes I didn't like it at all. But I knew I could discern the wheat from the chaff.

[Male, 53, Nonprofessional]

He didn't think I handled money with my patients properly. I lost 2 patients because I tried to do it his way and didn't follow my own gut feelings.

[Female, 57, Professional]

> If I wanted be taught it felt fine. If I didn't, it was irritating.
>
> [Female, 50, Nonprofessional]

> Sometimes he would and I would interrupt him.
>
> [Female, 52, Nonprofessional]

Patients may experience the therapist's teaching as critical of their own abilities.

> He would say things in a way that presupposed that I was as adept at doing things as he was. He's very good at handling people, and he presupposed that I was too, and it made me feel terrible. It took me a lot of years before I could tell him that I wasn't as good at it as he thought.
>
> [Male, 50, Professional]

The patient doesn't always understand what the therapist is trying to teach.

> In a sort of Socratic way, he would ask questions where he had a point in mind. Sometimes I didn't get what he was trying to show me, and he would tell me directly.
>
> [Female, 41, Nonprofessional]

> It was more that she was trying to show me something. I thought it was fine, but I didn't always get what she was trying to show me.
>
> [Female, 45, Nonprofessional]

Sometimes the patient wants to be taught but the therapist declines to do that.

> I remember having that feeling at different times. I wanted more of that, a more directive therapy.
>
> [Female, 47, Nonprofessional]

> I wanted him to teach me something but he wouldn't.
>
> [Female, 48, Nonprofessional]

NUMERICAL DISTRIBUTION

Professionals: Eighteen said that the therapist was trying to teach them something; 2 said that had not happened. Of those who said yes, only 2 did not find it useful, positive, or pleasant.

Nonprofessionals: Twenty-five said the therapist was trying to teach them something; 18 said that had not happened. Of those who said yes, only 4 said they did not like it or want it.

COMMENTS

The therapist is, in various ways, always trying to teach something: by investigating, by offering interpretations, by modeling, by challenging assumptions and beliefs. But sometimes a didactic role is useful in describing and explaining something specific and concrete. As the therapist, I try to ask if the patient wants to hear such material before I offer it, since otherwise it can so often feel condescending or parental.

As the patient, I don't mind learning something from the therapist, but I don't want to feel it's being offered because of the therapist's agenda. I will usually ask for specific information if I want it.

RELATED READING

DeJong, P., and Miller, S. D. (1995). How to interview for client strengths. *Social Work* 40(6):729–736.

Holmes, J. (1996). Values in psychotherapy. *American Journal of Psychotherapy* 50(3):259–273.

Renik, O. (1995). The role of the analyst's expectations in clinical technique: reflections on the concept of resistance. *Journal of the American Psychoanalytic Association* 43(1):83–94.

Salerno, M., Farber, B. A., McCullough, L., and Winston, A. (1992). The effects of confrontation and clarification on patient affective and defensive responding. *Psychotherapy Research* 2(3):181–192.

᠗᠗᠗᠗

Question 61: Did your therapist ever do anything that made you angry?

In general, therapists try to avoid an adversarial relationship with the patient, but sometimes what the therapist says or does makes the patient angry.

Patients get angry as a result of feeling mistreated in some way.

Once she let me walk out of her office in hysterics, crying. She said she wouldn't have done it if she thought I couldn't handle it, and I thought that was a lame excuse.

[Female, 48, Nonprofessional]

I've been going to therapy for the same thing since I was a kid, and the fact that I still have panic attacks, and I don't feel that there was ever any real answer, that makes me angry. Maybe I need some kind of medication, and that was never even brought up.

[Female, 28, Nonprofessional]

Several people remembered getting angry when they felt misunderstood, or when their experience seemed to be dismissed.

He didn't see my need for support in separating from someone, and said that I was trying to control him.

[Male, 42, Professional]

I got angry when she didn't understand. The whole thing about the institute built up to the point where, in the last year, I was screaming at her.

[Female, 62, Professional]

A couple of times I told her that I had been upset earlier about something she had said that made it seem that she wasn't listening or didn't understand, and she said that she wished I had told her, and she was listening and did understand.

[Male, 52, Nonprofessional]

When she said things that showed she didn't know me, I was frustrated and angry. I thought, "How can she still not get this?" I told her and she didn't react.

[Female, 50, Professional]

A few times I had something horrible happen with my supervisor, and if it was about my father he would be interested, but if it was about my supervisor the implication was that it was all my own issue and not them. I felt dismissed. My anger was not legitimate.

[Female, 48, Nonprofessional]

There were a couple of times when I felt he didn't understand me and I felt very betrayed. He listened and tried to make some interpretations about it, relate it to other things.

[Female, 59, Professional]

Others said that an interpretation or comment by the therapist made them angry.

> She said that I may have been depressed all of my life. I just couldn't deal with that. I still can't. It's such a shocking thing to say. Also she compared my mother to Eleanor Roosevelt, who saw all the problems out in the world but didn't see them in her own family. It's too strong to accept.
>
> [Female, 50, Nonprofessional]

> When I wanted to stop and he said I was running away, that pissed me off.
>
> [Male, 30, Professional]

> I got irritated a couple of times. One was her insistence that I find the good in my father. There was one point when she kept asking what something reminded me of in my childhood, and I said that my childhood was over and it didn't matter. But she explained what she was doing.
>
> [Female, 39, Nonprofessional]

Often the trigger for an angry reaction is money.

> I went through this whole thing with the insurance coverage, first submitting it to my company, then to my husband's company—it was very confusing. Then I found out that my therapist was actually a participating therapist in their plan and he didn't tell me that, so there was a whole year I could have been covered with him and just paid $10 a session. He said that he never thought about what kind of insurance I had.
>
> [Female, 42, Nonprofessional]

> The biggest anger I had was about money—not his fee, which I thought was fair, but whenever I talked about something that was a reality problem he would turn it into a psychological issue. That was really offensive to me. Not that he was wrong, but not to acknowledge the reality made me really angry.
>
> [Female, 58, Professional]

> I called her recently because I wanted to see her again, and the fee was so high that I couldn't afford it. I felt like, "It's nice to know that you really care, that you can give me a break." Her husband's a doctor,

she's a doctor, she's making a hundred dollars off of everybody. She knows me, why can't she give me a break?

[Female, 26, Nonprofessional]

A firm cancellation policy, strictly enforced, can also elicit angry responses.

I thought he was being exploitive about missed sessions when my husband was so sick.

[Female, 48, Professional]

Sometimes she wouldn't be able to reschedule if I was sick, and she would charge me for the appointment.

[Female, 42, Nonprofessional]

When I was hospitalized, she charged me for missed sessions. I had a very hard time with that.

[Female, 47, Nonprofessional]

Some people reported getting angry at the therapist's style.

I was very angry the night he failed to protect me in group. I'm a very very polite, easing-around-the-edges kind of person, and he's much more of a New Yorker. Sometimes I would tell him that he just wasn't tactful. Or he would say something that was just too simplistic. It was mostly around these kinds of style issues.

[Female, 50, Professional]

He was very challenging and it made me angry and I told him.

[Female, 48, Nonprofessional]

I was angry all the time at her not reciprocating or sharing feelings.

[Male, 44, Professional]

Therapist lateness is sometimes the issue.

She was always late, sometimes as much as 10 minutes, either because the previous session ran over or she got hung up on something. It would make me crazy. Finally I confronted her about it and she was very responsive.

[Female, 50, Professional]

A few people reported feeling used by the therapist, when the therapist's needs took precedence over the patient's.

After I had been out of treatment for a while, a year, I got a phone call from him inviting me to come back for a session. I felt he was calling because he was soliciting business, not because I might need it. We spoke and I told him I would be happy to come in but I wouldn't pay for it. He said that was all right, and I did come and we chatted and I left.

[Female, 48, Nonprofessional]

She canceled our group, which had been meeting for 5 or 6 years. She just didn't want to do it anymore.

[Female, 47, Nonprofessional]

I got angry when she would get into her own stuff in the middle of the sessions.

[Female, 50, Nonprofessional]

Sometimes the patient's anger is dispelled by discussing it.

I know that I've had feelings of anger toward her, and I can't remember why. We would talk about it and it would sort of go away.

[Female, 45, Nonprofessional]

A number of people mentioned specific situations that made them angry.

I think she referred someone to me, and it didn't seem to me to be a good idea, and I was angry about that. She said that she thought I was right and that we could undo the referral.

[Female, 52, Professional]

I was in therapy and my brother was seeing her too, and she called me to minister to him, to go to his apartment and take care of him.

[Female, 45, Nonprofessional]

She would often be eating in the session. It made me angry but I didn't tell her.

[Female, 51, Professional]

The only time was when she would accept a phone call during the session.

[Female, 42, Nonprofessional]

She gave away my time to the woman I referred to her. I didn't have a set specific time, there were two times I would see her, and she gave one away to her without asking if it was all right. She apologized and acknowledged she was wrong.

[Female, 39, Professional]

I left her a note asking her to give me a call, and I got a call from the secretary. I told her I was really annoyed, and she explained what she had understood.

[Female, 45, Professional]

NUMERICAL DISTRIBUTION

Professionals: Seventeen said that something the therapist did made them angry; only 3 said that had not happened.

Nonprofessionals: Twenty-three said that something the therapist did made them angry; 17 said that had not happened.

COMMENTS

It's curious that so many of the nonprofessionals said that nothing the therapist did made them angry; perhaps they didn't know they were allowed to get angry at the therapist, or perhaps they expected less than did the professionals. Some of the responses above indicate that even when the patient knows about the anger, he or she may not tell the therapist. As the therapist, I expect that patients will sooner or later get angry at something I say or do, and watch carefully for signs that this may be unexpressed.

As the patient, I may get angry at many different kinds of behavior, any of which indicate a failure of some sort on the part of the therapist. I'd like to think I would always tell the therapist, but I know that sometimes I have not, at least not for a while, during which I need to think over how important it is to me.

RELATED READING

Anchor, K. N. (1977). Personality integration and successful outcome in individual psychotherapy. *Journal of Clinical Psychology* 33(1): 245–246.

Buckley, P., Karasu, T. B., and Charles, E. (1979). Common mistakes in psychotherapy. *American Journal of Psychiatry* 136(12):1578–1580.

Buffone, G. W. (1991). Understanding and managing the litigious patient. *Psychotherapy in Private Practice* 9(2):27–45.

Clark, F. C. (1995). Anger and its disavowal in shame-based people. *Transactional Analysis Journal* 25(2):129–132.

🔰🔰🔰🔰

Question 62: Did your therapist ever do anything that made you mistrustful or suspicious?

Patients, especially at the start of treatment, are carefully watching the therapist and monitoring for signs of danger.

Some people said they were hesitant to trust the therapist at the beginning of treatment.

> I never doubted her sincerity. At the very beginning I was somewhat cautious and reserved, and we had to spend a good deal of time getting familiar with each other and with me getting comfortable with her.
>
> [Male, 48, Nonprofessional]

Some people said certain remarks by the therapist made them suspicious.

> He was trying to talk to me about relationship stuff, and he was bringing in an issue from his own relationship. He told me that his wife would complain that he gave more compassion to his patients than he did to her and the kids, and he made the mistake of saying that his response to her was, "Yes, but I don't care about them." I said to him that I knew what he meant, but it was a very weird moment. He popped the delusional bubble that psychotherapy patients have about the therapist. You think that they really care and they're looking at the clock or thinking about a movie.
>
> [Female, 48, Nonprofessional]

> I remember once having a terrible sense of betrayal, and I was going to leave, and we worked on trying to stay in the therapy while I had such feelings and trying to understand what they were.
>
> [Female, 59, Professional]

A couple of times I told her that I had been upset earlier about something she had said that made it seem that she wasn't listening or didn't understand, and she said that she wished I had told her, and she was listening and did understand.

[Male, 52, Nonprofessional]

Others reported that they got suspicious when the therapist's behavior seemed inappropriate or unusual.

He didn't do anything in the session, but I felt that about his distant aloofness.

[Male, 46, Nonprofessional]

I've gone through periods, especially when he got into some of the flakier stuff, like the rebirthing therapy, when I got suspicious.

[Male, 50, Professional]

In the end when he was having trouble with my relationship with someone I really loved, I was sad that he couldn't make the transition, and disappointed that he didn't realize when the analysis should have ended.

[Female, 45, Nonprofessional]

Several people said they had questions about the therapist's competence.

I was mistrustful in terms of whether he knew what he was doing.

[Female, 48, Nonprofessional]

She came in once and brought up certain issues that had nothing to do with the flow of our therapy, as if she had had a consult with someone and was told to bring these things up.

[Female, 50, Professional]

A few people said the therapist had made a questionable recommendation that raised concerns about competence.

She recommended a doctor to me that I had a very bad experience with, and it made me suspicious of her judgment.

[Female, 45, Nonprofessional]

NUMERICAL DISTRIBUTION

Professionals: Six said they had felt mistrustful due to something the therapist did; 14 said they had not.
Nonprofessionals: Six said they had felt mistrustful or suspicious at times; 34 said they had not.

COMMENTS

Many of the questions in this section suggest that the professionals judged their therapists more harshly than the nonprofessionals. The professionals were more likely to find fault with the therapist, probably because they were more knowledgeable and expected more from the therapist.

As the therapist, I am, of course, trying not to do anything that will make a patient mistrustful or suspicious. Over the years I have learned what these things are likely to be (for example, rigid, arbitrary, or inconsistent behavior) and have adjusted my behavior accordingly.

As the patient, I'm always watching for signs of incompetence or failure to keep the agreements and the rules. Any irregularity makes me suspicious.

RELATED READING

DiRienzo-Callahan, C. (1994). Competence and credentials. *Hospital and Community Psychiatry* 454(5):500.
Perlin, M. L. (1996). Power imbalances in therapeutic relationships. In *The Hatherleigh Guide to Psychotherapy*, pp. 215–229. New York: Hatherleigh.
Prochaska, J. O., and Norcross, J. C. (1983). Psychotherapists' perspectives on treating themselves and their clients for psychic distress. *Professional Psychology: Research and Practice* 14(5):642–655.
Rhodes, R. H., Hill, C. E., Thompson, B. J., and Elliott, R. (1994). Client retrospective recall of resolved and unresolved misunderstanding events. *Journal of Counseling Psychology* 41(4):473–483.

⬧⬧⬧⬧

Question 63: Did your therapist ever do anything that seemed like a mistake? (See also Questions 61 and 62)

Therapists are human, and sometimes make mistakes. Patients react differently.

Some remarks by the therapist demonstrate to the patient a lack of knowledge, understanding, or support.

> On occasion she would go with an angle on something that didn't feel like it was on the center of the issue. Especially around the work situation she made some mistakes.
>
> [Female, 45, Professional]

> A couple of times I thought that she wasn't defending me, or wasn't seeing things that I saw so clearly.
>
> [Male, 52, Nonprofessional]

> There were times when I was dating someone and he thought I should be with a doctor or a lawyer. He didn't take my point of view about why I wanted out of a relationship, he thought I was just pushing them away.
>
> [Female, 59, Professional]

> She kept insisting that what I was experiencing was my grief, and I knew that it wasn't, that it was about who I am as a person.
>
> [Female, 45, Professional]

Sometimes the therapist says the wrong thing to a patient, something that indicates that the therapist doesn't know who the patient is.

> I had been in therapy for quite a while and she said something about my mother having plastic covers on the furniture. My mother would never have plastic covers on the furniture in a million years. That was not my mother. I can't imagine who she was thinking of. It made me especially upset because I had a previous therapist who had no idea who I was, and here it was happening again.
>
> [Female, 50, Professional]

> Only once, early in therapy. She forgot that my father had killed himself, and I thought that was something she shouldn't forget.
>
> [Female, 46, Nonprofessional]

Late in treatment, she referred to something from the past and it wasn't me, it was some other patient. I didn't say anything because I thought it was funny. I smugly sat there feeling like I had caught her.

[Male, 44, Professional]

Sometimes the therapist will do something that feels wrong to the patient.

Very often when we stood up for me to leave, she would throw some fresh ideas at me, or say something thought-provoking, or sometimes just provocative, and that was troublesome for a couple of reasons. One was because the session was supposed to be over, and what was this? This was sort of an after-session. But it was troublesome also because she very often brought up fresh issues or fresh ideas or fresh insights or questions that I would then be burdened with the rest of the week or until I had the next session.

[Male, 48, Nonprofessional]

When she billed me an extra $10 for a session, after not telling me that her fee had gone up, I called and left a message on her machine and I was really upset because it felt to me like the $10 was more important to her than I was. I was upset with myself for doing that. But she never called me. I sent her the $10, and she sent it back with a note apologizing and saying that it wasn't the $10 that was important, and she was sorry I was upset about it. It really bothered me that she had never called me back. I would have called immediately.

[Female, 62, Professional]

Some people mentioned boundary violations.

She would accept a phone call in the middle of a session.

[Female, 42, Nonprofessional]

My brother saw her, my husband saw her, my mother saw her father. Even a cousin started to see her. There were no boundaries.

[Female, 45, Nonprofessional]

Some people said that they felt the therapist revealed too much.

She told me too much about herself.

[Female, 45, Nonprofessional]

> He was talking about his daughter when I was having problems with my own.
>
> [Female, 50, Nonprofessional]

> Occasionally it would happen in the session that she would start talking about herself, and I would be conscious that it was on my nickel.
>
> [Female, 50, Nonprofessional]

Sometimes the patient may feel initially that the therapist is making a mistake, and later see it differently.

> When she insisted on my paying the balance I owed her, I thought that was a mistake, but I later came to see that it was right.
>
> [Female, 51, Professional]

> In the beginning, some of his techniques felt that way, but it turned out that they really were helpful.
>
> [Male, 43, Nonprofessional]

Many people said the therapist was willing to acknowledge mistakes.

> I told him that something he said was a mistake and he shouldn't have said it, and he said I was probably right.
>
> [Female, 52, Nonprofessional]

> A couple of times he did, and I told him so. There were times he admitted that I was right.
>
> [Male, 53, Professional]

But therapists don't always react well to hearing that they have made a mistake.

> She got kind of defensive whenever I would express negative things about her.
>
> [Female, 55, Professional]

NUMERICAL DISTRIBUTION

Professionals: Fourteen said that the therapist had made mistakes; 6 said not.

Nonprofessionals: Eleven said that the therapist had made mistakes; 29 said not.

COMMENTS

Again, a much larger percentage of the professionals found fault than did the nonprofessionals, probably because of greater awareness of what constitutes a mistake. Any therapist can make a mistake; even the silent analyst can fail to speak. Inevitably I will do something that feels wrong to the patient (and maybe to me, too), and I can only hope that the mistake is not too egregious and that the relationship has become strong enough to survive the damage.

As the patient, I don't mind most mistakes, unless they indicate some real pathology in the therapist. What is crucial, however, is the therapist's reaction when I point out a mistake: don't argue with me and tell me why it wasn't a mistake; understand and accept my experience.

RELATED READING

Brody, E. M., and Farber, B. A. (1996). The effects of therapist experience and patient diagnosis on countertransference. *Psychotherapy* 33(3):372–380.

Field, N. (1992). The way of imperfection. *British Journal of Psychotherapy* 9(2):139–147.

Koeske, G. F., Koeske, R. D., and Mallinger, J. (1993). Perceptions of professional competence: cross-disciplinary ratings of psychologists, social workers, and psychiatrists. *American Journal of Orthopsychiatry* 63(1):45–54.

Overholser, J. C., and Fine, M. A. (1993). Defining the boundaries of professional competence: managing subtle cases of clinical incompetence. In *Issues in Clinical Psychology,* ed. J. A. Mindell, pp. 94–103. Dubuque, IA: Brown and Benchmark/Wm. C. Brown.

Owen, I. (1995). Core skills for psychotherapy. *Counselling Psychology Review* 8(2):15–23.

🔊🔊🔊🔊

Question 64: Did your therapist ever do anything that seemed unethical?

Patients these days are more sophisticated and knowledgeable about the rules and ethics of psychotherapy. What kinds of behavior seemed unethical to them?

One woman reported an obvious violation of the rules.

I had been in treatment for 2 years, and he ended up proposition-ing me. He had gone through a crisis in his life, a divorce, and he settled on me. And this guy had been recommended by the head of the department of psychiatry at a major hospital. I was pretty disappointed by that. Thank God I had the judgment not to fall for it.

[Female, 45, Nonprofessional]

Boundary problems were mentioned by 2 people.

There were things he got involved in with other patients in the group that at times I thought were unethical. When I first started with him 20 years ago, the boundaries were very fuzzy about dual relationships.

[Male, 50, Professional]

I think he had boundary problems. I got to know him and many of the people who worked with him, and there were many boundary issues.

[Male, 46, Nonprofessional]

One person mentioned billing.

He would sometimes bill sessions on days that sessions didn't occur. It wasn't dishonest in that would make money for me or for him, it was in dealing with the insurance company in anticipation of them denying our longer sessions, so we would bundle them.

[Male, 53, Professional]

Even something not strictly unethical can feel that way to the patient.

He asked me if he could write about me for a book. Technically it's not unethical because he asked me, but I still felt like I was being used.

[Female, 48, Professional]

NUMERICAL DISTRIBUTION

Professionals: Three said the therapist had done something that seemed unethical; 17 said not.

Nonprofessionals: Two said the therapist had done something that seemed unethical; 38 said not.

COMMENTS

Again, more professionals saw ethical problems than did nonprofessionals, and the ethics of some of these situations are ambiguous. Boundary violations are a fairly common problem, and some people mentioned these in response to other questions without identifying them as such.

As the therapist, I know what the boundaries are, and have to think long and hard about any impulse to modify them. Many studies have shown that one step over the line often leads to other more egregious steps in the wrong direction.

As the patient, I regard anything that smacks of ethical uncertainty or flouting of the rules as a real danger sign.

RELATED READING

Chodoff, P. (1996). Ethical dimensions of psychotherapy: a personal perspective. *American Journal of Psychotherapy* 50(3):298–310.

Ciardello, J. A. (1996). Therapist–patient sexual contact. *Psychoanalytic Review* 83(5):761–775.

Pepper, R. S. (1991). The senior therapist's grandiosity: clinical and ethical consequences of merging multiple roles. *Journal of Contemporary Psychotherapy* 21(1):63–70.

Pope, K. S., and Vasquez, M. (1991). *Ethics in Psychotherapy and Counseling: A Practical Guide for Psychologists.* San Francisco: Jossey-Bass.

ೞೞೞೞ

Question 65: Did you ever think that your therapist was trying to control you or get you to do something?

Therapists sometimes have an agenda that differs from the patient's goals. Patients can experience the therapist as trying to control them. They usually don't like feeling pressured.

Sometimes the therapist seems to be trying to encourage a particular course of action in the patient's life.

> It was her suggestion to take the personal ad. I don't work that way as a therapist so I was a little shocked. But I did it and it was a good thing.
>
> [Female, 51, Professional]

She had a bias toward getting married and having children. I wanted to do that, but she was also pressuring me to.

[Female, 45, Nonprofessional]

He tried to get me to continue dating someone and I knew it wasn't going to work out.

[Female, 59, Professional]

The whole behavioral kind of approach lends itself to feeling that I was getting an assignment and I have to do it.

[Female, 44, Nonprofessional]

She was trying to get me to stay in the institute.

[Female, 62, Professional]

For years she had suggested that I belonged in AA, that this would be a good move for me. Whenever the issue of drinking would come up, she would mention AA, it was a constant theme, and she was very glad when I finally did.

[Male, 49, Nonprofessional]

He told me to have an affair, but there was no real pressure to do it.

[Male, 53, Nonprofessional]

Sometimes the therapist seems to want the patient to behave a certain way in the sessions, to do therapy the way the therapist wants.

She was trying to get me to be in touch with my own feelings. If I got angry at her, it was a great success. In that sense, she was "egging me on," but very subtly.

[Female, 50, Nonprofessional]

I went for months at one point refusing to speak at all.

[Male, 53, Professional]

I felt that when we were talking about what I would do after she left, and using the couch was an issue. She really was urging me to undergo what she was calling "psychoanalysis." I was rather resistant to this, and in fact I haven't called any of the people whose names she gave me.

[Male, 48, Nonprofessional]

There was the rebirthing therapy that he wanted me to do.

[Male, 50, Professional]

She pressured me about staying in therapy. I was having a lot of anxiety about not being able to afford the sessions, and she didn't help me with that.

[Female, 28, Nonprofessional]

He called me after treatment to get me to come in again.

[Female, 48, Nonprofessional]

As a group leader, he had definite ideas about what we were supposed to be doing.

[Male, 43, Nonprofessional]

Some people said they didn't object to the therapist having specific goals in mind, or even pressuring for certain behaviors.

He would give me homework assignments, which were part of the treatment.

[Male, 30, Professional]

Broadly speaking, I knew that she had certain goals for me, but I never felt like she was manipulating me.

[Female, 42, Nonprofessional]

That's what she's supposed to do.

[Female, 56, Professional]

One person found the therapist's lack of an agenda a real problem.

As a matter of fact it was the opposite. It was his utter lack of need for me to do anything that made me suspicious that he didn't really care.

[Male, 46, Nonprofessional]

Some people found the pressure extremely objectionable.

His obsession with getting paid immediately made me extremely angry with him. He also tried to get me to stick with my relationship, which isn't psychoanalytically neutral.

[Female, 57, Professional]

I had this feeling almost right from the beginning of being in some sort of a power struggle with him. I felt like I was being coerced or manipulated. And that's what ended our therapy. He became so controlling that if I didn't do what he wanted me to do then he couldn't be my therapist. He said that. I wasn't conscious of provoking it in any way.

[Female, 45, Nonprofessional]

NUMERICAL DISTRIBUTION

Professionals: Eleven said they had not felt the therapist was trying to control them; 9 said they had.

Nonprofessionals: Thirty said they had not felt the therapist was trying to control them; 10 said they had.

COMMENTS

Once again the professionals report more instances of this kind of behavior. Perhaps the nonprofessionals expect this as part of treatment, and therefore don't find it so objectionable. As a therapist, I try not to have an agenda of my own, but to follow the patient's lead. At times, this is difficult; when the patient is doing something risky or self-destructive I sometimes feel I have to say something challenging the patient's position and beliefs, and may even pressure the patient to stop. This sometimes works and sometimes leads to the patient quitting therapy.

As a patient, I don't want my therapist in a parental role and I don't want to be told what to do, unless I ask for input, and even then the decision has to remain mine. On some level, I may appreciate the therapist questioning behavior that seems self-destructive, but in spite of that I may not be ready to stop doing it.

RELATED READING

Dolliver, R. H. (1986). Counselor directiveness and client task-readiness reviewed. *Counseling Psychologist* 14(3):461–464.

Goodstein, L. D. (1975). Self-control and therapist-control: the medical model in behavioral clothing. *Journal of Abnormal Psychology* 84(2): 178–180.

Heatherington, L. (1990). Family therapy, control, and controllingness. *Journal of Family Psychology* 4(2):132–150.

Morrison, J. K., Libow, J. A., Smith, F. J., and Becker, R. R. (1978). Comparative effectiveness of directive vs. nondirective group therapist style on client problem resolution. *Journal of Clinical Psychology* 34(1):186–187.

Woody, J. D. (1990). Clinical strategies to promote compliance. *American Journal of Family Therapy* 18(3):285–294.

᠍᠍᠍᠍

Question 66: Did you ever have an argument with your therapist?

Although therapists try to avoid serious conflict with patients, some disagreement inevitably arises. When conflict escalates, arguments may occur.

It is common for patient and therapist to have discussions, sometimes heated ones, when they disagree.

> They weren't arguments. It was intellectual rational disagreement that was laden with feelings.
>
> [Female, 47, Nonprofessional]

> We did, in the way that you argue with a therapist. I was never enraged, but certainly we had some animated discussions.
>
> [Female, 50, Professional]

> We had some lively discussions. We discussed some movies that we didn't agree about.
>
> [Male, 48, Nonprofessional]

Sometimes the therapist and the patient disagree so strongly that the discussion becomes an argument.

> We would argue about things sometimes. I would say I couldn't do something, and I would have a whole stack of reasons, and she would take the devil's advocate position and challenge me.
>
> [Female, 46, Nonprofessional]

> We would have arguments frequently in the group. I was a dominant member of that group, and I would frequently take a position against him in the group.
>
> [Female, 48, Nonprofessional]

The patient can get upset by something the therapist says.

> Once we had an argument and I went ballistic because she was saying something supportive of my mother.
>
> [Female, 51, Professional]

The therapist's policy regarding fees and money can make the patient angry.

> We argued over missing a session because of the blizzard and having to pay for it.
>
> [Male, 44, Professional]

Sometimes the therapist's style or way of responding can make the patient furious.

> We would be screaming. When my mother was deteriorating and I desperately needed some help, I asked him if he knew of organizations that dealt with that condition; he knew nothing and he wouldn't try to find out. He didn't want to talk about it. I was having so much stress, and he just kept going on with the usual thing. I finally said, "I have to go every day to the hospital, and I'm going crazy here, and I don't want to talk about this stuff, I want help."
>
> [Female, 48, Nonprofessional]

When the patient feels pressured to do something by the therapist, she may fight back.

> She pressed me to find some accommodation with my father.
>
> [Female, 39, Nonprofessional]

The patient may see the argument as a test of his or her own strength.

> I did later on in the therapy, but I think they were tests, finding something to argue about with her to see what would happen, to see if I could hold my own.
>
> [Female, 45, Professional]

> When I thought I had things figured out, he came from a different angle, and sometimes I stuck to my position and tried to argue with him. Ultimately the whole thing crumbled, and I saw that they're just positions.
>
> [Male, 30, Professional]

NUMERICAL DISTRIBUTION

Professionals: Twelve said they had argued with the therapist; 8 people said they had not argued.

Nonprofessionals: Seven people said they had argued with the therapist; 5 said they had not argued but had heated discussions; 28 said they had not argued.

COMMENTS

A much greater percentage of professionals reported arguments with the therapist than did the nonprofessionals, perhaps because the professionals were more aware that this was allowed and were less afraid of the consequences. As the therapist, I try not to paint myself into a corner and get myself into a position that I have to defend so vehemently that an argument occurs. On the other hand, I do want the patient to feel free to express anger and hostility. Provoking an argument may sometimes be the only way to get to this material, though I don't like doing anything that feels artificial or contrived.

As the patient, I may be afraid of the consequences of a fight with the therapist, but eventually I will probably test this area to see what happens. I'm not sure I want the therapist to fight back, though, and would wonder more about what's going on with him than I would about my own behavior, which is, after all, why I am there.

RELATED READING

Hartley, D. E. (1993). Therapists' contribution to negative therapeutic reactions. In *Clinical Challenges in Psychiatry,* ed. W. H. Sledge and A. Tasman, pp. 393–421. Washington, DC: American Psychiatric Press.

McDougall, J. (1989). The anti-analysand in analysis. In *Essential Papers on Character Neurosis amd Treatment,* ed. R. F. Lax, pp. 363–384. New York: New York University Press.

Rice, L. N. (1973). Client behavior as a function of therapist style and client resources. *Journal of Counseling Psychology* 20(4):306–311.

Teitelbaum, S. (1994). Treatment issues of patients who engage in power struggles. *Clinical Social Work Journal* 22(3):263–276.

ॐॐॐॐ

Question 67: Did you ever feel that your therapist didn't like you?

For most patients, the esteem and caring of the therapist is important. Usually patients experience the therapist as liking them and caring about them. But sometimes it may be hard to believe that the therapist, who is getting paid, cares about the patient as a person.

> I always had a problem with that, going to a therapist and thinking, "I'm paying this person to listen to me, they don't really care about me." I worked through that.
>
> [Female, 48, Nonprofessional]

> Sometimes I thought that she felt that I was just a patient, or that she thought I made mountains out of molehills.
>
> [Female, 39, Nonprofessional]

A therapist who tries to be completely neutral may be perceived as not liking the patient.

> His affect was not suited to me. He was kind of deadpan, and I never felt that he really cared about me. I don't know what he thought. With my previous therapists, I felt that they had regard for me, and he showed no affect toward me.
>
> [Female, 48, Nonprofessional]

> I never felt that she didn't like me, but I never felt that she liked me either.
>
> [Female, 28, Nonprofessional]

> I never got the feeling that he liked me. He was completely neutral, and it troubled me. I wish I had gotten some feeling one way or the other.
>
> [Female, 41, Nonprofessional]

Sometimes patients can feel as if no therapist could like them.

> In the many early years of my therapy I was a pretty unlikable and difficult client.
>
> [Female, 50, Professional]

Some people said they were unsure about whether the therapist liked them.

It was important for me that he like me, but I never had a sense of certainty.

[Female, 46, Nonprofessional]

When I first started seeing her, I was anxious about it.

[Female, 42, Nonprofessional]

And a few people were certain that the therapist did not like them.

I felt that way a lot. It was part of the intense relationship.

[Male, 44, Professional]

I had a sense right from the beginning that this person did not like me. I often wondered who I reminded him of. I often felt in sessions that he was working something out that had little to do with me.

[Female, 45, Nonprofessional]

NUMERICAL DISTRIBUTION

Professionals: Four people said they thought at times that their therapist didn't like them; 16 said they had not felt that way.

Nonprofessionals: Eight people said they thought at times that their therapist didn't like them; 32 said they had not felt that way.

COMMENTS

The same percentage (20 percent) of professionals and of nonprofessionals said they had felt at some point that the therapist didn't like them. This is obviously a disturbing feeling and puts the whole therapy into question.

I think there has to be some genuine affection between patient and therapist for therapy to happen. As the therapist I want to like the patient, and usually have no difficulty doing so. When I have trouble liking someone, it's a countertransferential reaction that has real significance. Occasionally I have had this reaction to a very suspicious and distant patient; in this case my reaction fades over time as the patient comes to trust me more. It sometimes indicates a very narcissistic patient to whom I am not even a real person, and in this case my feelings don't change much.

As the patient, feeling that the therapist didn't like me would make me wonder why he or she was working with me and what the value would be of our work together. I could tolerate this feeling briefly, but only if the therapist could show me very soon that it was not true.

RELATED READING

Bongar, B., Markey, L. A., and Peterson, L. G. (1991). Views on the difficult and dreaded patient: a preliminary investigation. *Medical Psychotherapy: An International Journal* 4:9–16.

Meissner, W. W. (1996). *The Therapeutic Alliance*. New Haven, CT: Yale University Press.

Rinaldi, R. C. (1987). Patient–therapist personality similarity and the therapeutic relationship. *Psychotherapy in Private Practice* 5(2):11–29.

Smith, R. J., and Steindler, E. M. (1983). The impact of difficult patients upon treaters: consequences and remedies. *Bulletin of the Menninger Clinic* 47(2):107–116.

▨▨▨▨

Question 68: Did you ever feel eager and excited to see your therapist?

Both patients and therapists hope that the patient will feel enthusiasm and happy anticipation about coming to therapy.

Most people reported feeling good about going to therapy, especially in the beginning of treatment.

> There were times in the beginning when I felt that it was working.
>
> [Female, 44, Nonprofessional]

> I did, particularly when I was in pain. It was like an oasis.
>
> [Female, 50, Professional]

> I was always happy to be there. I never skipped a session and was never late.
>
> [Male, 52, Nonprofessional]

> In the beginning I especially looked forward to seeing her because she was helping me control my panic attacks.
>
> [Female, 51, Professional]

I looked forward to going, and knowing I could tolerate almost anything that went on during the week because I could deal with it there.

[Female, 52, Nonprofessional]

I did when there was something very heavy going on, or when something very interesting happened during the week and I couldn't wait to share it with him.

[Female, 58, Professional]

At the beginning of treatment it was very important to me to be there. And also when I had a little crush on him I would be excited to be going to see him.

[Female, 48, Nonprofessional]

Often I was really looking forward to seeing him.

[Female, 59, Professional]

I always felt that I could dump whatever I was carrying there, that I could relax there.

[Female, 53, Nonprofessional]

Of course, some people, who were unhappy with their therapy, did not look forward to being there.

Sometimes something really good had happened, but it could have been anybody I was telling about it.

[Female, 48, Nonprofessional]

And even when the therapy is working, people can feel apprehensive about going.

Maybe I did toward the end when I was used to it. I'd rather do something else, because it was always painful.

[Female, 40, Nonprofessional]

NUMERICAL DISTRIBUTION

Professionals: Seventeen people said they looked forward to going with some eagerness or excitement, especially at the beginning of treatment; 3 said they did not.

Nonprofessionals: Thirty-three people said they looked forward to going with some eagerness or excitement, especially at the beginning of treatment; 7 said they did not.

COMMENTS

The same percentage of both groups said they looked forward to going to therapy, so knowledge and experience are not relevant parameters here. Even a positive experience of the therapy and the therapist are no guarantee that the patient will always look forward to going.

As the therapist, I want the patient to want to be there: therapy is hard enough even then and virtually impossible when the patient consistently does not want to come to sessions.

As the patient, I hope to be always excited about the process of self-discovery and the freedom that often results. What could be more interesting than my own inner workings?

RELATED READING

Bader, M. J. (1996). Altruistic love in psychoanalysis: opportunities and resistance. *Psychoanalytic Dialogues* 6(6):741–764.

🔊🔊🔊🔊

Question 69: Did you ever dread going?

Just as people can look forward to seeing the therapist, they can also have other feelings about it.

Many people admitted there were times that they didn't want to go to therapy. Sometimes that was because there were things they didn't want to discuss.

> I did when I knew I had to 'fess up to something or talk about something uncomfortable.
>
> [Male, 30, Professional]

> I did when I had difficult issues and didn't want to talk about them.
>
> [Female, 45, Nonprofessional]

> Never dread, but sometimes I didn't feel like it, there was stuff I didn't want to deal with.
>
> [Male, 53, Professional]

> I had things on my mind that I was very hesitant to bring up.
>
> [Male, 50, Nonprofessional]

I did because there were some things I didn't want to work on.

[Female, 51, Professional]

Sometimes going to therapy made them anxious about what might happen, or what might come up.

Usually I got very anxious about going. Partly as I was learning all the things that therapists were doing and thinking I would get quite anxious before I would see him. It was like I was sitting in both chairs. I also got very anxious before group.

[Female, 50, Professional]

There was always some amount of trepidation and tension about going. It had nothing to do with her; it was the notion of what was going to happen.

[Male, 52, Nonprofessional]

Some people dreaded not having things to say or issues to talk about.

I did when I didn't feel like I had anything to say.

[Female, 44, Nonprofessional]

Sometimes I felt, "Who needs this? There's nothing to talk about today."

[Female, 59, Professional]

Not dread, but sometimes I didn't feel like it and wondered how productive it was going to be.

[Female, 41, Nonprofessional]

Some people reported feeling pressured to produce or to work hard.

There were stresses in my life with implications that there were certain things I had to do, and I knew I had to think about them there, and sometimes I didn't want to do that.

[Female, 52, Professional]

There were times I didn't want to go because I didn't want to do the work—it was exhausting.

[Female, 50, Nonprofessional]

I didn't feel like working that day.

[Female, 39, Professional]

> Sometimes when I was in a mucky place, feeling hopeless about ever getting out of the stuff I had been avoiding for a long time, I would feel like I couldn't go any deeper. The dread would usually disappear by the time I got into the session.
>
> [Female, 46, Nonprofessional]

> It was uncomfortable, because I felt like I had to produce, and that always made me freeze up a little.
>
> [Female, 50, Professional]

Sometimes just getting to therapy felt burdensome.

> I was feeling interrupted in the work I was doing to have to drive over there, and feeling I really didn't need to do that.
>
> [Female, 39, Nonprofessional]

> There were many times when I felt incredibly tired and fatigued after work and I really didn't want to go. It felt like one more obligation.
>
> [Female, 58, Professional]

> There were times when I was too depressed to get out of the house or I was just too tired.
>
> [Male, 46, Nonprofessional]

> It was only that I had the first appointment in the morning and if I had been up late the night before.
>
> [Female, 45, Nonprofessional]

> I had 2 sessions: Tuesday evening and Friday morning, and I was okay about the evening session, because that was part of the day and I didn't have to make a special effort, but Friday morning it was the first thing I had to do, and that was sometimes hard.
>
> [Female, 50, Nonprofessional]

When the relationship with the therapist is turbulent, going to the session can be frightening.

> I dreaded being dragged back into the same old morass of unresolved feelings about her.
>
> [Male, 44, Professional]

Patients who are conflicted about even being in treatment may dread going.

I resented the whole setup.

[Female, 55, Professional]

At the very end, when I was deciding whether she was helping at all, I kept going each time feeling like I didn't want to anymore.

[Female, 50, Nonprofessional]

At the end I did, because I knew I wasn't going to feel good.

[Female, 48, Professional]

NUMERICAL DISTRIBUTION

Professionals: Fourteen said they did dread going at times or didn't want to go; 6 people said they never dreaded going.

Nonprofessionals: Eighteen said they did dread going at times or didn't want to go; 22 people said they never dreaded going.

COMMENTS

A higher percentage of professionals said they had dreaded going to therapy at times than did the nonprofessionals. This may be a sign that the professionals knew better what to expect, or that they were somehow going deeper into themselves than the nonprofessionals.

As the therapist, I know that the patient doesn't look forward to digging up painful memories or confronting frightening thoughts and feelings. Sometimes the patient is going to avoid therapy, or at least avoid working in therapy, and I'll try not to apply pressure when this happens. If the feelings persist, then we'll have to find out what's going on.

As a patient, I may be afraid of certain material, or worried about the consequences of uncovering it. I can tolerate a lack of enthusiasm for brief periods, but extended feelings of dismay at going will probably lead to termination.

RELATED READING

Bischoff, M. M., and Tracey, T. J. (1995). Client resistance as predicted by therapist behavior: a study of sequential dependence. *Journal of Counseling Psychology* 42(4):487–495.

McGuff, R., Gitlin, D., and Enderlin, M. (1996). Clients' and therapists' confidence and attendance at planned individual therapy sessions. *Psychological Reports* 79(2):537–538.

Safran, J. D., and Muran, J. C. (1996). The resolution of ruptures in the therapeutic alliance. *Journal of Consulting and Clinical Psychology* 64(3):447–458.

⊠⊠⊠⊠

Question 70: Did you ever feel dependent on your therapist?

Patients often feel dependent on the therapy and the therapist. Sometimes this feels good, and seems right.

> There was a time, the time when she was being most helpful, when we were talking about things that were really rocking my world, things that were enormously painful for me to uncover about myself and to admit, and I felt very dependent on her then. I felt enormously vulnerable, but I was never scared about it. I really did trust her.
>
> [Female, 45, Nonprofessional]

> At the time I wasn't at all together, so I needed something to keep me grounded. At the time it was fine because it was what I needed.
>
> [Female, 26, Nonprofessional]

> It felt fine because his nonverbal behavior and feeling tone conveyed a sense of safety and acceptance.
>
> [Male, 42, Professional]

> I was pretty dependent on her. I had these moments where I would just lose it, and I called her up a lot. I was glad that she was there.
>
> [Female, 42, Nonprofessional]

> For a long time she was my lifeline, and I was dependent on her.
>
> [Male, 49, Nonprofessional]

> There was the period when I was first in therapy where it was very, very important to me. That got me through the week. There was a period of time when I was totally overwhelmed and unable to remember things, and we would tape my sessions and then I had to listen to them during the week. It was tedious, but I did it because I was that dependent on the process.
>
> [Female, 48, Nonprofessional]

It was a good thing. It felt like progress for me.

[Female, 45, Professional]

It felt okay because I thought that was part of what I was learning how to do, to trust and be dependent on someone.

[Female, 41, Nonprofessional]

Sometimes feelings of dependency can be frightening or disturbing.

There were times when things were not going well, and I did during those times. I was reluctant to become dependent on her because of her rigid boundaries.

[Female, 62, Professional]

Especially at the beginning I did. I didn't like it because I didn't want to be dependent on any man.

[Female, 50, Nonprofessional]

It was troublesome to me.

[Male, 44, Professional]

When I was going through my divorce, it felt good that I had someone to depend on, but it didn't feel good to be so needy because I hadn't felt so needy prior to that.

[Female, 48, Nonprofessional]

It felt okay, but there were times I berated myself for that, particularly when I was younger. Before turning 30, not being self-sufficient and being less than fully emancipated was very hard for me to tolerate.

[Male, 53, Professional]

It was terrible to be dependent, scary.

[Female, 39, Nonprofessional]

Dependent feelings that seem appropriate during the treatment can be disturbing in retrospect.

I was glad that she was there. There were a couple of hard times that came up while I was seeing her, and if I hadn't been in therapy with her I'm not sure what I would have done. When I stopped therapy, I felt very bad about it because I had gotten a lot closer to her than I had realized. It was hard.

[Male, 45, Nonprofessional]

It wasn't disturbing at the time—it felt right. Looking back now I'm a little disturbed by how powerful it was.

[Female, 45, Professional]

Some people said they wouldn't call what they felt "dependent," but acknowledged that the therapist had become significant in their lives.

It wasn't so much dependent on her as feeling that this was an immensely valuable relationship. I felt that my therapy was a continuous presence in my awareness, in my life. In fact, she made a comment around the time we were working on the termination that I seemed to have the ability to sustain the therapy from one session to the next to an unusual degree. I would come in and it was as if we were immediately continuing the prior session, and I knew exactly what we had been talking about, what the issues were, and was able to just continue it. And that's the way I felt about it, that I was in therapy all the time while I was seeing her.

[Male, 48, Nonprofessional]

I found that what we were learning together was very useful. He was a very important ingredient in my life, but I wouldn't say dependent.

[Female, 45, Nonprofessional]

Some people said they never felt a dependency or need for the therapist.

I asked myself that a lot, about how I would feel about not seeing him again, and I never felt that it would be tragic.

[Female, 48, Nonprofessional]

I didn't feel dependent, and she didn't encourage it at all.

[Male, 52, Nonprofessional]

NUMERICAL DISTRIBUTION

Professionals: Seven people said they had not felt dependent; 13 said they had felt dependent, especially in the beginning of treatment. Of these, 5 said it was a disturbing or unpleasant feeling; 8 said it felt positive in some way.

Nonprofessionals: Fifteen people said they had not felt dependent; 25 said they did feel dependent, especially in the beginning of treatment. Of these, 2 said it was a disturbing or frightening feeling; 8 said it felt positive in some way.

COMMENTS

Again we find the same percentage of both groups feeling dependent, though more of the professionals found such feelings disturbing. As one professional said, it can be hard to give up the role of therapist and be the patient.

As the therapist, I don't mind having patients feel dependent on me—I am a dependable and reliable person—but I don't encourage it either, because it's not necessary to the therapy.

As the patient, if I'm in some sort of crisis I will feel very dependent on my therapist for stability, grounding, and guidance. If things improve and the crisis abates, the dependency will recede. I need to see that the therapist isn't overwhelmed by my feelings and doesn't resent giving me what I need.

RELATED READING

Abramson, P. R., Cloud, M. Y., Keese, N., and Keese, R. (1994). How much is too much? Dependency in a psychotherapeutic relationship. *American Journal of Psychotherapy* 48(2):294–301.

Bornstein, R. F. (1993). Dependency and patienthood. *Journal of Clinical Psychology* 49(3):397–406.

Coen, S. J. (1992). *The Misuse of Persons: Analyzing Pathological Dependency*. Hillsdale, NJ: Analytic Press.

de Jonghe, F., Rijnierse, P., and Janssen, R. (1992). The role of support in psychoanalysis. *Journal of the American Psychoanalytic Association* 40(2):475–499.

🔊🔊🔊🔊

Question 71: Did you ever call your therapist to talk between sessions?

The therapist tries to contain the patient's material in the sessions, but sometimes the patient needs contact between appointments.

Usually this occurs in some kind of crisis.

I called 2 or 3 times when there was a really difficult period. He was available, accessible, helpful.

[Female, 45, Nonprofessional]

I called only when I thought I was going to have a panic attack. She was helpful and nice. Just having the contact would really calm me down.

[Female, 51, Professional]

Not infrequently, I would have some kind of panic that I would need to talk to her about. She would talk to me until I felt better.

[Female, 48, Nonprofessional]

I did that twice in 10 years. Both times were a crisis. She was very helpful and supportive. It took major effort for me to do it, but it felt like a good thing that I was letting myself do it.

[Female, 45, Professional]

I used to have these psychotic moments where I'd be walking in the street and I'd just lose it and be crying and I'd call her a lot. I'd call her from home too. She was helpful, and she was quite clear that I could leave messages and she would get back to me when she could. One time she did give me her home number on the weekend in Connecticut. But I didn't use it very much.

[Female, 42, Nonprofessional]

The therapist will usually spend a short time on the telephone, and save the real work for the next session.

On occasion, if I was very upset about something that had happened, he would talk for a few minutes and then ask if I wanted to have another session.

[Female, 50, Professional]

She'd call me back and have a little conversation and then postpone it to the session, saying something like, "That'll give us something to talk about."

[Female, 50, Nonprofessional]

Whenever he could he would give me a little time, and then arrange for a session.

[Male, 53, Professional]

Sometimes the therapist spends a long time on the phone, and the patient may wonder about the fee for that time.

> Once or twice I did during periods of enormous crisis for me, and she was very generous with her time and she never charged me.
> [Female, 45, Nonprofessional]

> I remember being on the phone with her one time for an hour, and she didn't charge me for that.
> [Male, 49, Nonprofessional]

The patient sometimes wants more than therapist is willing to give.

> I remember early in therapy almost demanding a session on the phone, and he said no, that he would see me the next session in the office, and I was furious about it.
> [Female, 50, Nonprofessional]

> I remember calling once because I was really on edge, and she talked to me, but I remember feeling that she should have checked in with me a few days later.
> [Female, 39, Professional]

A few people revealed that they sometimes wanted just to hear the therapist's voice.

> Sometimes I would call her machine just to listen to her voice—it was very soothing.
> [Female, 50, Nonprofessional]

> A few times at the very beginning I called to listen to his voice on his machine.
> [Female, 48, Professional]

Patients are usually aware that calling is an imposition.

> Only once did I need to speak to her before a session. In that sense I was a good client: I colored inside the lines.
> [Female, 50, Professional]

> A couple of times I called her, but I didn't have a real sense that she was there for me and willing to talk. She's so formal that I had some reluctance to call her, but she was good when I did call.
> [Female, 62, Professional]

One time he stayed on the phone with me for quite a while; other times he kept it kind of short. There was a period of time when I would leave a lot of very long messages on his machine.

[Male, 50, Professional]

In spite of invitations from the therapist to call in a crisis, sometimes the patient decides not to call.

Once she was a little perturbed that I hadn't, because I had been mugged. I didn't feel a need to call.

[Female, 50, Professional]

She said I could, but I never did.

[Female, 28, Nonprofessional]

NUMERICAL DISTRIBUTION

Professionals: Fourteen said they had called the therapist between sessions; 6 said they had not.

Nonprofessionals: Twenty-five said they had called the therapist between sessions; 15 said they had not.

COMMENTS

There was no major difference between groups on this question. Patients call in crisis, and that can happen to anyone. Since many of the people in both groups had been in many different therapies and were discussing only their most recent experience, many were perhaps past the early crises that often lead someone to seek therapy at all.

As the therapist, I want to be available when patients need me, but I also want to help them contain their distress. I will always call back, as soon as I can, and then will try to make the phone conversation as brief as possible and still help the patient regain a feeling of calm and control.

As the patient, I will try to manage whatever I can myself, and expect the therapist to realize that if I call it's because I really need to speak with him—it's not just a whim. This means I expect a response in a reasonably short time. We don't have to talk all night, but I don't want to feel any resentment or sense of imposition from the therapist.

RELATED READING

Canning, S., Hauser, M. J., Gutheil, T. G., and Bursztajn, H. J. (1991). Communications in psychiatric practice: decision making and the use of the telephone. In *Decision Making in Psychiatry and the Law,* ed. T. G. Gutheil, H. J. Bursztajn, A. Brodsky, and V. Alexander, pp. 227–235. Baltimore, MD: Williams & Wilkins.

Daugird, A. J., and Spencer, D. C. (1989). Characteristics of patients who highly utilize telephone medical care in a private practice. *Journal of Family Practice* 29(1):59–63.

Hymer, S. M. (1984). The telephone session and the telephone between sessions. *Psychotherapy in Private Practice* 2(3):51–65.

🔁🔁🔁🔁

Question 72: Did you ever have a full session on the telephone?

When circumstances prevent a session in the office, the therapist may arrange a telephone session as a substitute. Most people didn't like the distance they felt with phone contact, but accepted it as better than no session at all.

Sometimes this happens when the therapist or the patient is out of town.

> We did when he was out of town. It wasn't as good, but it was helpful. I didn't feel the personal connection in the same way.
>
> [Male, 30, Professional]

Sometimes a phone session happens when the patient is ill and can't travel.

> We did it twice when I was sick. It's not as good, because I like to look at people, but it was helpful. Frankly, a big part of it was that I was paying for it anyway so I might as well have a session. And it was fine. It worked.
>
> [Female, 40, Nonprofessional]

> Only if I absolutely couldn't be in the city. It was kind of a rare thing. At one point I was pregnant and had medical complications, so that was when we did some phone sessions. It was fine.
>
> [Female, 50, Professional]

> We did when I was sick. It wasn't the same, but it was pretty close.
>
> [Female, 42, Nonprofessional]

Sometimes the weather makes a phone session necessary.

> We did that when the weather was so bad I couldn't get there, and she interpreted that as meaning I was more comfortable with the distance. I really don't like it as well, because I miss the contact.
>
> [Female, 62, Professional]

Sometimes phone sessions are the usual normal structure, as when one or the other person has relocated.

> He was very comfortable with telephone sessions, as I am, when it's practical. Every session for the last couple of years was over the phone.
>
> [Male, 53, Professional]

Some people don't experience much difference between a regular session and one on the phone.

> It didn't make much of a difference because I was on the couch anyway. I was grateful that he had the flexibility to do that.
>
> [Male, 42, Professional]

One person had difficulty with the transition when she was at work.

> Once I was at work and that was awful, because I was very uptight talking about personal things, and then I had to just hang up the phone and be completely ready to work but still feeling left with all my stuff.
>
> [Female, 39, Professional]

Another person expressed strong feelings against phone sessions.

> I would never have a session on the phone—it would be like 30 percent.
>
> [Male, 46, Nonprofessional]

NUMERICAL DISTRIBUTION

Professionals: Seven said they had a session on the phone; 13 said they had not.

Nonprofessionals: Three said they had a session on the phone; 37 said they had not.

COMMENTS

A much greater percentage of professionals reported telephone sessions, and this too may be due to a more relaxed attitude on the part of their therapists. Most patients seem to appreciate the usefulness of a phone session when circumstances don't permit a session in the office, and perhaps also appreciate some flexibility on the part of the therapist.

As the therapist, I will try to schedule phone sessions when patients are sick, out of town on business, or recently relocated. My feeling is that it's better than no session at all, whatever the drawbacks. Some modification in my style is required, but overall I have had good experience with these sessions.

As the patient, I hate the idea of missing my session unnecessarily, and I appreciate having the alternative of a telephone session. It's harder to talk without being able to see the therapist—it's almost like being on the couch—but I can tolerate it for a week or two.

RELATED READING

Grumet, G. W. (1979). Telephone therapy: a review and case report. *American Journal of Orthopsychiatry* 49(4):574–584.

Haas, L. J., Benedict, J. G., and Kobos, J. C. (1996). Psychotherapy by telephone: risks and benefits for psychologists and consumers. *Professional Psychology: Research and Practice* 27(2):154–160.

McLaren, P. (1992). Psychotherapy by telephone: experience of patient and therapist. *Journal of Mental Health U.K.* 1(4):311–313.

Spiro, R. H., and Devenis, L. (1991). Telephone therapy: enhancement of the psychotherapeutic process. *Psychotherapy in Private Practice* 9(4):31–55.

🔊🔊🔊🔊

Question 73: Did your ever feel like you weren't making any progress?

Patients can feel as if nothing is happening, that the therapy is not working and not helping them feel better. This can be a difficult time for both the patient and the therapist.

That's one of the frustrations: you just talk about the feeling that you're stuck, which just makes you feel more stuck.

[Female, 46, Nonprofessional]

I did, and I told her, but I was blaming myself for not making any progress.

[Female, 50, Nonprofessional]

The therapist may interpret such a feeling in various ways.

It was a reality check for me, and he said that I was going to have to accept that some things aren't going to change.

[Female, 41, Nonprofessional]

The basic interpretation was that I was being self-critical again, striving and expecting.

[Male, 30, Professional]

Her interpretation was that those were the times when something was about to happen, that there was some kind of defense going on. I sometimes thought that meant it was really time to stop.

[Female, 50, Nonprofessional]

Sometimes the therapist simply accepts such feelings, and this can be reassuring.

We both felt that way at the same time and said, "Hey, we're not getting anywhere." We just kept banging away at it.

[Male, 52, Nonprofessional]

There were times when I was really at an impasse. It was noted, but it was part of the process.

[Female, 45, Professional]

She basically gave me some options: going deeper, although she had the sense that I didn't want to go deeper in that issue, or continue working on some other issues in some way. She gave me a choice about how I wanted to proceed.

[Female, 46, Nonprofessional]

We would try to go with that feeling and see where it led us. Those were often the days when the most significant breakthroughs would happen.

[Male, 46, Nonprofessional]

Sometimes the patient accepts the feelings too.

> I did, but only in the sense that I realized that it takes a long time to make progress and I'd get frustrated that I wasn't, that I would still have some of the same reactions as before.
>
> [Female, 48, Nonprofessional]

> There were times when I didn't see where we were going, but I have enough understanding of educational and imaginative processes to know that that's the way it is sometimes.
>
> [Male, 50, Nonprofessional]

> For short periods of time I did, but I have a lot of patience with the process.
>
> [Female, 51, Professional]

> I didn't try to do anything; I was just patient.
>
> [Female, 48, Nonprofessional]

> At the beginning I sometimes felt that way. I knew that we were just beginning.
>
> [Male, 51, Nonprofessional]

> I never told him. I kept it to myself for a while, because in the beginning I didn't want to open up and didn't think that it was doing any good but I wanted to give it a chance.
>
> [Male, 43, Nonprofessional]

Sometimes when the patient feels stuck and tells the therapist, that can lead to a change in the way of working.

> We discussed it and talked about another way to approach things.
>
> [Female, 56, Professional]

> Sometimes I would sit with the feeling, sometimes it might have led to a change in the work.
>
> [Male, 53, Professional]

When the therapist fails to accept such feelings, trouble can result.

> I told him, and told him, and he just kept doing what he was doing. Eventually, he said, "But that's not what I do." And I said that other people do, so maybe I should be with somebody else. And he said

he could refer me outside the EAP, but not to someone inside it. But it was so convenient, and it was free; it was hard to go elsewhere.

[Female, 48, Nonprofessional]

I would bring it up, say we were in a stalemate, an impasse. She would say no, that we had to keep working on what it was I wanted from it. We'd go around in circles.

[Male, 44, Professional]

Sometimes the therapist tries to convince the patient that progress actually is occurring.

He would remind me of things that were changing.

[Female, 52, Nonprofessional]

I would talk to him about it, and he would say, "It took you 35 years to get to this point, and it takes a while to change that. I see progress. Sometimes it feels like you take one step forward and one step back."

[Female, 50, Professional]

Mostly she tried to explain how she thought we were making progress, even if I didn't see it. She also tried to explain the process: you don't feel you're making progress because this is where we are in the process.

[Female, 39, Nonprofessional]

At various periods of time I did. We'd look at it and see if it was a matter of me being stuck in something, a point of impasse, and then we would try a different route. Or we would talk about where she saw me progressing, which were sometimes things I hadn't seen. Sometimes I thought she was saying that just so I'd stay in therapy.

[Female, 45, Professional]

Patients may be able to see progress without the therapist reminding them.

I'm sure there was dead air from time to time, and I would sometimes feel I wasn't making progress, but then all I had to do was look back 2 years.

[Male, 49, Nonprofessional]

When treatment seems at an impasse, therapists often seek consultation, but patients can do that too.

I had a few consultations with other therapists, and discussed them with him. He was very welcoming of any additional input, and wasn't at all threatened by it.

[Male, 42, Professional]

Often, the feeling of making no progress leads to ending the treatment.

I finally felt that my work with him was done and gave him some notice.

[Female, 41, Nonprofessional]

I kept telling him about it but the whole last year I don't think I made any progress. The only progress was leaving him.

[Female, 57, Professional]

It was usually right before I would stop for a while. I would say, "This isn't going anywhere," and I would stop. That happened 2 or 3 times in 5½ years.

[Female, 45, Nonprofessional]

I did all the time. I decided to terminate and he beat me to the punch.

[Female, 48, Nonprofessional]

Some patients who wanted to terminate treatment were waiting for the therapist to make that decision.

I feel that I stayed in treatment too long, and I'm sorry I couldn't say something. I was afraid of hurting her feelings.

[Female, 50, Professional]

We had done a lot, and the rest was the fine tuning that one does on one's own. It was at that point that I would have expected him to terminate the sessions.

[Female, 45, Nonprofessional]

NUMERICAL DISTRIBUTION

Professionals: Eighteen said they had at times felt like they weren't making progress; 2 said they had not felt that way.

Nonprofessionals: Thirty-one said they had at times felt like they weren't making progress; 9 said they had not felt that way.

COMMENTS

A similar percentage of both groups felt at times that they were not making progress, and this is understandable and normal; in any such long process there are going to be plateaus where the work of the previous period is assimilated and internalized before the next stage begins. Sometimes, however, this feeling refers to an impasse between patient and therapist, which must be acknowledged and resolved if treatment is to continue.

As the therapist, I want to be patient with anyone resting between rounds, and not pressure for more progress. Usually it's the patient who becomes dissatisfied, not the therapist, and I have to be responsive when they're ready to get back to work.

As the patient, I always want to feel that I get something out of every session, and that I'm not just marking time. The idea that I need a pause between efforts may be hard to accept. If I feel stuck in a problem with the therapist, that's a different story, and I will not be able to make any further progress until that is dealt with.

RELATED READING

Bernstein, P. B., and Landaiche, N. M. (1992). Resistance, counter-resistance, and balance: a framework for managing the experience of impasse in psychotherapy. *Journal of Contemporary Psychotherapy* 22(1):5–19.

Curtis, H. C. (1992). Impasses in psychotherapy. *Psychiatric Annals* 22(10):500–501.

Hill, C. E., Nutt-Williams, E., and Heaton, K. J. (1996). Therapist retrospective recall of impasses in long-term psychotherapy: a qualitative analysis. *Journal of Counseling Psychology* 43(2):207–217.

Pulver, S. E. (1992). Impasses in psychodynamic psychotherapy. *Psychiatric Annals* 22(10):514–519.

◪◪◪◪

Question 74: Did you ever cry in therapy?

A common stereotype of therapy shows the box of tissues on the table for the patient in tears.

Most people said they had cried in therapy. Some said it happened quite often, and the therapist was supportive.

Often it felt relieving. I felt he understood and was very empathetic.

[Female, 59, Professional]

I cried almost all the time. It was painful, and a release. I didn't worry about the effect on her.

[Female, 40, Nonprofessional]

It felt good and I liked it. It felt cleansing. I think it touched her heart.

[Female, 50, Professional]

It was a tremendous release. She stayed right there with me.

[Female, 47, Nonprofessional]

It felt very good. She felt I needed to cry and was glad I was doing it.

[Female, 62, Professional]

I was depressed so I was always ready to cry. She was very patient with me.

[Female, 42, Nonprofessional]

It felt great. Before I went into therapy I wondered if I would, because I'm not much of a crier, and I started crying very early on in therapy. Looking back now, I'm surprised how hard I cried even at the very beginning. It touched her heart. Sometimes I cried because I thought I was supposed to be crying, and she would call me on that.

[Female, 45, Professional]

Others said it happened rarely.

For me it's generally a relief because I don't do it very often.

[Female, 51, Professional]

Some people consciously tried not to cry.

I did, but not much. I do that privately—that's who I am. There were times that I wanted to cry but I wouldn't allow it. He would have been perfectly happy for me to do it.

[Female, 50, Nonprofessional]

I remember tearing up, but not full-fledged crying. It felt like she felt sorry for me, and I don't like that feeling.

[Female, 39, Professional]

I did once right after a car accident on the way there. She pulled it out of me. I didn't like it—I felt ugly.

[Female, 44, Nonprofessional]

I never liked crying in therapy; it wasn't comfortable. I had such low self-esteem that I was afraid she would think I was a total asshole because I was crying and looked like a jerk. I hope she was thrilled that I was crying, and would see it as a sign of movement.

[Female, 42, Nonprofessional]

I tried not to show it, and then was annoyed that she didn't notice.

[Male, 44, Professional]

Many people found it a relief to cry.

It was difficult but also wonderful at times.

[Male, 30, Professional]

It felt good, because she seemed at her most sympathetic when I would cry.

[Male, 42, Nonprofessional]

It felt cathartic, and felt good to be able to cry when I felt like crying.

[Male, 42, Professional]

Others found it painful or disturbing.

I didn't like having it happen, but it didn't feel like a bad thing to have done. It helped demonstrate the extent of my depression and the things that I was upset about.

[Male, 51, Nonprofessional]

It felt like an ache in my throat. I think she was touched by my pain.

[Male, 49, Nonprofessional]

It was usually out of incredible frustration, so it didn't feel good. I think he was also frustrated.

[Female, 48, Nonprofessional]

It felt yucky.

[Female, 41, Nonprofessional]

It was a cathartic release, but it was very painful.

[Female, 48, Nonprofessional]

Most people thought the therapist was comfortable with their tears, and was able to connect with the feelings.

> It felt great, because she was so supportive and so much there with me, which I hadn't felt with previous therapists. It was a release, it was therapeutic, it was very good.
>
> [Female, 41, Nonprofessional]

> His response was a therapeutic one, although during major tragedies, like when my brother committed suicide, he was really there, feeling my pain.
>
> [Female, 50, Professional]

> It felt okay. It felt safe to cry there. She would well up with tears herself. It felt good that she was in tune with me.
>
> [Female, 45, Nonprofessional]

Some people thought the therapist liked the tears, and regarded them as a sign of therapeutic effectiveness.

> It made her feel that she had hit a nerve of some kind, maybe in a good way.
>
> [Female, 45, Nonprofessional]

> She was probably delighted that she got that out of me.
>
> [Female, 55, Professional]

> She was probably glad to see it, another level of emotion and psychic involvement brought out.
>
> [Male, 50, Nonprofessional]

> In some ways she felt that I had gotten to something important, so perhaps it was a relief for her too.
>
> [Female, 46, Nonprofessional]

> For a while he wouldn't give anyone tissues, because that would stop the tears.
>
> [Male, 50, Professional]

> My therapist wanted to make me cry, all the time. That was her goal. She was constantly trying to make me cry. It made me really annoyed.
>
> [Female, 26, Nonprofessional]

I asked her how I would know that I had a breakthrough, and she suggested that it might be when I cried, and I said I would *never* cry in therapy. But I did, in one of the very last sessions. And I said, "Oh my God, I did it." It felt terrible. If she was purely professional, she would just think, "Good, we've gotten somewhere." I hope that because it was such a terrible moment that she felt bad for me.

[Female, 39, Nonprofessional]

A few people thought that tears made the therapist uncomfortable or anxious.

At first I thought he wasn't able to handle it, that he was embarrassed. Later I thought just that he felt sad along with me.

[Male, 53, Professional]

One person distinguished different kinds of tears.

There were times when it was very deep work when he would be very touched and really moved. If it was surface hysterics he would just be patient.

[Male, 46, Nonprofessional]

One person said the therapy never got to the level where such strong feelings would arise.

We never got deeply into anything.

[Female, 48, Nonprofessional]

NUMERICAL DISTRIBUTION

Professionals: Fourteen said they had often cried in therapy; 6 said they had cried only rarely. Fifteen said it felt good; 3 said it did not feel good; 2 said it was mixed.

Nonprofessionals: Twenty-one said they had often cried in therapy; 11 said they had occasionally cried in therapy; 8 said they had not cried at all. Of the 32 who had, 14 said it felt good; 9 said it did not feel good; 9 had mixed feelings.

COMMENTS

There were similar percentages in these responses, although only nonprofessionals said they consciously tried not to cry. Tears can be a sign of deep feelings, and can coincide with a release of painful memories. Most therapists seem to regard them as healing, although the experiences they accompany are not always pleasant.

As the therapist, I neither encourage nor discourage tears. I don't want the patient to feel that I derive any satisfaction from his or her tears and I don't want to convey to the patient in any way that I am made uncomfortable or awkward by his or her crying.

As the patient, I want to feel safe enough to say or do anything. Tears are just one aspect of that freedom, but an important one, because they indicate that I am at my most vulnerable. I want the therapist to remain calm and attuned, as always, and I really don't want to see any sign of satisfaction that we are finally getting somewhere.

RELATED READING

Labott, S. M., Ahleman, S., Wolever, M. E., and Martin, R. B. (1990). The physiological and psychological effects of the expression and inhibition of emotion. *Behavioral Medicine* 16(4):182–189.

Okada, F. (1991). Is the tendency to weep one of the most useful indicators for depressed mood? *Journal of Clinical Psychiatry* 52(8):351–352.

Schwartz, A. (1990). To soothe or not to soothe: or when and how: neurobiological and learning-psychological considerations of some complex clinical questions. *Psychoanalytic Inquiry* 10(4):554–566.

🌊🌊🌊🌊

Question 75: How did the therapist end the session?

It is part of the therapist's job to keep track of time and end the session. Many therapists have an habitual way of doing this.

He said, "We have to stop for today."

[Male, 42, Professional]

"That's time for today."

[Female, 52, Nonprofessional]

He ended by saying, "I guess we will not solve this today." When I left he always said, "Take care."

[Female, 57, Professional]

Lots of times he'd say, "Well, that's more grist for the mill."

[Female, 50, Professional]

"Well, we're out of time."

[Male, 30, Professional]

She would just say, "Okay." It was a very pleasant way of doing it.

[Female, 62, Professional]

Some therapists seemed to be trying to make the ending gentle.

She would usually say in a very soft, soothing voice, "Okay, I guess we're going to have to close now."

[Female, 41, Nonprofessional]

We would wind down our conversation and she would say something like, "So, next week this time, is that still good for you?" It was pretty impressive because it was always right at the end of the hour.

[Female, 39, Nonprofessional]

Some therapists try to review the session or summarize the themes.

She tried to tie it up somehow.

[Female, 50, Professional]

He pulled together, to a kind of closing. If we were getting into something new, he would stop us and draw it to a close.

[Female, 41, Nonprofessional]

He would sometimes sum up what went on, especially about the emotional aspect, and that was very useful.

[Female, 59, Professional]

Some therapists try to alert the patient to the time left.

She would say, a few minutes before the end, "We're almost out of time now," and then she'd say we had to stop.

[Male, 44, Professional]

There came a moment when she indicated that we had to move toward closure.

[Male, 49, Nonprofessional]

She'd say, "The time is up, but finish what you're saying." Or she'd say that we had about 5 more minutes, if it was a natural break near the end of the session, to warn me not to launch into some whole new thing.

[Female, 45, Professional]

Some therapists end the session nonverbally.

She didn't have to say anything; she just looked at the clock. I would watch her eyes, and when she looked at the clock we would just naturally start to wind up.

[Female, 45, Nonprofessional]

Sometimes she'd say, "Time is about up," but she always would take out my file at the end, sort of an indication that it was time to give her the check and go.

[Female, 39, Professional]

After a period of time, I could tell from her face; her face took on a particular look: a raised eyebrow.

[Female, 47, Nonprofessional]

She would get up, and begin to water her plants. It was sort of a ritual. It was the end of her workweek, and I was the last client, and this is what she would do before she left the office. It was also a transition time during which we might talk about something more casual.

[Female, 45, Professional]

After some time in treatment patients often know when the hour is up.

After a fairly short period of time, I just kind of knew when wrap-up was necessary. It was very rare that I was surprised by the end of the session. There would just be a kind of wrap-up, either by the therapist or by me.

[Female, 48, Nonprofessional]

Sometimes they just seemed to end naturally in some way, like we both somehow knew it was time to end. I don't know if it was some unspoken signal and I somehow got the message. There were a couple of times where she said very gently, "We have to stop now," but much more often we both seemed to know it was time.

[Female, 45, Nonprofessional]

I think it was just basically knowing that the time was up, like there'd be a lull, or we'd get to a point where she'd say that was a good place to stop.

[Female, 26, Nonprofessional]

A few patients said that they had taken on this responsibility.

Usually I did, by looking at the time and keeping track of the last 5 minutes.

[Female, 52, Professional]

I would always end the session, because I had been watching the clock. It turned out to be a whole treatment issue. We experimented with letting him end the session, but he totally flopped. He wasn't able to do it in a sensitive way. It was a difficult area for me, and I guess I was asking him to reinvent the wheel, in a way, and he basically refused.

[Female, 48, Professional]

I got to know when the end of the session was and I usually indicated that it was over.

[Female, 44, Nonprofessional]

Very often I would end the session. I would say I think I have to go, that time is up. Or she would say it. I had a lot of resistance to being there, but I don't think she reacted negatively to that particular thing.

[Female, 55, Professional]

I usually ended it. I'd see the clock and I'd get ready to go and I'd say, "Well, time's up."

[Female, 50, Professional]

Some therapists tried to give the patient something to work on until the next session.

He would remind me that we needed to stop, and if we were in the middle of talking about something he would ask me a question or two to think about for the next time, or ask if we could continue to talk about the same thing next time.

[Male, 51, Nonprofessional]

In the beginning he would give me some thought to work with, and he would tell me when he was going to see me again.

[Female, 48, Nonprofessional]

He ended with an assignment, which was very useful.

[Female, 44, Nonprofessional]

While most people said that the way the therapist ended the hour felt acceptable to them, some people had difficulty with the ending.

"Time is up." It felt a little abrupt.

[Female, 42, Nonprofessional]

There were times when I probably could have talked all night, and when she would say that was all the time we had it was disappointing. There were some sessions where I couldn't get going and I was waiting for the time to go by. When I would hear her say, "That's all for today," I was kind of disappointed in myself. I wished she could extend it for a while.

[Male, 45, Nonprofessional]

NUMERICAL DISTRIBUTION

Professionals: Seven said their therapist said that time was up; 3 said the therapist said "We have to stop"; 3 said the therapist used some other phrase; 2 said the therapist summarized the session; 1 said the therapist used a nonverbal signal. Four people said that they themselves had ended the session.

Nonprofessionals: Fourteen said the therapist said, "We have to stop"; 6 said that time was up; 5 said some other phrase; 6 said the therapist would summarize; 4 said there was a nonverbal signal; 1 said there was a homework assignment. Two people said they themselves had ended the session. Two people could not recall how the session ended.

COMMENTS

As the therapist, I want to end the session in a way that avoids feeling abrupt or rigid to the patient, and yet seems consistent and unsurprising, as well as containing of the material of the hour. A simple phrase, such as "We have to stop for today," or "Our time is up," accomplishes this in most instances. Little is gained by abruptly interrupting the patient who will finish up in a few moments.

As the patient, I know there's a time limit, but I don't want to feel that it's more important to the therapist to watch the clock than to listen to what I'm saying. I want to know that the therapist is relaxed and feels in control of the treatment, not that he's anxious and worried about the structure.

RELATED READING

Allman, P., Bloch, S., and Sharpe, M. (1992). The end-of-session message in systemic family therapy: a descriptive study. *Journal of Family Therapy* 14(1):69–85.
Johnston, S. H., and Farber, B. A. (1996). The maintenance of boundaries in psychotherapeutic practice. *Psychotherapy* 33(3):391–402.
Winestine, M. C. (1987). Reaction to the end of the analytic hour as a derivative of early childhood experience: couch or crib. *Psychoanalytic Quarterly* 56(4):689–692.

℞℞℞℞

Question 76: How much did you learn about your therapist's personal life?

Therapists disagree about how much to disclose or reveal to the patient, but every patient eventually learns something about the therapist. What kinds of things did they learn?

Often the patient learns about the personal life of the therapist. This can come directly from the therapist, sometimes intentionally and sometimes inadvertently.

> He told me he was a grandfather. His apartment was connected to the office, so in the waiting room I would sometimes see his wife going in and out. I knew he had several children.
>
> [Female, 59, Professional]

> I knew he was married, how old he was, and that he had a son who went to Dalton.
>
> [Female, 57, Professional]

> I knew a little bit about her because her living space was in the rear of her professional space, so I saw her name on two bells, and I would occasionally hear her child in the back room when I was in the waiting area. Also, I asked her if she had children, because I needed to understand her reactions to things I was saying as to whether she was a parent herself. A lot of things were revealed by her, in that she talked

a lot about where she was in her professional development, about some of her teachers, and about her move from New York and what that meant.

[Male, 48, Nonprofessional]

I learned a lot about him—from him telling me, and because I was involved with him outside therapy.

[Male, 50, Professional]

I learned a little because of doing some work in his house as a barter arrangement. I got to see his house, and to see him on more of a personal basis.

[Male, 43, Nonprofessional]

She was married to a therapist—I once heard his voice on her answering machine. I knew she had two daughters. I knew some about her divorce.

[Female, 51, Professional]

We ended up buying a house on the same street that she lived on, five houses away, and at the time I was seeing her at her house. We talked about it. I knew what her husband looked like and I knew where he taught. I knew she had a dog, and his name. I knew she didn't have children, and that her husband had kids from a previous marriage. When her mother died, I knew that. The reality was that she was so well boundaried and private that it was not a problem at all.

[Female, 45, Professional]

Sometimes others tell the patient about the therapist.

Sometimes she would talk about herself a little bit, but I learned more about her personal life because not only did I have friends who were patients of hers, I had friends who were friends of hers.

[Female, 42, Nonprofessional]

Some people said they enjoyed learning details of the therapist's life, which can become a way of connecting.

I knew she was married, and she made more money than her husband. They were offered because it came up in the context of my own situations and concerns. I knew she was a basketball fan, and we would talk about that. It was a sort of bonding that we had things in common.

[Male, 49, Nonprofessional]

> I learned that his daughter was in the same profession that I am, so
> I would hear progress reports about her career.
>
> [Male, 51, Nonprofessional]

> I knew she had at least one child, and she had a dog. She told me
> about the child, because I had a very difficult pregnancy.
>
> [Female, 39, Nonprofessional]

> I got little bits here and there. Things would come up in conversation.
> I knew where she came from. She took me up on her roof once and
> showed me her garden, because I was moving to the country and
> was planting a garden.
>
> [Male, 49, Nonprofessional]

The anticipated bonding doesn't always happen.

> I learned only that she was married. And she was pregnant during
> the time I saw her, so I knew she had a baby. I felt like that should
> make us a little closer, like bonding, because she was pregnant, this
> huge thing that was going on in her life, but it was kept kind of
> separate from everything else.
>
> [Female, 26, Nonprofessional]

Many people said they learned very little about the therapist, and
wished they had known more.

> I knew she didn't have any children. I knew she went to Cape Cod in
> August. She told me that. But that's all I know. I find it very difficult
> not to know anything about her. She's just a blank.
>
> [Female, 50, Nonprofessional]

> She had told me little by little about her children and her former
> marriages, and her schooling, and the man she was seeing then who
> lived in another state, and those kinds of things. The whole process
> works much better for me when the person tells me something about
> her life, so I know they are a real person and not a machine.
>
> [Female, 42, Nonprofessional]

> I saw her car once because I saw her drive up, and looked at what
> was inside, like a detective.
>
> [Female, 44, Nonprofessional]

Some people said that knowing more about the therapist improved the therapy.

> Over the years she started disclosing more, and I learned more about her. I felt it accelerated the therapeutic process as opposed to frustrating it.
>
> [Female, 47, Nonprofessional]

Patients may experience the therapist's anonymity as a kind of withholding.

> I would ask him things, like where he was going on vacation, and he would give very short answers, like "Florida." He would always answer the question but he would never give anything.
>
> [Female, 41, Nonprofessional]

Some people implied that details of the therapist's personal life were a kind of credential, a proof of success in the areas being discussed in treatment.

> It was very important for me to know about her success in her own relationships.
>
> [Male, 52, Nonprofessional]

> He very rarely offered little anecdotes about his life, and would reveal information very carefully and grudgingly. Toward the end, he became more trusting that my questions could be useful if answered, and was more likely to tell little stories.
>
> [Male, 53, Professional]

> She may have wanted to make a point. She would say that this is what happened when she did that, or this is what it was like for her. She would tell me about how she reacted to some situation.
>
> [Male, 45, Nonprofessional]

A few people said they were content to know very little about the therapist, that they had no great desire to know.

> I learned very little, but I was never concerned the way other members of my group were concerned about the details of the therapist's life. I remember one guy being really obsessed about the room in the suite

where the door was always closed, and about whether the therapist lived in the place that we met for group. I didn't care.

[Female, 48, Nonprofessional]

I knew who her husband was, and I knew she had kids, boys. I never asked her about herself because I don't want to know, and I don't want her to use me as her therapist. I know a lot of therapists who do that.

[Female, 62, Professional]

Sometimes what the patient is told is upsetting or disturbing in some way.

In his helplessness about my husband's illness, he gave me the name of a nutritionist. She was, depending on your point of view, either cutting edge or wacky.

[Female, 48, Professional]

A few patients said they were uncomfortable with what they learned because of the way they believed therapy was supposed to work.

There were pictures of his children on his desk, which I thought was weird.

[Female, 48, Nonprofessional]

There was a part of me that thought, *He's not supposed to tell me things,* but that was because I believed that. It wouldn't have been a problem if I didn't believe it.

[Female, 48, Nonprofessional]

NUMERICAL DISTRIBUTION

Professionals: Seven said they had learned a lot about the therapist; 7 said they had learned some things; 6 said they had learned very little.

Nonprofessionals: Four said they had learned a lot; 11 said they had learned some things; 19 said they had learned very little; 6 said they had learned nothing about the therapist.

COMMENTS

A higher percentage of professionals said they learned a lot about the therapist's personal life, and this may be due to some collegial feeling on the part of the therapist. It's clearly a matter of personal style how much the therapist reveals, and there are some reasonable justifications for personal disclosure, as well as plenty of arguments against it.

As the therapist, I always say that I want my patients to know me, which is different from knowing about me. I always try to be myself, though I reveal little personal data, and most patients seem to understand and accept this limit. I'm concerned that too much disclosure inhibits the patient from revealing opinions or behaviors contrary to my own.

As the patient, I am of course curious about my therapist, and interested to know as much as possible, but I also realize that this may be counterproductive. The focus is, after all, on me, and details of the therapist's life may not be relevant.

RELATED READING

Auvil, C. A., and Silver, B. W. (1984). Therapist self-disclosure: When is it appropriate? *Perspectives in Psychiatric Care* 22(2):57–61.

Berg-Cross, L. (1984). Therapist self-disclosure to clients in psychotherapy. *Psychotherapy in Private Practice* 2(4):57–64.

Derlega, V. J., Margulis, S. T., and Winstead, B. A. (1987). A social-psychological analysis of self-disclosure in psychotherapy. *Journal of Social and Clinical Psychology* 5(2):205–215.

Mathews, B. (1988). The role of therapist self-disclosure in psychotherapy: a survey of therapists. *American Journal of Psychotherapy* 42(4):521–531.

——— (1989). The use of therapist self-disclosure and its potential impact on the therapeutic process. *Journal of Human Behavior and Learning* 6(2):25–29.

Simon, J. C. (1988). Criteria for therapist self-disclosure. *American Journal of Psychotherapy* 42(3):404–415.

🖫🖫🖫🖫

Question 77: Did you ever learn something about the therapist that you didn't want to know?

Most patients want to know at least something about the therapist, but sometimes patients learn more than they want to know.

In some cases, the knowledge is general.

I've learned all sorts of things about him that I wish I didn't know. The last few years I was much more scrupulous about maintaining the boundaries from my end.

[Male, 50, Professional]

He shared a lot about his personal life. At times I thought that the extent to which he took those stories was unnecessary and inappropriate.

[Female, 58, Nonprofessional]

There was nothing specific. There's the seduction of wanting to know everything, but you don't want to see your therapist's clay feet.

[Female, 45, Professional]

She told me too much about her own life, and I learned how indecisive she was.

[Female, 50, Nonprofessional]

I don't remember what, but I do remember having that feeling. I remember feeling uncomfortable knowing what he would do in his personal life.

[Male, 30, Professional]

I knew way too much. Every time we would stop for a while, she would tell me more about herself. It was more like I was a friend.

[Female, 45, Nonprofessional]

When she broke with the institute where I was training, we had to talk about that, and I felt that I was learning more than I wanted to know.

[Female, 45, Professional]

In other instances, the patient learns something specific.

I learned more than I wanted to, because she shared with me that she was actually going through a very similar experience to me, which was trying to have a baby, in her case with rather disastrous results. It made me somewhat inhibited about talking about my own experience. If she had failed, it would have been hard for me to succeed.

[Female, 45, Nonprofessional]

She crossed the boundaries all the time. Her office was in her house, so I could hear noises from upstairs. She would talk about where she had shopped, about her life at the synagogue, and it made me very uncomfortable. I never told her due to fear of upsetting her. I didn't want to hurt her feelings. So I had to stop going because I didn't trust her anymore. She actually complained to me about her husband in regard to something he had done.

[Female, 48, Nonprofessional]

I learned that his wife was sharing the suite, and it was his second marriage and it became a real oedipal thing for me, since she was about my age.

[Female, 48, Professional]

One of my colleagues told me she was a lesbian.

[Female, 50, Professional]

He told me stuff about his daughter, who was so much easier than my own.

[Female, 50, Nonprofessional]

NUMERICAL DISTRIBUTION

Professionals: Ten said they had learned more than they wanted to know about the therapist; 10 said they had not.

Nonprofessionals: Six said they had learned more than they wanted to know about the therapist; 34 said they had not.

COMMENTS

A much higher percentage of the professionals said they learned more than they wanted to know about the therapist's personal life, and this, when taken with the responses to the last question, again suggests that therapists may feel more collegial with a patient who is also in the field and thus reveal more. These responses also suggest that therapists need to be more cautious about revealing personal details of life outside the office. Disclosure of therapist reactions and experiences in the session is very different, and more likely to be useful.

As the therapist, I am cautious about self-disclosure of personal details, since I have had such disclosures come back to bite me later. Most patients seem to appreciate my keeping the space clear of my own stuff and more available for theirs. Occasionally a patient will insist on an answer to a specific question and if I understand the reason for the question I will probably answer it.

As the patient, it makes me a little anxious when my therapist tells me personal information I haven't asked for; it makes the boundaries seem blurry and unstable. I don't want to be inhibited by the knowledge of my therapist's history, opinions, or circumstances, because I may hesitate to bring up my own if I think they contradict the therapist's and will lead to some sort of conflict. So unless I specifically ask for the information, I'd prefer that she keep it to herself.

RELATED READING

Berg-Cross, L. (1984). Therapist self-disclosure to clients in psychotherapy. *Psychotherapy in Private Practice* 2(4):57–64.

Johnston, S. H., and Farber, B. A. (1996). The maintenance of boundaries in psychotherapeutic practice. *Psychotherapy* 33(3):391–402.

Stricker, G., and Fisher, M., eds. (1990). *Self-Disclosure in the Therapeutic Relationship*. New York: Plenum.

🅱🅱🅱🅱

Question 78: Did you have any fantasies about your therapist beyond what you knew?

Because therapists try to focus on the patient, keeping themselves from intruding, patients may have little information about what therapists are like outside the office. What kinds of things do patients imagine?

Many people tried to imagine what the therapist's life was like outside the office.

> I tried to imagine her married, where she lived, how old were her kids, what was she like as a person.
>
> [Female, 39, Nonprofessional]

> I made some assumptions about him. I assumed he was heterosexual, because he wore a wedding ring. I assumed he was married, and that he had a young child, because whenever I would talk about early schooling he would seem very interested.
>
> [Female, 48, Nonprofessional]

> In the beginning I might have had the fantasy that he had the wonderful life with the two kids and the perfect wife.
>
> [Female, 50, Professional]

When I heard her child screaming in the other room, I would some-times imagine what was going on.

[Male, 48, Nonprofessional]

I read about her in a book, and I had a good time thinking about her in that era.

[Female, 52, Professional]

I never saw her in a relationship, because she was such a blank slate, and used to see her as devoted to her practice and going home at the end of the day by herself.

[Female, 40, Nonprofessional]

I imagined that she had a very rich, involved set of interests and social life, that she was multifaceted and very smart. I always wondered whether there was a significant other in her life.

[Female, 47, Nonprofessional]

The fantasy is not always a positive one.

She once told me a story about renovating her kitchen, and it put her in the light of a "fancy lady," and I didn't like seeing her in that light.

[Female, 51, Professional]

I had an image of her, what she was like outside of therapy, and that was that she was almost like an actress, that she had this role, and she was very theatrical, but there was no feeling of authenticity.

[Female, 44, Nonprofessional]

The sexual life of the therapist is sometimes the content of the fantasies.

Toward the end, I thought that she was lesbian, because she didn't understand some of my issues with men.

[Female, 50, Professional]

I made the assumption that she was a lesbian, though we never discussed it. Most of the examples she gave from her life made me think that was so.

[Female, 46, Nonprofessional]

Sometimes patients fantasized about a special kind of relationship to the therapist.

The fantasy I had was that he would have a friend that he would introduce me to, because I really liked him.

[Female, 41, Nonprofessional]

It was just the usual sexual fantasies, living with him, like that.

[Female, 48, Professional]

I think I fantasized that we would somehow transcend the therapist–patient relationship and become buddies.

[Female, 45, Nonprofessional]

I knew that he was a twin, as I am, and I think I had the fantasy that there would be some sort of bond that we would have, that he would understand something about me that I can't articulate myself.

[Female, 58, Professional]

I thought it was a pity he was my psychiatrist because it would have been nice to have a social relationship with him and his wife. We shared some cultural interests, and I don't have too many people in my life like that.

[Female, 45, Nonprofessional]

When the therapist is very open and disclosing, fantasy may become more difficult.

There wasn't a lot of room for that because I knew so much.

[Male, 50, Professional]

I had enough concrete information so I didn't have to fantasize.

[Female, 39, Professional]

Many other people said that they actively avoided fantasizing about the therapist.

I thought about it a little, but I really didn't want to go there.

[Female, 45, Professional]

I didn't have any interest in what their life was like.

[Female, 48, Nonprofessional]

I didn't let my mind go there. I wanted the therapy to be about me and not her.

[Female, 45, Professional]

If I did they were very limited. I avoided that. I wanted to keep her in her place.

[Female, 50, Professional]

NUMERICAL DISTRIBUTION

Professionals: Ten said they did have fantasies about the therapist; 10 said they did not.

Nonprofessionals: Eighteen said they had fantasies about the therapist; 22 said they did not.

COMMENTS

Similar percentages of the two groups acknowledged fantasies about their therapists' personal lives, and it's easy to understand wondering about what the therapists do when they're not working, whether they're married or have children, where and how they live. Many of those who said they had no fantasies were deliberately avoiding such thoughts.

As the therapist, I'm interested in any fantasies the patient has about me, for what they might reveal about her or about me. I try to make it safe enough for the patient to discuss those fantasies, though many patients will not bring them up no matter what I do.

As the patient, I may explore the ideas of what my therapist's life is like, and imagine some relationship outside of therapy, but I probably don't think it's very important or worth discussing. If I find the fantasy either very pleasant or very disturbing I might be more willing to reveal and discuss it with the therapist.

RELATED READING

Ganzarain, R. (1991). Extra-analytic contacts: fantasy and reality. *International Journal of Psycho-Analysis* 72(1):131–140.

Levenson, E. A. (1996). Aspects of self-revelation and self-disclosure. *Contemporary Psychoanalysis* 32(2):237–248.

Levin, K. (1993). *Unconscious Fantasy in Psychotherapy*. Northvale, NJ: Jason Aronson.

Levine, F. J. (1993). Unconscious fantasy and theories of technique. *Psychoanalytic Inquiry* 13(4):326–342.

🅡🅡🅡🅡

Question 79: Did other people you knew see the same therapist?

When the patient finds a good therapist and has a successful therapy, he or she often wants to share that with significant others. Much of the time this occurs without creating problems or conflicts.

> I brought my current girlfriend in and we went together for a while. I also knew people who saw her too.
>
> [Male, 49, Nonprofessional]

> A friend of my mother's asked me if he was a good hypnotist, because she was looking to stop smoking. She went to him for one week, and hasn't smoked a cigarette since.
>
> [Male, 53, Nonprofessional]

Some people had been referred to the therapist by someone already in treatment.

> I went to see her because they recommended her, so it was a positive thing.
>
> [Female, 56, Professional]

Therapists are often careful about which referrals they accept, and about scheduling patient hours.

> She would not see people who were in my inner circle.
>
> [Female, 47, Nonprofessional]

> Another person from my company had the hour right after me for a while, and the therapist was conscientious about making sure we never saw each other.
>
> [Female, 41, Nonprofessional]

> I was referred by someone I knew who was seeing him, and later I referred my best friend. He was very careful about not even scheduling us back to back.
>
> [Female, 50, Nonprofessional]

One person said the therapist's willingness to see people without concern for privacy and confidentiality created problems.

My brother saw her, my husband saw her, my mother saw her father. Even a cousin started to see her. There were no boundaries.
[Female, 45, Nonprofessional]

Patients often refer people close to them, and the emotions can get complicated.

It became triangulated a lot. It was a problem in that I wanted him to be more effective in making her the way I wanted her to be.
[Male, 50, Professional]

There was a friend who made a derogatory remark about him. He found him very unhelpful, and I was very angry at that friend, and I talked about it with the therapist and with the friend.
[Male, 48, Nonprofessional]

I referred my wife's roommate before we were married. It got entangling.
[Male, 53, Professional]

I had a friend who saw him very briefly while I did. It was a problem because she didn't like him and quit very soon, and wanted to talk about that.
[Female, 48, Nonprofessional]

There was a woman in my class who I couldn't stand and she was in therapy with my analyst, and she had the previous hour sometimes, and I wondered how my therapist could stand to listen to her.
[Female, 62, Professional]

Competitive feelings can arise.

My cousin referred me. It was a problem because I wasn't sure for a while if she was my cousin's therapist or mine.
[Female, 45, Nonprofessional]

I hated it, because it was like sibling rivalry.
[Female, 50, Professional]

I knew a lot of people who saw her, and we'd often compete for who she liked best, who had the closest relationship with her.
[Female, 42, Nonprofessional]

I had nothing to be jealous of because I knew I was one of her special clients. Other people probably had feelings about that.

[Female, 45, Professional]

I was very close with a woman who saw him, and we were also in group together, and I thought she was one of the biggest time-wasters in there, and she was a very seductive person. She would do her set routine. I couldn't imagine why he would allow her to do this when he didn't tolerate it from me or from the others.

[Male, 46, Nonprofessional]

Some people resented providing new patients (and additional income) for the therapist.

With my first therapist, I did it a lot and I feel like I built his swimming pool. I did it this time only with people who were very special to me.

[Female, 51, Professional]

Occasionally this kind of situation can lead to breaks in confidentiality.

I saw a fellow employee there, and I was a little shocked. I wasn't too concerned because she wasn't in my department, but what if I saw someone who was?

[Male, 42, Nonprofessional]

I recommended to one friend that she see him, and she saw him for 3 years. He told me something that was supposed to be completely in confidence. He warned me at one time, when I was extremely fragile and vulnerable, that she was feeling very sexually experimental and might be playfully proposing some kind of lesbian relationship, and he told me that wasn't something that I had to include in my friendship with her. I thought it was a protective comment.

[Female, 45, Nonprofessional]

NUMERICAL DISTRIBUTION

Professionals: Ten said nobody they knew saw the same therapist; 10 said it had happened. Of these, 3 said it was a problem in some way.

Nonprofessionals: Twenty-three said nobody they knew saw the same therapist; 17 said it had happened. Of these, 6 said it was a problem in some way.

COMMENTS

Similar percentages of the two groups had the therapist all to themselves. When the patient is having a good experience, he may want to give that experience to important people from his life, and the therapist has to evaluate the distance between these two people and decide whether to accept the new person or refer him or her to another therapist. Patients who make referrals don't always want the therapist to accept them, and motivations must be explored.

As the therapist, I have to weigh the advantages and disadvantages of accepting new referrals from patients. Knowing both may enlighten me about certain issues, but maintaining boundaries can become difficult. I have to be sure that I accept the referral because that's what's best for my current patient and not because I have an open hour to fill.

As the patient, if I am getting a lot from my therapist I may want to share the benefits with people I care about, and trust the therapist to keep us separate. If he or she says that isn't possible, I may be a little disappointed but I will also be relieved that the therapist has made my therapy a higher priority than his income.

RELATED READING

Klein, R. H. (1983). Some problems of patient referral for outpatient group psychotherapy. *International Journal of Group Psychotherapy* 33(2):229–241.

Roll, S., and Millen, L. (1981). A guide to violating an injunction in psychotherapy: on seeing acquaintances as patients. *Psychotherapy: Theory, Research and Practice* 18(2):179–187.

Tryon, G. S. (1983). Why full-time private practitioners refer patients to other professionals. *Psychotherapy in Private Practice* 1(2):81–83.

🔊🔊🔊🔊

Question 80: Did you ever see your therapist outside the office, either accidentally or by arrangement?

Because therapy takes place in the real world, patient and therapist sometimes encounter each other outside the office.

Some people said they felt awkward and uncomfortable when this happened.

We bumped into each other a few times in the street. It was a little awkward. I wasn't sure how to handle it, and looked to him to take the lead, and he was looking to me to take the lead. In recent years, I saw him at conferences. It felt a little strange but increasingly normal.

[Male, 53, Professional]

I saw him in a store and got completely freaked out and hid in the back of the store.

[Female, 48, Nonprofessional]

I met her once in a store and I was very uncomfortable. I saw her and I didn't even go over to her.

[Female, 48, Nonprofessional]

It was very awkward for me. She didn't seem to be but I was. Do I say hello or not?

[Female, 45, Professional]

I was a wreck, I was very uncomfortable. My inclination was to go over to her and say hello, which I did, but I didn't know if I was overstepping her boundaries.

[Female, 47, Nonprofessional]

We go to the same hair salon, and I ran into her maybe twice, and once in a restaurant. It was very awkward. It's very difficult to change gears.

[Male, 49, Nonprofessional]

Even when the therapist seems at ease, the patient may feel uncomfortable.

We live in the same town. I didn't like it. I felt awkward, but she seemed to be fine with it. I had a sense that she would have been more sociable but she could see that I didn't want that.

[Female, 50, Professional]

Others said they felt at ease in the situation, and the therapist did too.

We met on the street outside her office. It was fine. I was able to introduce her to my husband and daughter.

[Female, 39, Nonprofessional]

Once I ran into him in the subway and sat next to him. We chatted briefly. He seemed comfortable and I was too.

[Male, 42, Professional]

I did run into her. It was comfortable, and it was fun to see her in a situation that was outside the office. It was like seeing a friend. She didn't seem uncomfortable with it.

[Male, 45, Nonprofessional]

I found out he spent his summers in the same town where I was going, and we talked about what would happen if we met, how we would handle that. We never did but I felt comfortable with the possibility.

[Male, 51, Nonprofessional]

Some people said the therapist seemed uncomfortable.

It was pretty dreadful—awkward, uncomfortable. Her rigidity allowed her to be very calm and just smile, but she was the one who made an issue of it back in the office, enforcing the boundaries.

[Male, 44, Professional]

We met at a basketball game. It was very strange. She was sitting right behind me with her son. It felt very weird. I wanted to make contact. I felt that she wanted to make contact too, but she also wanted to be invisible.

[Female, 46, Nonprofessional]

Other people reported encounters in which the therapist seemed at ease.

We've met at various conferences. At first it was odd but he was kind of friendly and I got used to it.

[Female, 59, Professional]

Sometimes the therapist's discomfort seems to come from concern for the patient's privacy.

In the beginning he would just ignore me, pretend he didn't know me, because there were other people around who know what he does. I assume it was out of courtesy to me, and I didn't feel he was being rude.

[Female, 48, Nonprofessional]

> Once I ran into him where we have a country house, in an outlet store, and that was a little awkward because I was with a friend and he didn't know how much he should say or reveal.
>
> [Female, 50, Professional]

Depending on the situation, some people didn't like what they learned about the therapist.

> I met her at a singles function, and she was a single, and I didn't like to think of her as wanting to meet somebody, as if there was something wrong with that, because in my mind at that point it was pathetic that you wanted to meet somebody.
>
> [Male, 44, Professional]

> Once I saw him give a professional talk. He revealed that he had had several glasses of wine and was a little tipsy, and then he revealed stuff about his own analyst and the sexual fantasies that he had in analysis. It was so out of character, and he knew I was in the audience. I didn't know if it was the wine, or if he was doing some exhibitionistic thing with me.
>
> [Female, 48, Professional]

> He lives near here. It's not awkward but it raises questions about who I am to him.
>
> [Male, 46, Nonprofessional]

> I would see her, but I never approached her. It would make me aware of how elderly she was.
>
> [Female, 62, Professional]

> It was awkward and uncomfortable for me, although she seemed fine. It was because there were things I didn't want to know about her, and here it was in my face.
>
> [Female, 45, Professional]

NUMERICAL DISTRIBUTION

Professionals: Four said they had not met the therapist outside the office; 16 said they had. Of these, 11 said it was a little awkward or uncomfortable; 5 said it felt fine.

Nonprofessionals: Twenty-one said they had not met the therapist outside the office; 19 said they had. Of these, 8 said it was a little awkward or uncomfortable; 11 said it felt fine.

COMMENTS

A greater percentage of professionals had encounters with their therapists outside the office, and this is readily understandable, since this group would be more often in professional situations. Many patients feel a little awkward or uncomfortable, which is unpleasant enough, but when the therapists appear visibly distressed, this is clearly disturbing to their patients.

As the therapist, I sometimes run into current or former patients. In most cases I'm unaware of any discomfort on my part. I try to take my cues from the patients, so I don't initiate contact, especially if they are with other people. I don't want to inadvertently reveal something they don't want revealed.

As the patient, I don't mind running into my therapist unless she seems unhappy about running into me—then I have a problem.

RELATED READING

Gates, K. P., and Speare, K. H. (1990). Overlapping relationships in rural communities. In *Feminist Ethics in Psychotherapy*, ed. H. Lerman and N. Porter, pp. 97–101. New York: Springer.

Schank, J. A., and Skovholt, T. M. (1997). Dual-relationship dilemmas of rural and small-community psychologists. *Professional Psychology: Research and Practice* 28(1):44–49.

Sharkin, B. S., and Birky, I. (1992). Incidental encounters between therapists and their clients. *Professional Psychology: Research and Practice* 23(4):326–328.

Weiss, S. S. (1975). The effect on the transference of "special events" occurring during psychoanalysis. *International Journal of Psycho-Analysis* 56(1):69–75.

🌊🌊🌊🌊

Question 81: Who did you tell that you were going to therapy?

In the old days, patients were often advised not to discuss their therapy, with the explanation that it would dilute the effectiveness of the treatment. Today, most patients feel free to tell anyone what goes on in therapy.

Most people said they let those around them know they were seeing a therapist, and felt encouraged by the reactions they got.

I discussed it a little bit with people who were very close to me. Most people thought it was a wonderful thing to be doing.

[Female, 40, Nonprofessional]

I told everyone, because this is how therapists function: they talk about their unconscious. It's a form of intimacy.

[Male, 42, Professional]

I discussed it a lot. I was so positive about it that nobody said anything negative.

[Male, 46, Nonprofessional]

Occasionally they found that some of the people who knew didn't like it. Often parents (and other relatives) have some fears about what goes on in therapy.

My mother had a problem. When I started I had no money, and I asked my mother to pay for it. I remember her handing me a check and looking at me and saying, "When do you think you're going to be well?" It's not part of her world.

[Female, 50, Nonprofessional]

My father had a very negative reaction. I wasn't making much money, and I had asked him to help me out financially, to help pay for it. He didn't understand what therapy was or what it would do. He said he didn't mind lending me money for what he thought was right, but he never actually said what was wrong about therapy. He said I needed to get on with my life. He did give me some money for therapy that first year. My mom was pretty supportive, and my friends were, too.

[Female, 42, Nonprofessional]

My family had a problem with it; they never accepted it.

[Female, 52, Nonprofessional]

My mother wanted to like it, but she just couldn't. My relationship with her changed dramatically, and she didn't like the way it changed.

[Female, 45, Professional]

My mother had a problem. Her fear is that the therapist is leading me to believe that all my issues originate with her. Her view is that therapy leads to anger at parents.

[Male, 49, Nonprofessional]

My aunt and uncle are clinicians who are against everything that they don't do themselves, and they made nasty remarks about it. Every once in a while my mother would make a comment about how long I had been seeing him.

[Male, 50, Professional]

My mother never supported my seeing a therapist, because she was very threatened by it.

[Female, 53, Nonprofessional]

My mother thinks the whole thing is a complete waste of time and money.

[Female, 51, Professional]

Sometimes a parent may worry about what being in therapy means.

My mother did, because she felt that therapy was for crazy people, and she didn't want me to be crazy.

[Female, 45, Nonprofessional]

My family thought you'd have to be in desperate straits before you would see a therapist.

[Male, 48, Nonprofessional]

Sometimes the partner has difficulty.

A boyfriend said I should give the money to him and he'd take me to the movies and make me feel better.

[Female, 44, Nonprofessional]

My husband had an issue with my being in therapy, and how long it was going to take. The therapist brought him in to discuss it with him and reassure him.

[Female, 50, Professional]

I think my husband doesn't get therapy at all, so for him, the fact that it goes on and on, and you're paying and paying, he wonders what it's all about. He didn't tell me to stop, but he didn't understand my going.

[Female, 46, Nonprofessional]

My wife wanted me to not be so dependent. She was jealous of my attachment to him, and she would have liked to see me as being more self-sufficient. I thought that she saw me as damaged goods if I was going so long.

[Male, 53, Professional]

Some patients said they didn't tell specific people because they knew those people would have a problem with them being in therapy.

I didn't tell the people who would have had a problem, namely my parents, who would have been appalled to think that there was a problem, and might have worried that I was talking about them.

[Female, 39, Nonprofessional]

I wasn't sure how the family would react. I didn't want to burden them with the idea that I had a problem. It was something I wanted to deal with on my own.

[Male, 45, Nonprofessional]

I discussed it only with friends. My family doesn't believe in therapy.

[Female, 62, Professional]

Some friends knew but family did not. We don't talk about such things, and I thought they would have a problem with me going.

[Male, 45, Nonprofessional]

A few people didn't discuss being in therapy because of feelings of their own about it.

Parents and friends knew, but I never really discussed it. I felt some kind of embarrassment about being in therapy.

[Female, 28, Nonprofessional]

Friends knew, but not family. I thought that it would become public knowledge and be discussed through the family, and I didn't want that.

[Female, 48, Nonprofessional]

I never found it possible to recreate what went on in therapy, so I discussed it only in a general way. And I didn't want to turn into a therapy bore.

[Male, 49, Nonprofessional]

Occasionally someone questioned the need for therapy.

One friend didn't understand therapy, and would tell me I didn't need it.

[Female, 46, Nonprofessional]

Some of my good friends wondered why I wanted analysis.

[Female, 48, Professional]

Sometimes those who knew questioned not the process but the particular therapist.

Only my closest friend had a problem, and felt that he was not the right therapist for me because he was too rigid.

[Female, 57, Professional]

Friends thought I should terminate with her long before I did.

[Male, 44, Professional]

No one had a problem with my going to therapy, but many of my friends questioned whether this therapist was any good.

[Female, 48, Nonprofessional]

NUMERICAL DISTRIBUTION

Professionals: All 20 said that everyone knew they were in therapy. Thirteen said they discussed it with both friends and family; 7 said only with friends and not with family. Nine people said someone had a problem with their being in therapy.

Nonprofessionals: Thirty-five said that everyone knew they were in therapy; 5 said they did not tell family. Nineteen said they discussed it with those who knew; 21 said they discussed it only a little or not at all. Thirteen people said someone had a problem with their being in therapy.

COMMENTS

Obviously, professionals are more likely to tell people that they're in therapy, without attaching any stigma to it. Knowing that some people, mostly parents but also some spouses, may have trouble with it makes it harder to tell them. Parents are often afraid of what may be said about them, afraid of being blamed, or worried about estrangement from their children.

As the therapist, I hope no one today attaches any shame to being in therapy, although some patients still tell me that being in therapy means that they are "sick." Therapists used to advise patients not to discuss their treatment with anyone, but this seems unnecessary to me. I think that the more patients discuss whatever is going on in therapy, the more they are thinking about and processing that material.

As the patient, I want to feel free to tell anyone that I'm in therapy without getting any criticism or resistance to my being there. Anyone who seems negative about my getting what I need is not on my side, and our relationship is called into question, even (maybe especially) with a parent.

RELATED READING

Bankoff, E. A. (1994). The social network of the psychotherapy patient. *Psychotherapy* 31(3):503–514.

Bankoff, E. A., and Howard, K. I. (1992). The social network of the psychotherapy patient and effective psychotherapeutic process. *Journal of Psychotherapy Integration* 2(4):273–294.

Hobfoll, S. E. (1996). Social support: Will you be there when I need you? In *A Lifetime of Relationships,* ed. N. Vanzetti and S. Duck, pp. 46–74. Pacific Grove, CA: Brooks/Cole.

Sze, W. C. (1990). Ego strength and coping capacity: friend and social group affiliation. In *Stressors and the Adjustment Disorders,* ed. J. D. Noshpitz and R. D. Coddington, pp. 510–520. New York: Wiley.

℞℞℞℞

Question 82: Did you ever go as a couple?

Couples therapy is an option when the primary problem is a relationship conflict. Most of the people interviewed had been in couples therapy at some point. (Responses to this and the next two questions refer to all therapies, not just the one of the main interview.)

Most of the people who had been in couples therapy found it helpful.

> I liked her and thought that she got to the heart of things. My husband didn't like her at all, although I think she helped us. It's a place to go where there's somebody monitoring both of your behaviors and how you react to one another, and in a nonjudgmental way validating

your feelings and your spouse's feelings. It's a safe place to say what's on your mind.

[Female, 48, Nonprofessional]

It de-escalated the conflict and reframed things so we could solve what was going on.

[Female, 56, Professional]

Somehow it is more validating to express yourself to your spouse in front of someone else than when you express the same thing alone with your mate. The objectivity that I've gotten from the therapist makes it much easier to accept when I'm not right.

[Female, 53, Nonprofessional]

We went in thinking we knew what the issues were and that they would be solved, and what came out was a lot more subtle, namely a deeper understanding of each other and a sense that we could work out what the issues were.

[Female, 46, Nonprofessional]

Often people brought a spouse or partner into their own therapy.

It was useful for the therapist, because he got a better sense of my partner.

[Female, 50, Nonprofessional]

I went with a boyfriend. It was helpful for the therapist to know who I was talking about in our sessions.

[Female, 59, Professional]

It was great. It was good for my individual therapy to have my partner there.

[Male, 49, Nonprofessional]

Sometimes bringing the partner can clarify some issues.

When I first started therapy, I was having trouble separating from my ex-boyfriend, and he was too, and we kept seeing each other. It was useful because it showed me how hopeless the situation was.

[Female, 42, Nonprofessional]

I once went to her with a guy I was dating. It wasn't anybody I had a really serious relationship with. It was someone with whom I was thinking of having a child, someone who would be more of a donor than a father. We went once together, and it was enormously illuminating, and that was the end of that idea.

[Female, 45, Nonprofessional]

This arrangement is not always productive.

It wasn't helpful because we didn't go to a neutral person, we went to her therapist. She had no reason to be interested in my perspective on things.

[Male, 52, Nonprofessional]

The role shift of the therapist can be difficult for the patient.

It was very hard to see her change roles from being my individual therapist to advocating for both of us.

[Female, 45, Nonprofessional]

One person described being on both sides of this situation.

When I went as a couple to my own therapist, I always felt that here was someone that would be on my team, that would help me to clarify certain issues that I couldn't articulate on my own. When I went to my partner's therapist, I always felt that it was very important that I clarify what my position was, because this person didn't know me, and it was two against one, and I was the one.

[Female, 48, Nonprofessional]

Some people said it had saved the relationship.

For a while it was useful, then it stopped being useful. Things shifted to focusing more on my wife's individual issues, and I didn't want to have to sit there and listen. Eventually we decided that she needed her own therapy. But for a while it was very useful—I think it saved my marriage.

[Male, 50, Professional]

Some people said couples therapy helped for a while, but did not resolve the basic problems.

It was useful in temporarily defusing what was becoming overtly hostile, but it was very short-lived.

[Male, 51, Nonprofessional]

I think that my partner and I were too good, and didn't bring up the real problems. It was early in our relationship and we were too intent on making a statement that we were going to be a couple.

[Female, 51, Professional]

By the time a couple seeks therapy, it may be too late.

My husband thought that the therapist would tell me to stay in the marriage, but he didn't and I didn't, so it didn't help.

[Female, 50, Nonprofessional]

It was not useful, because we were so estranged and had so many intractable problems by the time we got there.

[Male, 42, Nonprofessional]

It was a disaster. It probably encouraged and exacerbated the problems that led to the divorce. I don't know that I should blame the therapist. It's just that the circumstance enabled the issues to come up more readily.

[Male, 44, Professional]

A few people had had negative experiences. Sometimes this is due to the therapist.

I was in marriage counseling with a therapist who was totally off the wall. He used to do his sessions in his apartment, which was filled with folk art, totally bizarre stuff, kinetic sculptures, so I was totally distracted. He used to do the sessions in T-shirts with logos on them and running shorts. Actually, he was very smart. Occasionally, the phone would ring and he would answer it, because it was his father, who was very old and sick. He'd only stay on the phone for a few seconds, but still. . . .

[Female, 40, Nonprofessional]

It helped with some issues, but by and large I felt frustrated because I became the identified patient. It was a male therapist and he couldn't see the problems because my husband is very low-key.

[Female, 50, Professional]

The guy was awful. My boyfriend at the time was older than me, and had his Ph.D., and the therapist would call him Dr.—— and call me by my first name. I was appalled.

[Female, 50, Nonprofessional]

> I felt that the person I was involved with had a lot of issues to deal with, and I don't think the therapist pushed hard enough with him.
>
> [Female, 41, Nonprofessional]

A skilled therapist can make the process work.

> At first it was difficult. Since I had a lot of therapy before, I began to see some things that were technical in nature, in terms of how she was trying to work. I could see that she knew that my husband was more resistant at first to being there so she focused on me. Then when he was more familiar with the process she could focus on him, and then on us as a couple.
>
> [Female, 44, Nonprofessional]

Sometimes a bad experience feels like it is a result of the process itself.

> The first time we went it made things worse. It can stir up issues, and if the therapist isn't good at positive reframing and connecting a couple with the basic ground of their relationship, the positive aspects, you can go away feeling worse.
>
> [Male, 30, Professional]

NUMERICAL DISTRIBUTION

Professionals: Nineteen had been to couples therapy; only 1 had not; Of those who saw a couples therapist, 13 had a positive experience and 6 had a negative experience.

Nonprofessionals: Twenty-eight had gone to couples therapy; 12 had not. Of those who went, 19 had a positive experience; 9 had a negative experience.

COMMENTS

Couples therapy is an important variation on the theme of psychotherapy. The numbers in this question suggest that many couples therapists are not very good: a third of both groups had a negative experience.

As a therapist, I like couples work for the immediacy of the material and the speed of the impact: many couples start making changes very quickly.

Since long-term relationship is challenging and often difficult, I like, as the patient, knowing that my partner and I can get some help. Unfortunately, my own experience has been that, of the 7 therapists I have seen with a partner, none has been very helpful.

RELATED READING

Basham, K. (1992). Resistance and couple therapy. *Smith College Studies in Social Work* 62(3):245–264.

Friedman, R. C. (1991). Couple therapy with gay couples. *Psychiatric Annals* 21(8):485–490.

Jacobson, N. S., ed. (1993). Special section: couples and couple therapy. *Journal of Clinical and Consulting Psychology* 61(1):5–93.

Vansteenwegen, A. (1996). Who benefits from couple therapy? A comparison of successful and failed couples. *Journal of Sex and Marital Therapy* 22(1):63–67.

🔊🔊🔊🔊

Question 83: Were you ever in family therapy?

Family therapy is another modality available when problems arise. Bringing in the whole family can have an impact on the entire system, not just the individual patient. (Again, these responses refer to all therapies, not just the one in the main interview.)

Some people remembered that, when they were young, the whole family had gone to therapy. This is not always successful.

> When I was very young, I went to therapy with my parents, and I felt that the therapist was taking sides with my parents. I felt that my self-esteem was brought down by that. I was having anger toward my parents about things, and she would say that they must be right because they're the parents. So it was very frustrating.
> [Female, 28, Nonprofessional]

> I went many years ago, for 1 session. It was for my brother, to deal with whatever problem he had. It was awful, because my father didn't want to be there and made it terribly uncomfortable.
> [Female, 42, Nonprofessional]

> I was in when I was an adolescent. It was awful. The therapist was the worst therapist I could possibly imagine. She never asked me a

direct question. If she had, I would have spilled the beans on everything. I was just sitting there waiting. I couldn't tell her until she asked
because that would have been breaking the family rules, but if she
asked I could have told her.

[Female, 45, Professional]

I didn't think we needed to be there. My parents thought it was a
good idea.

[Female, 26, Nonprofessional]

We went once when I was a teenager, and it wasn't very helpful,
because the therapist did not seem very competent. I remember my
parents brought us all when they were having some real difficulties,
and I walked out thinking, "This guy is an idiot."

[Female, 46, Nonprofessional]

We did some sessions with my daughter and my husband. I thought
it was helpful at the time, but I found out later that my daughter had
not been very honest.

[Female, 50, Nonprofessional]

Sometimes it is successful in some way.

We saw a therapist with our daughter a few times. It got her into
treatment for an eating disorder.

[Female, 50, Professional]

My sister saw a therapist when she was younger, and I went in once
or twice because he asked to meet the rest of the family. It was
interesting because I was 16 and had always wondered what went
on in there.

[Female, 39, Nonprofessional]

Other people said they had brought the children into their own
therapy.

He referred one of my kids to a psychiatrist for medication.

[Female, 41, Nonprofessional]

We've had some sessions with our kids.

[Male, 53, Professional]

We've gone with our kids. It's extremely useful. Everybody gets to say their piece without fear.

[Female, 48, Nonprofessional]

Sometimes parents will attend sessions as part of a child's therapy.

When my stepdaughter was living with us, her father and I went to her therapist with her once or twice. It was not helpful. When she and I went alone it was helpful, because it enabled her to say some things to me that she hadn't when her father was present.

[Female, 50, Professional]

We went because my son was having migraines, and although they told us it was medical, I wasn't quite convinced. The therapist said he thought it was due to marital problems, and the family therapy turned into couples therapy, which turned into a divorce.

[Female, 51, Professional]

Adult patients will occasionally bring a parent in.

My mother went with me twice. I think it was useful. If nothing else, I felt a little respect for her for trying.

[Female, 48, Nonprofessional]

NUMERICAL DISTRIBUTION

Professionals: Five had been in family sessions; 15 had not. Of the 5 who had, 3 had a positive experience and 2 did not.

Nonprofessionals: Eleven said they had been in family sessions; 29 had not. Of the 11 who had; 7 had a positive experience and 4 had a negative experience.

COMMENTS

Only a quarter of each group had been in family therapy, which suggests that this modality is somewhat underutilized, though it's not clear why this is so.

As a therapist who does not generally do family work but who has specialized in working with adolescents, I like knowing that it's possible to work in a way that will deal with the dynamics of the family and not stigmatize my individual patient.

As the patient, I like the idea that everyone will be included in the problem and the solution. My own experience as a patient in family therapy is that it was useful temporarily, but the effects did not last long. Perhaps we did not stay in long enough.

RELATED READING

Brown, P. (1990). The wisdom of family therapists. *Clinical Social Work Journal* 18(3): 293–308.
Gurman, A. S., and Kniskern, D. P. (1992). The future of marital and family therapy. *Psychotherapy* 29(1):65–71.

⬚⬚⬚⬚

Question 84: Were you ever in group therapy?

Group therapy is another option when problems reflect interpersonal anxieties or conflicts. Many people had been in group therapy, either adjunctive to individual treatment or separately, sometimes following an individual treatment. (Again, responses to this question refer to all therapies, not just the one of the main interview.)

Most people had a good experience.

> I love group. It moves things along faster, especially coupled with my individual therapy. You get different things from each, and I find that I work harder and am much more aware of movement.
>
> [Female, 42, Nonprofessional]

> I enjoyed it very much and learned a tremendous amount about myself.
>
> [Female, 57, Professional]

> It's great. I love it. I love the interaction. I discover a lot about myself in interrelating and listening to the group and giving them feedback. I find the connection with other people really helpful to my own therapy.
>
> [Female, 45, Nonprofessional]

I loved it because of the universality of it. I liked seeing therapy done, and I liked seeing people learn from other people's therapy.

[Female, 52, Professional]

It was extremely beneficial because it was my first experience in therapy and shattered a lot of misconceptions about therapy. It gave me permission to have a lot of feelings that I had thought were out of bounds.

[Male, 46, Nonprofessional]

It was a very useful, very positive experience, expanding on the individual therapy I was in at the time.

[Female, 55, Professional]

You got a diverse group of people giving you feedback, so you see how you affect other people.

[Male, 49, Nonprofessional]

It gave me a chance to see how I appear to other people and to examine my own role in things in a different way. It gave me an arena to resolve interpersonal conflicts with other people.

[Female, 56, Professional]

Some people said group enhanced the relationship with the therapist.

It added a lot of dimension to my view of him, because I could see him doing things with other people, and it added some vitality to my relationship with him. I had a different view of him, I was sitting up, I could look at him more, I had more sense of being part of a family.

[Male, 53, Professional]

Several people mentioned learning some specific things about themselves.

I learned something about myself and how people perceived me and how I get along in groups. It became sort of a family supportive atmosphere and that was nice.

[Male, 42, Professional]

They had those soft bats [batakas] and one time I whaled into one of those, and I scared the group with the way I went at it. I had dust flying everywhere. It was a surprise to see that they were afraid of me.

[Male, 43, Nonprofessional]

Patients usually join a group at the therapist's suggestion, but a few people said they had asked for group.

I was a very motivated patient, and I requested that she start a group. I wanted a group experience with the same therapist. The value of that group was the transference issues, the support, the ability to watch the therapist in a group situation and experience different parts of her that I could then work with in individual therapy.

[Female, 47, Nonprofessional]

My therapist wanted me to be in a group but none of her groups were suitable. Finally I asked her to recommend somebody that would be suitable. She was just waiting for me to say that; she practically leapt out of her chair.

[Female, 42, Nonprofessional]

Some people said their feelings about group therapy were quite complicated.

It's wonderful and miserable at different times. It's wonderful when there's a charge in the room and a dynamic of feedback that you'd never get in any other context, or interactions that would never happen any other place. I feel like I can experiment in ways that I wouldn't be able to elsewhere. It's miserable when it feels like we're analyzing the process so much that we're not doing as much.

[Male, 30, Professional]

And each group is different.

I thought it was helpful, but since then, I've been in other groups where the leader felt more helpful, and I've looked back and thought that he could have done a better job of leading it. I got something out of it, but it could have been more helpful if my therapist then was like he is now.

[Male, 50, Professional]

I was in 2 different groups for long periods of time, and I got a lot out of group. In the first group, during my depression, that became a group issue. The therapist took me out of the group for a while because my depression was disruptive to the group. In the second group, I was a dominant member, very much so, and I really enjoyed going to that group because I could really mouth off in that environment in a way I couldn't anywhere else.

[Female, 48, Nonprofessional]

Several people mentioned that their view of and feelings about the group changed over time.

I found it incredibly helpful for a short period of time, feeling that there were other people around who had some of the same feelings. After a while, though, I didn't feel like I was getting any more out of it.

[Female, 46, Nonprofessional]

During the time I was going, it didn't seem helpful, but it retrospect it was.

[Female, 41, Nonprofessional]

Group is very subtle. Sometimes I feel like I'm not getting anything out of it. You don't see immediate results like with individual.

[Female, 42, Nonprofessional]

Some people felt that they didn't fit well into the group.

I felt that the people in the group were dealing with very serious issues, and I felt that they were in another league. I really didn't have much to say, and the group criticized me about that. It was frustrating, and that's why I quit.

[Female, 41, Nonprofessional]

At first I thought that the group was a very depressed group, and I was very insulted that he would put me into such a group. I wanted to be in his other group, but it didn't fit my schedule, so I stayed.

[Female, 59, Professional]

And some people said they didn't feel safe in the group.

It was during a period when I was very depressed, and there was a guy in the group who was very attacking, and I was very passive and didn't defend myself. The therapist didn't defend me either, and said I had to develop those skills. The fact is I have those skills, I was just in a bad way, and he didn't help at all. I probably shouldn't have been in a group at all during that time, because I didn't have much to give other people then.

[Female, 51, Professional]

I joined the group and 2 weeks later another person joined, and I never felt safe from her. She was always attacking me. I hated it.

[Male, 44, Professional]

Some criticisms were directed at the therapist.

I don't think the therapist was terribly skilled. I don't feel it really led anywhere.

[Male, 49, Nonprofessional]

It was poorly run. It was a therapy support group for the staff of a center where I worked, and the therapist was doing it pro bono. He had very loose boundaries and his commitment was inconsistent.

[Female, 45, Professional]

It was pretty bad. It was completely nondirective, and it was like a crybaby session.

[Female, 45, Nonprofessional]

My husband and I were in a couples group together with 4 couples. I didn't find it useful, because I don't think there was a good mix of couples and the therapist didn't do well with the group.

[Female, 44, Nonprofessional]

Some criticisms were directed at the process itself.

I tried a group, a new group that was formed there once. It didn't last; the group fell apart.

[Female, 48, Nonprofessional]

I don't quite understand the dynamics or how it transfers out or how you're supposed to feel toward the people in the group.

[Female, 50, Nonprofessional]

One person described an unusual situation.

My therapist had a group, and asked me if I wanted to come into the group, and I was really very interested in doing that. I had been in individual for about 6 years. So I joined and was in the group for about a year and a half. It was a Gestalt group, one-on-one therapy with the therapist in front of the group. I enjoyed watching other people work because I was in training at that point. Then she decided that she didn't want to do group any more. So everyone went back into individual therapy. But the group continued to meet without her for 3 more years, once a month. She was kind of amazed that we did it.

[Female, 45, Professional]

NUMERICAL DISTRIBUTION

Professionals: Fifteen had been in a group at some point; 5 had not. Of those who had, 11 had a positive experience and 4 had a negative one.

Nonprofessionals: Twenty had been in a group; 20 had not. Of those who had, 15 had a positive experience and 5 had a negative experience.

COMMENTS

A much higher percentage of the overall sample had been in group therapy than in couples or family therapy. Many therapists will recommend group as an adjunct to individual treatment, and this combination can be extremely powerful: the therapist gets to see the patient interact with others; issues raised in group can be worked on in individual sessions. The two have a synergistic effect.

As the therapist, I love leading a group, and my weekly group has been running continuously for over 16 years. When doing group, I try to keep the focus on the interactions in the room, which offer the most immediacy and emotional energy.

As the patient, I love the variety of the different people in group, and the challenge of being open and direct in the moment. At its best, group is more exciting even than individual therapy.

RELATED READING

Derr, D. B., and Zimpfer, D. G. (1996). Dreams in group therapy: a review of models. *International Journal of Group Psychotherapy* 46(4): 501–515.

Kleinberg, J. L. (1995). Group treatment of adults in midlife. *International Journal of Group Psychotherapy* 45(2):207–222.

Lipsius, S. H. (1991). Combined individual and group psychotherapy: guidelines at the interface. *International Journal of Group Psychotherapy* 41(3):313–327.

Shapiro, E. (1991). Empathy and safety in group: a self psychology perspective. *Group* 15(4):219–224.

꧁III꧂
The Ending

This section covers the end of treatment and the period afterward. Patients evaluated the therapy as a whole, with the perspective of several months or years to absorb what had occurred. Often some kind of connection and relationship continued after treatment ended.

Most people were happy with their treatment and the results they saw in themselves and their lives. Opinions about how the process works varied greatly, and some said that the process does *not* work.

Question 85: What made you stop going to therapy?

Therapy goes on for a few sessions or several years. At some point, the treatment terminates. How and why do patients decide that they have had enough and therapy is finished?

Patients have many different reasons for discontinuing treatment. Patients who have been satisfied with the therapy normally stop when they feel finished, or feel that they have had enough.

> I felt that it just seemed like a natural end, like a plateau or ending.
>
> [Female, 45, Nonprofessional]

> I didn't feel like I needed to go anymore.
>
> [Female, 62, Professional]

> I felt well, and the sessions were no longer making much difference.
>
> [Male, 51, Nonprofessional]

> I felt as if I had finished. I had gotten married, so it felt like my relationship issues were resolved. I was bored with the people in the group.
>
> [Female, 59, Professional]

> I wanted to graduate. I was able to move in with my boyfriend into a new and larger apartment. I had gotten tenure. I felt better about myself as a woman and a career person. A lot of the issues were resolved.
>
> [Female, 50, Nonprofessional]

> I felt that I had gotten as much as I could, and in a peculiar way I remember thinking, "This could go on forever."
>
> [Male, 42, Professional]

> I felt finished. I got what I came for.
>
> [Female, 56, Professional]

> I had had enough therapy.
>
> [Female, 51, Professional]

> I was feeling better and handling situations better. I felt we had accomplished our mission.
>
> [Female, 52, Professional]

Some people said that their life situations had changed, and therapy was no longer a priority.

> I got involved in a relationship with a woman, and I felt that I needed my time to myself. It didn't seem as important anymore.
>
> [Male, 42, Nonprofessional]

> I stopped soon after adopting my daughter, because I felt that I was entering into a new phase. I could have continued talking about things, but I didn't feel like working on them.
>
> [Female, 46, Nonprofessional]

> I just felt like stopping. I had just adopted a child and I felt like I wasn't the focus anymore.
>
> [Male, 46, Nonprofessional]

Sometimes the patient feels he or she has outgrown the therapist.

> I felt that I had outgrown her. I thought she was wishy-washy. I felt that she didn't have any more to offer me, and I felt that I was more powerful than she was.
>
> [Female, 50, Nonprofessional]

> I felt like she took me as far as she could. It would have been easier if she had acknowledged that, but she didn't, so it made ending unpleasant.
>
> [Female, 50, Professional]

> I realized I couldn't talk to her about certain issues. She had her own relationship with my brother, so I never made any progress with her on that. I felt like everything was too mixed up together. When my mother died, that's what broke it open for me. I went to her for that, and when I would cry she would get even more emotional than me, and she would say, "You'll help me when this happens to me."
>
> [Female, 45, Nonprofessional]

Some people said they stopped because therapy, while it had once been productive, didn't seem to be helping anymore.

> I was only in group, and I felt that the group was no longer challenging to me.
>
> [Female, 48, Nonprofessional]

Some people stopped out of dissatisfaction with the therapist or the therapy.

> It wasn't what I wanted.
>
> [Female, 48, Nonprofessional]

> I didn't think I was getting much out of being there. He wasn't giving me any guidance. It was very nonpsychotherapeutic. It was more like I could be talking to anybody. There was no meat being exposed. I was thinking of ending it and that same day he said, "I don't see the need for you to be here."
>
> [Female, 48, Nonprofessional]

> I really felt that the treatment was going nowhere, and I think she knew it too, and I'm a little resentful that she wasn't able to say something. Notice I'm putting it on her.
>
> [Female, 50, Professional]

Sometimes a termination occurs because of one or the other person relocating.

> I moved out of the city toward the end of therapy. We were pretty much finishing up, but I came in once a week to see him and go to group.
>
> [Female, 50, Professional]

> My therapist relocated to another city.
>
> [Male, 48, Nonprofessional]

> He left town. When he came back I saw him monthly, but that wasn't satisfactory.
>
> [Male, 30, Professional]

Occasionally the therapy stops because insurance coverage is no longer available.

> I had to switch insurance companies. I knew months ahead of time so I felt prepared and we kind of tailed off.
>
> [Male, 49, Nonprofessional]

> The insurance ran out and I didn't want to spend the full fee. And also the distance that I had to travel. And part of it was her rigidity, her lack of warmth and responsiveness.
>
> [Female, 62, Professional]

> I had access to her through my wife's health plan and when we divorced I lost that.
>
> [Male, 50, Nonprofessional]

Some people stopped because of an impasse with the therapist, a feeling of betrayal and failure.

> I quit because he didn't trust me to pay him what I owed him.
>
> [Female, 57, Professional]

> There was another horrible medical situation, and once again I felt he was failing me.
>
> [Female, 48, Professional]

> I stopped because of despair, feeling very depressed and at an impasse.
>
> [Male, 44, Professional]

A few people said they stopped because the problems seemed external.

> A lot of what I was going for was external to myself, and no matter how much I worked on me, the situation wasn't going to change.
>
> [Female, 47, Nonprofessional]

> The basic change happened because I found out my whole family was alcoholic, and once that became evident, the problems that had been generated by that became comprehensible. And quitting drinking solved a lot of problems. And so there was no need to keep being there.
>
> [Male, 52, Nonprofessional]

Stopping treatment may be hard, especially after many years, and patients may stay longer than they want.

> I was ready to leave 2 years before that but he made no move to terminate.
>
> [Female, 45, Nonprofessional]

> It took me a while to work up to stopping. I didn't trust my own feelings. I kept thinking, "What do I know? He's the therapist."
>
> [Female, 45, Nonprofessional]

The initial problem that I had gone for we had pretty much resolved. Other things came up along the way, and then it just seemed like I was groping for things to say. I was running out of things, and I would almost dread going because I wouldn't know what we were going to talk about. I started to feel like I was wasting my time and wasting her time.

[Male, 45, Nonprofessional]

NUMERICAL DISTRIBUTION

Professionals: (Some people gave more than one response.) Seven people said they stopped because they had felt finished; 6 because of a disagreement or disappointment with the therapist; 3 because either they or the therapist relocated; 3 because they had had enough; 1 because she had finished training; 1 because of the cost. One person was still in treatment.

Nonprofessionals: (Some people gave more than one response.) Eighteen people said they stopped because they had felt finished; 9 because of disappointment with the therapist; 5 because either they or the therapist relocated; 5 because they had had enough; 5 because of the cost.

COMMENTS

The percentages in response to this question are similar in the two groups. Most people stop when they feel they have completed whatever tasks or accomplished whatever goals brought them to therapy in the first place. Sometimes, of course, goals are modified or expanded as therapy opens things up and it seems possible to go even further. It's unfortunate that a quarter of each group stopped because of a conflict or disappointment with the therapist—this is not a good batting average for the therapists.

As the therapist, I want patients to stay long enough to get all that therapy has to offer, much of which they may not know when they begin. When patients express a desire to stop, I try to avoid creating a conflict about that, knowing that if it is easy to stop it will be easy to return in the future.

As the patient, I want my decision to stop to be respected, and I don't want to be pressured to stay. If I need more work that will almost certainly become evident to me, and I will return a far more motivated patient than if I allow the therapist to convince me to remain in treatment.

RELATED READING

Abarbanel, A. (1995). Consultation when the patient terminates an impaired treatment. *American Journal of Psychoanalysis* 55(4):347–363.

Beckham, E. E. (1992). Predicting patient dropout in psychotherapy. *Psychotherapy* 29(2):177–182.

Lane, R. C., and Hyman, M., eds. (1997). Special section on termination. *Psychoanalytic Psychology* 14(3):143–270.

Tryon, G. S., and Kane, A. S. (1995). Client involvement, working alliance, and type of therapy termination. *Psychotherapy Research* 5(3): 189–198.

℞℞℞℞

Question 86: What happened when you first talked about stopping?

When the patient decides to end treatment, the decision is usually announced and discussed with the therapist. Therapists have different reactions to this announcement.

Once the decision to stop is made, the patient normally announces it to the therapist, and the therapist may simply accept the decision.

> His reaction was positive. He felt that things were better, and suggested that I discuss stopping with my wife, because she's such a good observer, to see what her thoughts were.
>
> [Male, 51, Nonprofessional]

> I told her I didn't know what else to talk about, what else I needed to work on, and she tossed it back at me. We agreed that I would stop and see if I wanted to come back.
>
> [Female, 46, Nonprofessional]

Occasionally the therapist suggests it.

> I had decided to terminate, and he beat me to the punch. And that was it— there was no progression to termination; it was just the last session.
>
> [Female, 48, Nonprofessional]

I'm sure he mentioned it before I did. I tapered off: every other week, then once a month.

[Female, 52, Nonprofessional]

She actually suggested it. I was surprised, but at the same time I felt ready. I was sorry not to be seeing her anymore.

[Male, 52, Nonprofessional]

Sometimes patients stop therapy when they feel they have gotten as much as possible from that particular therapist.

I probably talked about stopping for years before I actually did. In some ways it was resistance. We tapered off, so it was mushy. It wasn't as clean as it should have been. Part of it was that I was upset with her, and so I was really pulling back. I needed her to have been more supportive of me about it, but I felt protective of her, I didn't want to hurt her feelings, and that made it harder to leave. She wasn't reluctant to let me, but I didn't feel encouraged. I had to do it on my own.

[Female, 50, Professional]

Sometimes patients quit in anger or disappointment.

When he likened our financial transactions to shopping at ShopRite, I went for a consultation. Once I did that, my feelings changed. I realized I was a big portion of his income. As a result of being in treatment with him I was going deeply into debt, and he would never lower the fee. When I told him I was planning to stop, he called me on the phone twice, the only calls in 13 years, and started telling me how much more mature he was than I was. As soon as he started doing that, I knew that there was something very seriously wrong with him.

[Female, 57, Professional]

Occasionally the therapist may try to repair the damage.

He was reluctant, but in the normal way. I ended it because I was so angry. I basically walked out. Then I wrote him a long letter, and he called me immediately, saying that he felt terrible that I was feeling so badly about the treatment. He was very humane and offered me an hour and a half session at no charge to talk about everything, which I did. I was touched by that, and it did help.

[Female, 48, Professional]

Usually the therapist is supportive, even encouraging, of the patient's decision to stop treatment.

> She was very supportive. She said that she would miss me and would miss the fun we did have in sessions.
>
> [Female, 52, Professional]

> She was fine about it, and said I could always come back if I wanted.
>
> [Female, 44, Nonprofessional]

Sometimes the therapist cautions the patient about the risks of stopping therapy.

> She tried to stay neutral but I could see that she had some issues with it. And she brought them up. Her words were, "I'm not sure that this is such a good time, and this is what I'm afraid might happen."
>
> [Female, 44, Nonprofessional]

> She wanted to know why, and she kind of talked me into not ending just then. I don't remember what her reasons were at the time. We kind of went back and forth about that for a while. We wound up cutting the frequency to every other week. I wasn't too happy with that. I didn't seem like I was working as intensely. So we went back to once a week before we eventually decided to end. She seemed reluctant for a while to let me stop.
>
> [Male, 45, Nonprofessional]

Most therapists seem to feel that termination should be a gradual process.

> He was fine with it. He wanted to talk about it, to make a plan and have it be a gradual process.
>
> [Female, 46, Nonprofessional]

> The first time she said she wanted to set a date 6 weeks from then, and we'd talk about it because she didn't think it was a good idea to stop abruptly. When I finally stopped it was in only one session.
>
> [Female, 42, Nonprofessional]

> It was a very gradual process. We talked about it for a couple of months. She seemed very glad that I was ready to go.
>
> [Male, 49, Nonprofessional]

There were one or two false stops, where I agreed to come back and talk about stopping. She encouraged me to think about whether I had done enough work on a particular issue.

[Male, 42, Nonprofessional]

The therapist may try to explore the patient's reason for leaving.

She encouraged me to continue, and wondered if the money issue was due to something with my husband, which it was. She was reluctant but that was okay; I didn't feel it was that she needed to hold on to me.

[Female, 62, Professional]

But sometimes the therapist actively opposes the patient's decision to leave.

Whenever I brought it up he'd try to talk me out of it. At one point he couldn't come to a session—he said he couldn't make it—and having that 2 weeks enabled me to write a letter saying I was stopping.

[Female, 48, Nonprofessional]

He said I was running away. I got resentful and angry, and it didn't change my mind.

[Male, 30, Professional]

She was surprised. She came back from a long vacation and things had really changed. She was very cautious about what was going on and really wanted to explore that. She was disappointed that we didn't do that.

[Female, 45, Professional]

I talked about stopping a number of times, and I was talked out of it. He said there was more stuff that I could work on.

[Female, 48, Nonprofessional]

I think he wanted me to stay and still work on some other issues. He seemed a little reluctant, but I worked on it for about 8 months.

[Female, 59, Professional]

When I first talked about stopping, years before I actually did, she would say we were not at an impasse and we had to work it through. Finally I didn't announce it, I just didn't go—I left phone messages. Finally she called me, and that was when I saw a display of real affect, a real anger. I wrote her a long letter explaining the issues. She left a phone message saying she had gotten the letter.

[Male, 44, Professional]

When the therapist opposes termination, that can make it more difficult for the patient.

At different times she did seem reluctant. And I felt guilty for leaving.

[Female, 47, Nonprofessional]

The therapist can have difficulty with the loss of a patient.

She was very hostile to me when I said I was leaving, and she said, "It's easier for you to leave your therapist than to leave your husband."

[Female, 45, Nonprofessional]

He had trouble with my severing the relationship. He had a good deal of personal anguish over it. I would have expected him to know when the therapy should have ended, and that it would be initiated by him. He seemed pained and startled.

He made some inappropriate comments with some sexual content. His feelings were beyond what should have been expressed by a therapist. That was his job, to deal with those feelings. He was reluctant, not in a controlling way, but it was clear that he hadn't even considered having me stop. He urged me to have a few more sessions at the very least, which I did, but then, when the sessions became a little strained because his feelings were clearly not in control, I wrote him a carefully worded letter in which I recounted some of what he had said and my responses. I also referred to how much we had accomplished, so it was also a loving letter, but then I stopped.

[Female, 45, Nonprofessional]

The therapist who accepts the patient's decision to stop treatment can make it easier for the patient to return to treatment later on.

Over the years he's had different reactions, but lately he says that I know what I'm doing, and I can always come back.

[Female, 50, Nonprofessional]

NUMERICAL DISTRIBUTION

Professionals: Ten people said the therapist had seemed reluctant to let them stop; 10 said this had not happened.

Nonprofessionals: Eleven people said the therapist had seemed reluctant to let them stop; 27 said there was no reluctance. Two therapies ended when the therapist relocated.

COMMENTS

A much greater percentage of the professionals (almost double) felt their therapists were reluctant to let them leave. Maybe the therapists felt it was more crucial for the professionals to resolve all their "pathology" if they were going to be seeing patients themselves.

As the therapist, I don't want to convey to the patient any reluctance beyond being sorry to lose the connection and the relationship. Anything that implies that I know better than the patient what he or she needs has to be condescending and alienating. This can be hard to do, especially when I don't think that the patient has given the process a fair chance or when it seems obvious to me that much remains undone.

As the patient, I will react badly to any sense that the therapist is trying to keep me there, unless I am absolutely certain that it's based entirely on concern for me. I don't want to feel that the therapist needs me to stay for financial or emotional reasons. If I am free to go then I am free to come back.

RELATED READING

DeBerry, S., and Baskin, D. (1985). Termination criteria in psychotherapy: a comparison of private and public practice. *American Journal of Psychotherapy* 43(1):43–53.

Dickes, R., and Strauss, D. (1979). Countertransference as a factor in premature termination of apparently successful cases. *Journal of Sex and Marital Therapy* 5(1):22–27.

Guy, J. D., French, R. J., Poelstra, P. L., and Brown, C. K. (1993). Therapeutic terminations: how psychotherapists say good-bye. *Psychotherapy in Private Practice* 12(2):73–82.

Mohl, P. C., Martinez, D., Ticknor, C., et al. (1991). Early dropouts from psychotherapy. *Journal of Nervous and Mental Disease* 179(8):478–481.

🐚🐚🐚🐚

Question 87: Have you had any contact with the therapist since you stopped going?

Even though therapy has ended, contact between patient and therapist often occurs.

Professionals will often see their former therapists at work-related events.

> I see him occasionally in a workshop.
>
> [Male, 30, Professional]

> I still see him for supervision.
>
> [Male, 53, Professional]

Post-termination contact sometimes involves referral of a patient.

> She has since referred people to me, and has called me about different subjects to get information.
>
> [Female, 52, Professional]

> She called me once, with a referral.
>
> [Female, 55, Professional]

Even a nontherapist may get a professional referral.

> She called me to refer the boyfriend of one of her patients for my particular type of therapy.
>
> [Female, 50, Nonprofessional]

Sometimes the contact between patient and therapist is planned.

> There was a charity event we were holding and he wanted to be part of it.
>
> [Female, 41, Nonprofessional]

> I went to a book signing of his.
>
> [Female, 48, Nonprofessional]

Occasionally the therapist initiates the contact.

A few months ago she sent me something that said the center was going to have some kind of group, but I was busy when the announcement came in; plus I wasn't that thrilled with the center.

[Female, 28, Nonprofessional]

She called me last week to wish me a happy new year, in response to a card I sent her. She left me a message and it was very warm and very kind.

[Female, 45, Nonprofessional]

I never call her, but she would call me occasionally, and we would talk briefly. Occasionally I'll write her a note. She just called me a month ago to thank me for a referral.

[Female, 40, Nonprofessional]

Chance encounters sometimes lead to contact after treatment.

I saw her at the movies once. I said hi and gave her a hug.

[Female, 45, Professional]

I ran into him on the street. It felt great to see him.

[Female, 50, Nonprofessional]

Patients are often comfortable with such encounters.

A couple of times I've run into him. It was really neat. The first time was at a spiritual event and he was there with his wife. I wasn't sure if I should engage with him, because I didn't know if you were supposed to. I said hello to them and introduced them to my boyfriend. The second time I saw him it was in a bookstore, and I didn't say hello. He and his wife were avidly looking for something and I let it pass.

[Female, 48, Nonprofessional]

Therapists sometimes seem awkward or uncomfortable.

I met him at a friend's wedding. He was very awkward about it. It's been a long time since I was his patient. I've referred people to him, and he's never acknowledged that. He called me once to say that he was publishing a paper about me and another person, and he would send it to me before he submitted it, and he never did that. I still have a lot of questions about it, but I never asked him about it. That

was the only time he's ever spoken to me as a person. I know that
he's avoided parties where he knows I might be there. I'm not his
patient anymore and I'm never going to be again. What's wrong with
the guy?

[Female, 58, Professional]

I saw her in the neighborhood, on the subway platform, and it
appeared that she was commuting to her office. She was exactly the
same, just as aloof, and she had the same mask on as she had in the
office. I said hello to her, and she was cordial, but I had the distinct
feeling that she was not comfortable having that kind of casual social
contact with one of her former patients. I saw her again later on but
didn't approach her that time.

[Male, 42, Nonprofessional]

Post-treatment contact is often by mail. The therapist may or may
not write back.

I sent her a birth announcement, and she sent back a congratulatory
card. I also wrote her about my husband's experience with a therapist
that she had recommended, who had done something I considered
outrageously unprofessional and inappropriate, so I wrote to give her
feedback.

[Female, 39, Nonprofessional]

I've written her a couple of times and she has written me back.

[Female, 41, Nonprofessional]

I send her Christmas cards. I've never heard from her.

[Female, 42, Nonprofessional]

Even mail contact can get complicated.

We talked about whether we could have any sort of communication
after she moved, and I suggested that I might want to write to her
and she indicated that she would be comfortable with that. We were
a little unclear as to what sort of communication that would be. I
wrote her a letter soon after we terminated, and I didn't hear from
her for a long time, and I wrote her another letter saying that I felt
very bad that I hadn't heard from her and asking if I had completely
misinterpreted what we had discussed, if I had misunderstood. I got
a letter back saying that she was sorry to hear that her not replying

had engendered all these feelings, and that she had never received my first letter. It was a very nice letter, and I wrote her another letter after that and didn't get a reply to that second letter, so I concluded that she's not as comfortable corresponding with me as she had thought she would be, and I'm a little hurt by that.
[Male, 48, Nonprofessional]

Occasionally there is telephone contact after treatment ends.

I did speak to him twice on the phone for some concrete advice, for his opinion about what I should do in a particular situation.
[Female, 46, Nonprofessional]

Something came up and we had a phone session.
[Female, 39, Professional]

Many people said they would go back for brief periods, often a single session.

I see her every 2 months or so. It's a support system.
[Female, 48, Nonprofessional]

I had one or two sessions afterward.
[Female, 59, Professional]

I'd like to set up a session and maintain the contact and fill her in on what's going on, to touch base. I'd like to do that on an occasional basis, every 6 months or so.
[Male, 49, Nonprofessional]

I would occasionally go back for "tuneups," for a session or two, to discuss a particular issue.
[Male, 42, Professional]

After I left and had my child, I had a very bad postpartum period, and it took me a while to realize what was happening. I called him and we had a few sessions, and he referred me to the therapist I started seeing in my new location.
[Female, 50, Professional]

Some people said they had some feelings about the question of contact with the former therapist.

I feel guilty about it, and have a fantasy that she died and I didn't even know about it.

[Female, 62, Professional]

I think about it sometimes. This is the awkwardness of it: I don't feel it's okay. I know she'd be happy to hear from me, but I never had that relationship with her. She always seemed a bit like a cipher, like a blank. If I were to do it now, I'd want it to be reciprocal. I think about going back to see her, but would it be a session? Would I have to pay for it? It's weird.

[Female, 50, Nonprofessional]

NUMERICAL DISTRIBUTION

Professionals: Twelve people said they had some contact with the therapist after termination; 7 said they had no contact. One person was still in treatment.

Nonprofessionals: Twenty-four people said they had contact after termination; 16 said they had not.

COMMENTS

Exactly the same percentage of each group answered this question affirmatively. In the professional group, contact often occurs in a professional context, and former therapists vary in their ability to make the shift to the new role. Social contacts can occur at any time (see also Question 80), and after termination patients will more often initiate these.

As the therapist, I enjoy hearing from former patients, learning how they are doing in life, reminding them of my availability. I keep a mailing list to let ex-patients know about my new book or a public presentation, and everyone gets a Christmas card. Most never respond, which is what I have learned to expect.

As the patient, I will send a former therapist a card when something significant happens in my life, and always appreciate some response when I do. I like getting mailings from previous therapists and finding out what they're up to. I might make a referral if I think they will work well together.

RELATED READING

Ryan, C. J., and Anderson, J. (1996). Sleeping with the past: the ethics of post-termination patient–therapist sexual contact. *Australian and New Zealand Journal of Psychiatry* 30(2):171–178.

Schachter, J. (1990). Post-termination patient–analyst contact: I. Analysts' attitudes and experience: II. Impact on patients. *International Journal of Psycho-Analysis* 71(3):475–486.

———(1992). Concepts of termination and post-termination patient–analyst contact. *International Journal of Psycho-Analysis* 73(1):137–154.

Wzontek, N., Geller, J. D., and Farber, B. A. (1995). Patients' post-termination representations of their psychotherapists. *Journal of the American Academy of Psychoanalysis* 23(3):395–410.

🕮🕮🕮🕮

Question 88: Have you ever made referrals to your former therapist?

Therapists depend to large degree on former patients as referral sources, and a satisfied customer is usually willing to recommend the therapist to others.

Many of the interviewees had referred new patients to their former therapists.

> I referred a friend of my mother.
>
> [Male, 53, Nonprofessional]

> The person I referred had the exact same reaction to the therapist as I did, but she didn't like it and didn't stay.
>
> [Male, 42, Nonprofessional]

> I've referred friends to her.
>
> [Female, 56, Professional]

> I referred one particular person, but that person is scared to death of therapy, which is why I referred her to this therapist—she's so non-threatening and accepting.
>
> [Female, 50, Nonprofessional]

Many others had not referred anyone yet but would if the situation arose.

> I haven't but I definitely would.
>
> [Male, 48, Nonprofessional]

> I haven't had occasion to, but I wouldn't hesitate for a second.
>
> [Female, 45, Nonprofessional]

Even when the therapy was not entirely successful, the patient may still be willing to make a referral.

> Once, when I thought it was helpful. As much as I have my reservations about her, she was still helpful.
> [Female, 44, Nonprofessional]

Several people said they would be very careful about making referrals.

> I don't know if I would—it would depend on who was asking.
> [Female, 44, Nonprofessional]

> I worry that I wouldn't be making a good referral, because so many people want quick fixes and this guy was not a quick fixer.
> [Male, 53, Professional]

> I would, but I wouldn't refer anyone with whom I was closely involved, because then they wouldn't be dealing with an impartial listener.
> [Female, 26, Nonprofessional]

And the therapist may be careful about accepting referrals.

> He won't take people that are connected, so when I referred someone who was, he saw them once and then referred them to someone else.
> [Female, 52, Nonprofessional]

But a few people would not make referrals, and explained why they would not.

> I wouldn't, because he's too rigid and compulsive.
> [Female, 57, Professional]

> He's just too rigid.
> [Female, 48, Professional]

> I don't think I would, because of the dual relationships that she's so comfortable with and I'm not.
> [Female, 45, Professional]

> My friends wouldn't be able to afford it. I could recommend her to someone more like her than I was. It seemed like we were from different worlds.
> [Female, 28, Nonprofessional]

I wouldn't, because he didn't help me.

[Female, 48, Nonprofessional]

I probably wouldn't, because I found someone better.

[Female, 41, Nonprofessional]

I would definitely not, because I didn't think he was a real therapist.

[Female, 48, Nonprofessional]

NUMERICAL DISTRIBUTION

Professionals: Thirteen said they had made referrals; 4 said they had not but would; 3 said they had not and would not.

Nonprofessionals: Twenty-five said they had made referrals; 11 said they had not but would; 4 said they had not and would not.

COMMENTS

Again there are similar percentages in the two groups. Most people either had made a referral or would if the situation came up. I wonder if many nonprofessionals realize how much the therapist depends on former patients for referrals of new patients.

As the therapist, I welcome referrals from ex-patients partly because I need them to stay in business. While I also get referrals from other professionals, I like a referral from an ex-patient because it confirms that the person had a good experience and wants someone important to her to have it, too.

As the patient, I want to share the benefits of good therapy with my friends and loved ones. I may also want to give the therapist to whom I feel grateful the gift of another patient.

RELATED READING

Cheston, S. E. (1991). *Making Effective Referrals: The Therapeutic Process.* New York: Gardner.

Haas-Wilson, D. (1990). Quality signals and patient referrals in the market for social workers' services. *Administration and Policy in Mental Health* 18(1):55–64.

Mayer, E. L., and deMarneffe, D. (1992). When theory and practice diverge: gender-related patterns of referral to psychoanalysts. *Journal of the American Psychoanalytic Association* 40(2):551–585.

⬚⬚⬚⬚

Question 89: What did the therapist do or say that was most helpful?

Most people said that the therapist had been helpful overall, but some special aspects of the therapist's behavior or particular moments stood out.

Several people mentioned the therapist's calm acceptance and support as significant.

> She absolutely believed in me. I felt her respect for my experience. Her constancy, dependability, and reliability.
>
> [Female, 45, Professional]

> It was her loving acceptance and sympathy.
>
> [Male, 49, Nonprofessional]

> It was the way that he listened. He always looked like he was 100 percent present.
>
> [Female, 59, Professional]

> He nurtured and he taught me to listen to and nurture my "inner child." He pointed out that, no matter how bad I was, no matter how depressed I was, he made me see that I had a spirit in me that was beautiful, and it manifested itself in ways that I had previously judged to be bad. He showed me that I had a great spirit and that I should honor it and listen to it and pay attention to it.
>
> [Male, 46, Nonprofessional]

> He listened well and didn't get rattled, even when my life took very extreme turns, and really stayed with me emotionally.
>
> [Male, 53, Professional]

Many people said that this attitude helped them accept themselves.

> She provided an extremely accepting, uncritical, nonjudgmental environment. We spent a lot of time talking about issues relating to the "false self," and I think she created a situation in which I could become very grounded and rooted in an authentic self. We talked a lot about my parents and their many inadequacies, and she helped me work through a lot of them. She was relentlessly, consistently on my side. Even when I was negative and judgmental, she refused to

be. She absolutely refused to join me in self-criticism. She was always consistently finding the sympathetic and nonjudgmental interpretation for things in me or my behavior that I was negative about. She reframed those things. But also by the way she was responding, she was demonstrating a different way to feel and think about myself.

[Male, 48, Nonprofessional]

One time when I told him I was really feeling like a piece of shit, he held my hands and told me he didn't think I was a piece of shit. He was really there for me. He absorbed a lot. He believed in me.

[Male, 50, Professional]

It was his general attitude of letting me off the hook, because I tend to beat myself up a lot.

[Male, 48, Nonprofessional]

I tend to feel very guilty and blame myself for things that are not going well in my life, and she helped me to objectify that.

[Female, 62, Professional]

The most helpful thing was to bolster my self-esteem and talk about the whole process subtly changing the voice inside, so that I wouldn't hear that critical voice so loud.

[Female, 42, Nonprofessional]

When I wasn't aware of how horrendous something was, she would point it out, things that she thought were just unacceptable. She also confirmed my emotions, that it was okay to be sad, that I had every reason to be angry.

[Female, 50, Nonprofessional]

She encouraged me to tell her the truth of how I was experiencing her, not just the facts but the feelings. She really made it safe for me to delve into all of my feelings.

[Male, 52, Nonprofessional]

One of the things he talked about was that I tend to do too much in life. Like when I shovel snow off the sidewalk I would have to fight the urge to shovel all the way to the end of the block. My life is filled with all sorts of obligations and responsibilities. One of the things we worked on was getting to the point where I could feel comfortable doing what I had to do and not doing more than that.

[Female, 41, Nonprofessional]

Other people said that the therapist's attitude helped normalize what they were feeling.

> She gave me the feedback that my perceptions were appropriate, accurate, and valid, and that was what going on for me was real.
> [Female, 48, Nonprofessional]

> She tolerated the experience of all my stuff for all those years.
> [Male, 44, Professional]

> When she gave me some things to fill out, it made me feel that there were other people who had similar problems. She also gave me a handout on anxiety, and that was helpful, because it explained a lot of what was going on.
> [Female, 28, Nonprofessional]

> There were certain guidelines that were very useful to me in gauging how crazy I am in a particular situation, and a look from him that reassured me that I was okay.
> [Female, 52, Nonprofessional]

> When she asked me why I was going, why I needed her, I told her what was going on and she said it sounded to her like everything was fine and she didn't see why I needed to be there. It was reassuring, and it stimulated me to look closer at my situation.
> [Female, 53, Nonprofessional]

> He told me that all the weird stuff I was thinking was normal weird stuff, which made me feel comfortable about the process. At one point, I had a lot of stuff on my mind, and he told me that he would keep it for me, that I could leave it in his office.
> [Female, 48, Nonprofessional]

Some people said the therapist helped them understand themselves better.

> She made me aware of relationships in my childhood that very much affected my adult relationships. She helped me realize a lot of things that I was just oblivious to.
> [Female, 45, Nonprofessional]

> He helped me understand how certain traumatic events in my childhood history surrounding my parents' separation and divorce affected

me, and affected my identity in ways that I hadn't realized, and he made connections with that for me.

[Male, 42, Professional]

She guided me through a lot of the childhood stuff, which was very helpful. She really helped me understand the difference between going in to try to get a specific answer to a specific question, and unraveling a set of issues and complexities, and made some very good characterizations or definitions of my own psychic processes.

[Male, 50, Nonprofessional]

He provided a rationale for my issues, a pattern that was insightful.

[Female, 48, Nonprofessional]

I got a real understanding and ability to make connections between my early illness as a child and who I am today.

[Female, 47, Nonprofessional]

Several people said the therapist was especially helpful in the area of relationship.

Before I was dating my husband, I was in a relationship with a man who was not emotionally available, and he helped me get out of that relationship. Then when I was dating my husband, I was afraid that he wasn't available either, and my therapist said that he was available, so I stuck it out and ultimately married him.

[Female, 57, Professional]

It was very specific. She said that I absolutely had to have a separate space from my boyfriend, that it never could work with just one space.

[Female, 50, Nonprofessional]

She helped me deal with one of my kids, and showed me how I was being rigid, and I think she helped me save that relationship.

[Female, 51, Professional]

She was able to draw from conferences and books, to bring in fact-based stuff relevant to feelings I was having. She was able to draw me a diagram of a relationship pattern, or a sibling pattern, that helped me. It provided a conceptual framework that was very helpful.

[Female, 39, Professional]

Several people said the therapist helped them deal with certain behaviors or symptoms that were troubling them.

> I always had a lot of difficulty in elevators, and he related that to certain sexual fears, and the connection became so obvious to me at that point that I haven't been afraid in an elevator since.
>
> [Male, 53, Nonprofessional]

> He showed me how to let my anger out in different ways than I had been using.
>
> [Male, 43, Nonprofessional]

Others said that the therapist became a role model for certain behaviors and feelings.

> It was the way she was, very unassuming and down-to-earth. She didn't have a lot of money and wasn't into material things, and that was appealing to me.
>
> [Female, 42, Nonprofessional]

> I had parents who never admitted that they made any mistakes, although they made lots of them, and the first time I called him on something where I thought he was wrong, he listened and said, "Yes, I think that wasn't the right thing to say. I'm sorry, I made a mistake." That was a big deal, and was very powerful.
>
> [Female, 50, Professional]

> There was a certain kind of patience that I learned from.
>
> [Male, 51, Nonprofessional]

> She was a great role model for me in getting angry. She would get very angry about things I was telling her that my father had done.
>
> [Female, 45, Professional]

Some people mentioned specific ways of working that the therapist used.

> She worked a lot with fantasies, not dreams but conscious fantasies, and I had never really wanted to touch that kind of material, but I trusted her enough to look at it, and it was very fruitful.
>
> [Female, 51, Professional]

> This happened almost every session. I would get going, get talking, and she would stop me, tell me to sit back in the chair and close my eyes and breathe, and it was her way of telling me I was stuck in my head and not touching what it really was.
>
> [Female, 46, Nonprofessional]

One thing really stands out in my mind. When I was in a lot of passive resistance and withholding she sent me home in the middle of a session, and it was intense. I don't know if it would be appropriate for everyone but it was for me. It really made me bring up a whole lot of other issues.

[Female, 45, Professional]

She was very consistent in her way of putting me on the spot so I had to talk. Otherwise we would have had long silences that would have been very uncomfortable. She had a good sense of humor, was always willing to laugh, and would put me at ease that way.

[Male, 42, Nonprofessional]

He took a sledgehammer to my rigid thinking. Every time I think I have things figured out, or have a perspective, then he moves and I fall over.

[Male, 30, Professional]

A few people mentioned specific suggestions that the therapist made.

It was when she suggested antidepressants.

[Female, 44, Nonprofessional]

It was her idea to take out a personal ad, through which I met my current partner.

[Female, 51, Professional]

NUMERICAL DISTRIBUTION

Professionals: Six people mentioned caring and supportiveness; 5 said the therapist helped them understand something important; 3 said useful interpretations; 3 said listening and understanding them; 1 said the therapist was a role model; 1 said the therapist challenged their beliefs and assumptions; 1 said the therapist was able to admit a mistake.

Nonprofessionals: Twelve people said the therapist provided safety and support; 12 said the therapist helped them understand something specific; 4 said it was the way the therapist listened and understood them; 4 said they felt validated; 2 said the therapist helped them set boundaries; 2 said the therapist taught them a specific skill; 1 said it was the caring of the therapist; 1 said the therapist was a role model. Two people said they could not select anything.

COMMENTS

The two groups had similar responses to this question—not surprising, since people are people and need what they need no matter what kind of work they may do.

As the therapist, I'm trying to provide whatever the patient needs, though I may be surprised when something specific has special meaning or impact. It's always different for each person—what is special to one patient won't necessarily have any special impact for the next one—so it's not possible to develop a collection of sure-fire interventions. Trying for the clever intervention and the dramatic moment raises the risk of making a major mistake.

As the patient, I prefer consistency and dependability to bold strokes, but there will probably be something I'm not expecting that will touch me in some special way. Looking back, these moments will stand out for me as turning points in the therapy.

RELATED READING

Allison, K. W., Crawford, I., Echemendia, R., et al. (1994). Human diversity and professional competence: training in clinical and counseling psychology revisited. *American Psychologist* 49(9):792–796.
Blau, T. H. (1988). *Psychotherapy Tradecraft: The Technique and Style of Doing Therapy*. New York: Brunner/Mazel.
Greenberg, J. (1996). Psychoanalytic interaction. *Psychoanalytic Inquiry* 16(1):25–38.
Kron, T., and Friedman, M. (1994). Problems of confirmation in psychotherapy. *Journal of Humanistic Psychology* 34(1):66–83.

℞℞℞℞

Question 90: What did the therapist do or say that was not helpful?

Not everything the therapist says is going to have the desired effect. In spite of the best intentions, therapists can offer things that simply don't work.

Several people said that when the therapist took a position that felt rigid to them it was not useful.

It wasn't any one thing he said. It was his rigidity. I chose him only because he was so good as my supervisor. We had so much in common, so many interests, and when he became my therapist all of that stopped. It was as if we didn't know these things about each other. And the warm relationship we had as supervisor/supervisee disappeared. That was not helpful at all.

[Female, 57, Professional]

I drove an hour to get there and an hour back, and I was the first appointment of the day and this particular day I was in a hurry to get back. I saw her in the coffee shop before the session and asked if we could possibly start early so I could leave early, and she wouldn't do it.

[Female, 62, Professional]

When my husband got very sick, I was very scared and he was being classically analytical and said nothing about it. He just didn't react.

[Female, 48, Professional]

Sometimes the patient can feel abandoned or unsupported by the therapist.

She genuinely had difficulty addressing my feelings for her.

[Male, 44, Professional]

It was ironic, because my major issue was having confidence in my own decision making, and I felt that every time I would say anything he would ask, "Well, what makes you think that?" Which could have been a good exercise, a reality check, but it never felt that way, so I felt undermined.

[Female, 48, Nonprofessional]

Her support of the institute was really not helpful at all.

[Female, 62, Professional]

I remember there was one session where she said one word, and I don't remember what the word was, but I remember that I brooded about it all week and then I came in and discussed it. I had taken it as a judgment and I was wounded by it, and she was really quite upset to hear that, because she had meant it in a nonjudgmental way. It was very sobering for her, because I'm extremely sensitive to language and she had used a word thoughtlessly. She was quite surprised to see how much effect that had had. She didn't get defensive. I think she dealt with it very well.

[Male, 48, Nonprofessional]

Others mentioned situations in which they felt misunderstood or let down by the therapist.

> There was one point where I was involved with someone, a woman who did something that I thought was really very disturbed behavior. I was very upset by it and I needed his feedback and needed him to validate my perceptions of what was going on in order to feel stronger about separating from this person, and he said that he felt I was trying to control him. I got very angry that he said that, because even if it was true, he was missing the level of anxiety that I was feeling, and my need for his support in being able to separate from someone who had exhibited very disturbed behavior that could be hurtful to me, but to whom I was still attached. His reaction undermined my striving to do that. I told him that and we spent a number of sessions talking about it.
>
> [Male, 42, Professional]

> She said after I had been seeing her a while, after the terrible breakup between me and a particular woman, that she had always thought we were such a terrific couple, a natural relationship. It bothered me that after that amount of time she could say something like that.
>
> [Male, 52, Nonprofessional]

> He minimized the real elements in what was upsetting me, and focused only on the psychological aspects without acknowledging the facts. Also, he never validated feelings that I was having about him.
>
> [Female, 58, Professional]

> There was one night in group where I was about to go in for surgery and I said at the beginning of the session that I didn't even want to be there, and he let the group attack me. I felt very wronged by him. It was the only time I felt that way. When I got home from the session, he called me that night, and said that he felt he should have stopped them and he was sorry.
>
> [Female, 50, Professional]

> In couples therapy, he would always focus on how my partner didn't feel safe and therefore couldn't make a commitment, and I always felt that was the wrong path. Years later my partner acknowledged that it wasn't the real issue, it was his anger. We spent so much time on the feeling safe issue, and it wasn't at all helpful.
>
> [Female, 41, Nonprofessional]

Some people said the therapist made recommendations that either did not seem right for them or turned out badly.

> There have been times when I've been frustrated, because he has been repetitive with suggestions about how to be with myself, and he kept giving me those suggestions in many different ways in many sessions.
>
> [Male, 30, Professional]

> One of the issues I had was about my daughters from whom I am estranged, and he suggested writing again to the younger one. I did, but it turned out she had moved, and I felt bad when the letter came back.
>
> [Male, 51, Nonprofessional]

> There was a period where he got involved in a mixture of bodywork and spiritual stuff, postural integration, rebirthing, and I couldn't relate to it at all. It came to a point where I told him I couldn't do those things, and he was treating that as resistance, and I told him we couldn't deal with it that way. I told him he had to work with me in a primarily verbal way, and he had to make sure that I was not left with the feeling that I was getting a second-rate therapy because I wasn't doing the other stuff.
>
> [Male, 50, Professional]

> Sometimes she would go into these discussions about things that she had read that she thought might be relevant, but I didn't think that was helpful.
>
> [Female, 44, Nonprofessional]

> Sometimes when I would talk about my work, which was in advertising, she never really got it, and I felt that she didn't understand the demands of that kind of work, and would say things like, "You don't need to do that," but if I didn't do it I wouldn't have a job. She was a little naive about the business world. So I stopped talking about that stuff.
>
> [Female, 45, Professional]

> When I really wanted to end my marriage, and I was feeling like that's it, I want out of here, she encouraged me to stay and work, and sometimes I wonder if she wasted 6 months for me.
>
> [Female, 40, Nonprofessional]

> He was a proponent of Albert Ellis and rational-emotive therapy, and he thought I needed assertiveness training, and it was true. I would

not do the things he wanted me to do. He wanted me to randomly call phone numbers and talk to whoever answered. He wanted me to go into a store and get change for a $20 bill and then go into the next store and get a $20 bill for the change. I really don't enjoy doing those things, and I didn't see the value of doing them. Also he was in his fifties and unmarried, so I wasn't interested in his advice about marital relationships. He thought I was repressed and suggested that I go out and have an affair. I thought that was really inappropriate.

[Male, 53, Nonprofessional]

Several people said they reacted badly when the therapist seemed to be advancing his or her own agenda.

She became a real feminist over the time we were working together, and when she got into a sociopolitical interpretation of my behavior, I really got pissed.

[Female, 50, Professional]

She did a lot of work with incest survivors, and fairly early on in therapy, I thought she was leading me in that direction. It didn't ring true for me, and I was a little bothered to think that might be her agenda. She let it go when I said it wasn't resonating for me.

[Female, 46, Nonprofessional]

There were moments that she would go a little ahead of me. It was usually out of enthusiasm, and not a pressure.

[Female, 45, Professional]

She told me that I wasn't going to get better unless I could start loving my father again, or forgive him, and I didn't then and don't now find either of those tenable solutions.

[Female, 39, Nonprofessional]

Several people said their therapists talked too much, about themselves or about others.

There were times when I just didn't want to hear about his daughter and how wonderful her life was when my kid was having a hard time.

[Female, 50, Nonprofessional]

Sometimes she would talk about herself, and I didn't need that. I was always curious, so I would listen, but I didn't need it.

[Female, 51, Professional]

She shared too much information with me about herself.
[Female, 45, Nonprofessional]

The references to other patients really turned me off.
[Female, 39, Professional]

NUMERICAL DISTRIBUTION

Professionals: Five people said it was a lack of understanding, acceptance, or support over a particular issue or in general; 3 said it was the therapist's rigidity; 3 said it was a particular intervention or technique; 2 said the therapist was controlling or pressuring; 2 said the therapist disclosed too much; 1 said the therapist failed to protect her in group. Four people could not specify anything.

Nonprofessionals: Five people said the therapist showed a lack of understanding, acceptance, or support at some point; 4 said the therapist tried to get them to do something that felt wrong for them; 3 said the therapist disclosed too much; 3 said the therapist wasted time on his or her own agenda; 2 said the therapist used an intervention or technique that was of no help; 1 said the therapist had poor boundaries. Twenty-one people said the therapist never did anything that really did not help, and 1 person said that nothing the therapist did was of any help.

COMMENTS

Any therapist can misjudge the effectiveness or impact of a remark, interpretation, or suggestion. Most of these complaints above, however, seem to refer to situations in which the therapist was told that an intervention was not useful and yet he or she persisted in it.

As the therapist, I want to hear when something I do works or fails to work, and the reasons for the outcome. I can't imagine continuing in a particular behavior after being told that it was objectionable, unless it is so much part of who I am that I simply can't stop.

As the patient, I need to feel free to say when I don't like what the therapist is doing, and I will watch carefully what happens after that. I will give the therapist I trust some latitude, but I need to see that he is at least trying to incorporate my feedback and modify his behavior. Otherwise, we are going to have a problem.

RELATED READING

Bader, M. J. (1994). The tendency to neglect therapeutic aims in psychoanalysis. *Psychoanalytic Quarterly* 63(2):246–270.

Basescu, S. (1990). Tools of the trade: the use of the self in psychotherapy. *Group* 14(3):157–165.

Faimberg, H. (1995). Misunderstanding and psychic truths. *International Journal of Psycho-Analysis* 76(1):9–13.

Schwaber, E. A. (1992). Countertransference: the analyst's retreat from the patient's vantage point. *International Journal of Psycho-Analysis* 73(2):349–361.

ಜ಼ಜ಼ಜ಼ಜ಼

Question 91: What was the best thing about your therapist? (See also Question 89.)

Every therapist has many different qualities, personality traits, habits and behaviors, knowledge and experience. What was valued most by the patients?

Many people mentioned the therapist's warmth and caring.

> She was very receptive and soft, and sympathetic. She's the only therapist I really felt accepted by. She had a lot of empathy.
>
> [Female, 50, Nonprofessional]

> He always gave me the impression that he really cared and took it very seriously and that it was purposeful and encouraging and important.
>
> [Female, 46, Nonprofessional]

> It was her warmth. She really gave off such humanity and sincere caring. It made it possible for me to be so trusting of her as to visit some very dark places. I felt very safe.
>
> [Female, 45, Nonprofessional]

> Generally the feeling that she listened and valued who I was. I really appreciated that.
>
> [Male, 52, Nonprofessional]

> She was very reassuring through the entire time I saw her. She was very calm and soft.
>
> [Female, 53, Nonprofessional]

It was her loving acceptance.

[Male, 49, Nonprofessional]

Others said the therapist's calm acceptance and flexibility.

It was her centeredness. She seemed solid and centered and wasn't jolted by anything.

[Female, 50, Professional]

It was her consistent relentless acceptance.

[Male, 48, Nonprofessional]

It was his composure, his comfort with talking about anything and everything.

[Male, 53, Professional]

I felt that I could really say anything. He was completely unimposing of his own agenda. He was uncontrolling, soothing, accepting.

[Female, 48, Professional]

It was her endurance and tolerance.

[Male, 44, Professional]

Some mentioned the therapist's intelligence and cognitive skills.

She was very smart, and I liked the way she practiced therapy. I knew what she was doing, but it was wonderful that she could do it the way she did.

[Female, 62, Professional]

He always seemed to have a good sense of picking up where we left off. I guess it was his memory. It led to a kind of seamless progression from session to session.

[Female, 41, Nonprofessional]

She's brilliant, absolutely brilliant. She understands process in a very deep way. She brings a dimension of humanness into the therapy that deepens the work and is very growthful.

[Female, 45, Professional]

Others focused on the therapist's ability and experience.

He had the talent or the gift to use whatever was happening in a way that worked.

[Male, 46, Nonprofessional]

He had a very good knowledge base. He was very well-trained, and intelligent.

[Female, 57, Professional]

He seemed to really know what he was doing, and he was really competent.

[Male, 48, Nonprofessional]

She was wise.

[Female, 52, Professional]

Some mentioned the therapist's integrity and trustworthiness.

I felt her to be extremely solid and extremely ethical, and I trusted her very much.

[Female, 47, Nonprofessional]

He was so honest and straightforward.

[Female, 52, Nonprofessional]

She was very decent, she was trustworthy, and she tried hard.

[Female, 55, Professional]

Several people said it was the therapist's encouraging support.

He was able, without being laid back or easygoing, to help me focus on my own needs. He told me that if I were more aware of my behavior I would be better able to make decisions about how to conduct my life that would make me a more responsible and ethical person. Since that's a worthy goal, I went for it.

[Female, 45, Nonprofessional]

He was willing to take into consideration what I thought would be best for me. He had a capacity to relate to me as a colleague and an equal while at the same time treating me like a patient.

[Male, 42, Professional]

Some people mentioned some quality of the therapist's personal style.

She was very unassuming and down-to-earth. She didn't have a lot of money and wasn't into material things, and that was appealing to me.

[Female, 42, Nonprofessional]

It was her sensitivity, and her ability to work on a level that wasn't intellectual.

[Female, 46, Nonprofessional]

She's a very thoughtful person. She never made flip comments—she would think about things.

[Female, 42, Nonprofessional]

She had a good sense of humor, and was able to laugh with me.

[Male, 42, Nonprofessional]

NUMERICAL DISTRIBUTION

Professionals: (Some people gave more than one response.) Five people mentioned the therapist's calm presence; 5 mentioned the therapist's intelligence; 4 people said the therapist's openness and acceptance; 3 said experience or skill; 3 said warmth and caring; 3 said consistency and reliability; 2 said gentleness and flexibility; 2 said trustworthiness; 2 said integrity; 1 said the effort.

Nonprofessionals: (Some people gave more than one response.) Fourteen people said the therapist's warmth, caring, and supportiveness; 10 said the therapist's skill and experience; 7 said the therapist's openness and acceptance; 4 said intelligence; 4 said the therapist's calm presence; 2 said the therapist's integrity. One each said: gentleness; trustworthiness; consistency; responsiveness; patience; memory; and sense of humor.

COMMENTS

Again there were similar responses from the two groups, although the professionals didn't seem to need the therapist to be warm and caring as much as the nonprofessionals did, and emphasized more the therapist's calm self-assurance and skill. All of the qualities mentioned are important, and all appear in good therapists in various proportions.

As the therapist, I value most in myself my calm and my confidence, which are a result of the other qualities (skill, experience, openness, etc.), and which seem to allow the patient to calm down, too. My lack of distress or disturbance at whatever the patient tells me normalizes that material for the patient and allows him to look at it with more objectivity and less shame.

As the patient, I value all the qualities mentioned above, especially skill, intelligence, warmth, experience, and sense of humor—whatever makes the therapist a genuine human being inside the role of therapist.

RELATED READING

Blatt, S. J., Sanislow, C. A., Zuroff, D. C., and Pilkonis, P. A. (1996). Characteristics of effective therapists: further analyses of data from the National Institute of Mental Health Treatment of Depression Collaborative Research Program. *Journal of Consulting and Clinical Psychology* 64(6):1276–1284.

Mahrer, A. R. (1996). Lessons from 40 years of learning how to do psychotherapy. *Psychotherapy* 33(1):139–141.

Miller, L. (1993). Who are the best psychotherapists? Qualities of the effective practitioner. *Psychotherapy in Private Practice* 12(1):1–18.

Owen, I. (1995). The personalities of psychotherapists. *Counselling Psychology Review* 8(3):10–14.

⬙⬙⬙⬙

Question 92: What was the worst thing about your therapist?

Therapists have good qualities and some not-so-good qualities. The range of those qualities mentioned varies quite a lot.

Some people mentioned the therapist's rigidity or inflexibility.

> The worst thing about him was his pathological, unresolved obsessive-compulsiveness.
>
> [Female, 57, Professional]

> It might have been nice if I could have sometimes gone past the 50 minutes. She was really very rigid about the time thing. I hear people talk about how their therapy session was so heavy and it ran over, and I think she was very rigid about that. Sometimes I wonder if she's just a rigid human being.
>
> [Female, 40, Nonprofessional]

She was a stickler for procedure, rigid in her way of approaching therapy.

[Female, 62, Professional]

Others mentioned a passivity, a cautiousness, or a lack of courage.

He could never be definite about anything.

[Male, 30, Professional]

She didn't give me any guidance about how to do therapy.

[Female, 44, Nonprofessional]

At times she could be tentative. I wanted her to tell me what to do, or say that this was exactly what was going on, and she couldn't do that. At first I found that very difficult. Later I came to value that she wasn't going to tell me what to do, and she was going to make me decide things for myself.

[Male, 52, Nonprofessional]

There was a certain cautiousness or tentativeness that you would expect to see in someone who had a British upbringing, a certain reserve. I never felt he was cold or distant or detached—there was always warmth and friendliness—but it was a cautiousness that probably affected his analytic technique and made him a little more careful and tentative in the way he worked. There were times when I would have preferred that he just come out and share what he was thinking in a more spontaneous free way.

[Male, 42, Professional]

Some people said that the therapist was not a real person with definition and presence, and identified the worst quality as distance and anonymity.

She didn't share enough of herself.

[Female, 47, Nonprofessional]

Sometimes she seemed too ethereal.

[Female, 50, Professional]

There was no depth, no presence.

[Female, 44, Nonprofessional]

Maybe it would have helped if she did talk a little more about herself, to give some insight, or even examples of other people she knew, so I wouldn't feel like I was the only one.

[Female, 28, Nonprofessional]

Maybe that she didn't share more of her personal life with me, though I've come to understand that's not necessary or productive.

[Female, 48, Nonprofessional]

I would have liked him to talk more.

[Male, 48, Nonprofessional]

Sometimes he was too quiet and hard to read. I'm not sure he addressed my aggression explicitly enough.

[Male, 53, Professional]

I had trouble with his nonreactivity. I think if I were to go back to him I would be more confrontational and more direct, and insist that he discuss things more.

[Female, 41, Nonprofessional]

Sometimes this came across to the patient as artificiality.

Particularly in the early sessions, she smiled too much. It was a very false, uncomfortable, social smile, and I told her about it, and we spent a good deal of time on this.

[Male, 48, Nonprofessional]

Several people mentioned a lack of skill, an inability to provide what the patient needed.

She couldn't cut through. In hindsight, she could have given me a different way of looking at things. If she could have role-played with me it would have been helpful.

[Female, 50, Professional]

What most frustrated me about the experience was that I thought we could have gotten deeper, that we didn't get as deep as we might have.

[Male, 49, Nonprofessional]

She had certain blind spots. I kept trying to discuss psychoanalytic theory with her, and she was very limited. She knew her one way, which was actually excellent technique, but her whole rationale for it was a very limited Freudian one, so you couldn't really discuss anything with her. She always had a very ready answer for everything, and the subject was closed.

[Female, 62, Professional]

There was only a certain point you could go to with him. He was limited.

[Female, 46, Nonprofessional]

She would tell me specific things, she wouldn't help me learn. I thought she was going to help me understand my problems better, but I ended up having to sort it out myself. I would have enjoyed getting more input: advice, suggestions, ideas.

[Male, 42, Nonprofessional]

She was lacking in the kind of insight I needed. She was limited.

[Female, 55, Professional]

He was completely ineffective.

[Female, 48, Nonprofessional]

Some mentioned structural violations of various sorts.

She had no boundaries.

[Female, 45, Nonprofessional]

Even though I had the fantasy that we would become friends, I think the lines got a little sloppy.

[Female, 45, Nonprofessional]

She was too mushy and wishy-washy. She told me too much about how hard it was for her to make decisions.

[Female, 50, Nonprofessional]

He didn't have enough insight into himself to manage his feelings toward me.

[Female, 45, Nonprofessional]

Some people found the therapist's attitude toward money a problem.

The worst thing was her greediness about money.

[Female, 26, Nonprofessional]

> She had a very high fee.
>
> [Female, 56, Professional]

Keeping to the schedule was sometimes a problem.

> She was late sometimes.
>
> [Female, 45, Professional]

> Sometimes he started late.
>
> [Female, 50, Professional]

Some people mentioned a quality of the therapist's style or personality.

> He had a temper, and he could switch moods in a moment.
>
> [Male, 43, Nonprofessional]

> He got caught up in himself.
>
> [Male, 50, Professional]

> She was impatient at times.
>
> [Female, 46, Nonprofessional]

> She could be a little finicky, a little fussy or stuffy sometimes.
>
> [Female, 51, Professional]

> Sometimes he was pedantic.
>
> [Female, 50, Nonprofessional]

> He was definitely on his own planet, and he had these ideas about the real world that were impractical or just odd.
>
> [Male, 46, Nonprofessional]

> There was a narcissistic need for dependency.
>
> [Female, 45, Professional]

> He was somewhat opinionated.
>
> [Male, 53, Nonprofessional]

> She tended to repeat herself a little bit.
>
> [Male, 50, Nonprofessional]

> She talked too much.
>
> [Female, 39, Professional]

NUMERICAL DISTRIBUTION

Professionals: Six people said the therapist's rigidity; 5 said the therapist's lack of presence, definition, or assertiveness; 2 said the therapist's self-centeredness; 2 said lateness; 1 said the fee; 1 said the therapist was not smart enough; 1 said the therapist talked too much. Two people said there was nothing negative about the therapist.

Nonprofessionals: Twelve people said the therapist was too distant, too undefined, and not a real person; 8 said the therapist's lack of skill in some area; 4 said the poor personal boundaries; 3 said the therapist was not supportive in some way; 2 said the therapist did not talk enough; 2 said the therapist was bad at dealing with the fee or the insurance forms; 2 said the office was unpleasant. One each said: the therapist's rigidity; his self-centeredness; her inauthenticity; his temper; his impatience; her repetitiousness; and her location.

COMMENTS

There were similar responses from the two groups, except that more than a quarter of the professionals chose the therapist's rigidity as the worst quality, while only one nonprofessional mentioned it. None of the professionals mentioned a lack of skill, which probably reflects their greater knowledge and greater selectivity in choosing the therapist.

As the therapist, I can see that none of the qualities mentioned is anything I want to project to the patient. It might be difficult for me to imagine what my patients would say is my worst quality, but if pressed I would guess they would say that I can be smug when proven right.

As the patient, I hope that the worst thing about my therapist is comparatively minor, and not something serious like rigidity or passivity or lack of skill. If that quality, whatever it is, creates problems for him, that's one thing, but if it creates problems for me I'm probably going to find another therapist.

RELATED READING

Canter, J. S., and Schwebel, M. (1997). Well-functioning in professional psychologists. *Professional Psychology: Research and Practice* 28(1): 5–13.

Cummings, N. A. (1991). Ten ways to spot mismanaged mental health. *Psychotherapy in Private Practice* 9(3):79–83.

Kelly, J. L. (1996). *Psychiatric Malpractice: Stories of Patients, Psychiatrists, and the Law*. New Brunswick, NJ: Rutgers University Press.

Mahoney, M. J. (1997). Psychotherapists' personal problems and self-care problems. *Professional Psychology: Research and Practice* 28(1): 14–16.

🖎🖎🖎🖎

Question 93: What was the hardest part of therapy?

Therapy can be hard work. Which aspect of the work did the patients identify as the most difficult?

Many people mentioned the pain of returning to traumatic childhood memories.

> It was hard to explore things about my childhood, very painful things.
>
> [Female, 45, Nonprofessional]

> It was the pain of going back to the time in my life when I was terribly mistreated.
>
> [Female, 57, Professional]

> It's really delving into your feelings, sometimes feelings that are very painful. So much of the stuff we uncovered were fears that I had, and my childhood, and it was hard.
>
> [Female, 40, Nonprofessional]

> It was hard sticking with painful feelings.
>
> [Male, 30, Professional]

> It was hard going back and digging up all the terrible childhood years.
>
> [Female, 50, Professional]

Others said that accepting painful truths about themselves was most difficult.

> It was hard facing the dark side. The parts of myself that were like my father, for example, the sadistic pieces. I didn't like that one bit.
>
> [Female, 45, Professional]

> It was hard facing up to what goes on inside of me.
>
> [Male, 50, Professional]

When I had some medical problems, it was very difficult to look at the psychogenic aspect of them.

[Female, 45, Professional]

It was hard facing imperfections in myself and my relationships.

[Female, 39, Professional]

Some people mentioned some difficult feelings about what was discovered.

Facing my shame was very hard.

[Female, 50, Professional]

I had a hard time admitting certain things to her, which meant admitting them to myself.

[Male, 50, Nonprofessional]

Several people mentioned the pace and structure of treatment.

It was hard not getting to the real center of whatever the problem was at the time, the frustration of knowing I was skipping along the surface.

[Male, 46, Nonprofessional]

It was the frustration that I wasn't getting anywhere.

[Male, 49, Nonprofessional]

I felt the danger of being at the mercy of another person's personality who isn't going to be clear or honest or validating about his or her actual personality.

[Female, 48, Professional]

It was the settling in to the extent of it.

[Female, 52, Nonprofessional]

It was the tedious slowness of progress: the very slow rate of progress, how difficult it is to change, even though you might intellectually understand the root and the cause of the problems and your contribution to maintaining the problems.

[Male, 42, Professional]

I was frustrated that I wasn't moving along faster.

[Male, 48, Nonprofessional]

I had trouble facing things that I thought were solved and they weren't solved.

[Female, 59, Professional]

The process was very painful sometimes. I would go and it would be very hard because there were times when I felt very stuck, and I couldn't seem to get untangled. I would go to a session, and I would work and work and work. I spent a lot of time in my sessions figuring out what the therapist wanted and what I should be doing.

[Female, 44, Nonprofessional]

The hardest thing was the open-endedness, the lack of structure, never fixing something definitively.

[Male, 53, Professional]

It was hard being indirectly forced to think about things that I wouldn't necessarily have thought about, in a way that I wouldn't have thought about them.

[Female, 26, Nonprofessional]

Several people mentioned the difficult transition between the session and the rest of life, at both the beginning and the end of the hour.

It was hard going in and not having any idea of what I want to talk about, no topic. If I'm going in with a dream or something, then I have an agenda and that makes it easier to start.

[Female, 46, Nonprofessional]

I had trouble going in at the beginning of the session and having to start talking.

[Female, 48, Nonprofessional]

Sometimes I came out of the session feeling like I had open wounds on my body, because it was emotionally very painful.

[Female, 41, Nonprofessional]

The hardest thing was reentering the world after a session. You might go through the wringer and then have to come back to the real world. Especially first thing in the morning.

[Female, 42, Nonprofessional]

Some people found the relationship with the therapist difficult.

The relationship between me and the therapist had always been the hardest part, how I felt about having that kind of relationship.

[Female, 53, Nonprofessional]

It was hard addressing the intense feeling about my therapist.

[Male, 44, Professional]

Certain specific topics were a problem for some people.

It was difficult when there was an issue I wanted to bring up but was too afraid to. I regret not discussing that with her.

[Female, 42, Nonprofessional]

Dealing with the experiences with my father was the hardest part.

[Female, 39, Nonprofessional]

Talking about sex was almost impossible.

[Female, 50, Nonprofessional]

For some the logistics of time and schedule were most difficult.

I had a hard time keeping the appointments. I knew I was going to be working during the day, and I don't have a lunch break that allows me an hour to get there and an hour to get back, plus the time of the session.

[Female, 28, Nonprofessional]

I started seeing her when I was living nearby, but after I moved it was very hard to get there.

[Female, 45, Nonprofessional]

It was hard physically finding the time to be there, fitting it in to the rest of my life.

[Male, 53, Nonprofessional]

I had trouble just getting there. It was a long drive.

[Female, 62, Professional]

It was never convenient. I have a full life, and it was hard to find time for it. The logistics and the stress of getting there.

[Male, 49, Nonprofessional]

Some people said starting treatment, admitting that they needed help, or learning to be a patient was the hardest part.

> The hardest thing was admitting that I needed to go. I thought I had to be really crazy to go. It was a revelation to learn that I could go just because I wanted to.
>
> [Female, 46, Nonprofessional]

> It was very hard getting started, picking up the phone and saying that I needed help. Once I got into it there was nothing difficult about it.
>
> [Male, 45, Nonprofessional]

> Opening up was very difficult.
>
> [Male, 43, Nonprofessional]

> Learning to think about and talk about myself took a long time.
>
> [Female, 45, Nonprofessional]

> It was very hard for me to let go of the therapist role and be the patient.
>
> [Female, 58, Professional]

> Not knowing how to do it was very hard, not seeing how what I was talking about would help.
>
> [Female, 44, Nonprofessional]

Others said the hardest part of therapy was leaving.

> It took me the longest time to tell her that's what I wanted to do, to leave.
>
> [Female, 50, Professional]

NUMERICAL DISTRIBUTION

Professionals: Eight people said the hardest part was facing something in themselves; 3 said it was painful feelings or memories; 2 people said feelings about the therapist; 2 said terminating was the hardest part; 1 person said the lack of structure; 1 said the pace of therapy; 1 said the cost; 1 said the distance to the therapist's office. One person said no aspect of therapy was difficult.

Nonprofessionals: Eleven people said the hardest part was painful feelings or memories; 5 people said it was finding time in their schedules; 4 people said it was facing something in themselves; 3 said the pace of therapy; 2 people said the lack of depth of the process; 2 said the distance to the therapist's office; 2 people said learning how to be in therapy; 2 people said making the initial call; 2 people said starting the session; 2 people said revealing themselves to the therapist; 1 person said feelings of dependency; 1 said reentering the world after the session. Two people said no aspect of therapy was difficult, and 1 person said everything was difficult.

COMMENTS

This question elicited similar kinds of responses from both groups, although more nonprofessionals had trouble with the process itself. Different people interpreted the word "hard" differently: some in the sense of "most difficult to do" and others in the sense of "most difficult to tolerate." Therapy is hard at times, in both senses of the word, and all of these answers apply at different times to most patients.

As the therapist, I see that reexperiencing painful memories is very hard for most patients, and facing unpleasant truths about themselves is equally difficult. Overall I think the most difficult thing for the patient is to stick with the process, no matter what comes up, to stay present through it all and not back away from thoughts, feelings, or issues.

As the patient, I am willing to do very hard work if I see that the result will be improved mood, higher self-esteem, enhanced relationships, or better overall functioning. I may need the support of the therapist at times, but I can do whatever it takes if I have some confidence in the outcome.

RELATED READING

Deutsch, C. J. (1984). Self-reported sources of stress among psychotherapists. *Professional Psychology: Research and Practice* 15(6):833–845.

Duncan, B. L., and Moynihan, D. W. (1994). Applying outcome research: intentional utilization of the client's frame of reference. *Psychotherapy* 31(2):294–301.

Lamprell, M. (1989). The paralysis of indecision. *British Journal of Psychotherapy* 6(2):227–234.

Myerson, P. G. (1979). Issues of technique where patients relate with difficulty. *International Review of Psycho-Analysis* 6(3):363–375.

🐚🐚🐚🐚

Question 94: What was the most fun in therapy?

Although the stereotype of therapy is that it's often painful and always hard work, somehow patients do manage to have fun sometimes. The discovery of oneself can be exciting and joyful.

> It was great to realize a lot of good things about myself that I hadn't been conscious of.
>
> [Female, 45, Nonprofessional]

> It was analyzing my dreams and seeing things that should have been obvious, and suddenly it was right there.
>
> [Female, 58, Professional]

> I loved breaking through the nonsense and the roles. Experiencing the connection with the person in me that I liked, that I loved, and not only experiencing the me who was in pain, who was suffering, who was torturing himself.
>
> [Male, 46, Nonprofessional]

> The best part was discovering the lightness around some pretty heavy issues, discovering that I had a goofy side that didn't make me an airhead.
>
> [Female, 46, Nonprofessional]

Feeling healed can be joyful.

> I loved the better feeling that I ended up with about myself.
>
> [Male, 45, Nonprofessional]

> It was the tremendous relief of realizing that I wasn't such a bad person.
>
> [Female, 45, Professional]

> The best part was letting go of the pain.
>
> [Female, 47, Nonprofessional]

> The most fun was coming alive.
>
> [Female, 50, Professional]

Some people expressed this as a sense of progress.

I loved seeing progress, making small breakthroughs.

[Female, 48, Nonprofessional]

The progress was the best, seeing that things didn't have to be as miserable as they were. There was always some incremental progress, sometimes a lot and sometimes a snail's pace, but I can look back now and see that my life has changed, and this is the main cause of it.

[Male, 49, Nonprofessional]

Some people mentioned the pleasure of feeling understood by another person.

When you really feel understood and it's exciting and there's this incredible flow, and you don't feel judged or blocked, but just heard for where you are and who you are.

[Female, 45, Professional]

The most fun was to be in a place where someone was focused on me and seeing me and hearing me, and paying attention.

[Female, 62, Professional]

This has its counterpart in the pleasure of understanding oneself.

I loved the Freudian moments, where an event suddenly reveals its symbolic meaning.

[Male, 50, Nonprofessional]

I loved having things make sense.

[Female, 48, Nonprofessional]

I enjoyed getting the answers.

[Male, 52, Nonprofessional]

The best part is when the light goes on, when you have the "aha" experience.

[Female, 46, Nonprofessional]

The most fun were the moments of insight, making some connections.

[Female, 39, Nonprofessional]

The high of getting a real insight was great.

[Female, 45, Nonprofessional]

Many people enjoyed the freedom to say anything, to explore, to be spontaneous.

> I loved the open-endedness, the lack of structure and rules.
> [Male, 53, Professional]

> The best was having someone to talk to with whom there are no dynamic consequences.
> [Female, 50, Nonprofessional]

> The most fun was the moments of acting really silly, the freedom to do that.
> [Male, 42, Professional]

> I loved the release of being able to say anything.
> [Female, 53, Nonprofessional]

> The freedom to say whatever you want was the best part.
> [Female, 48, Professional]

New ideas about how the mind works can be stimulating.

> I enjoyed talking theory.
> [Male, 50, Professional]

> My therapist's perspectives were fun to learn about.
> [Female, 55, Professional]

Many people enjoyed the relationship with the therapist.

> I loved entertaining her.
> [Male, 48, Nonprofessional]

> When the relationship with my therapist was really clicking, that was wonderful.
> [Female, 57, Professional]

> It was really fun to have somebody so interested in me and to have somebody to talk about things with. One of my fondest memories is of talking about books we were both reading.
> [Female, 42, Nonprofessional]

We had fun talking about the men I was dating. I would tell her about them and we would laugh a lot.

[Female, 41, Nonprofessional]

I loved talking about shopping.

[Female, 39, Professional]

I always looked forward to spending the time with her, because I knew I would always come out of there feeling something.

[Female, 42, Nonprofessional]

Many times he and I could enjoy something together. We have so much in common in our situations, and we really understood each other.

[Female, 50, Nonprofessional]

Patients and therapists often laugh together.

Occasionally stuff would come up, and we'd just laugh, so hard that my stomach would hurt. And I can't tell you what we were laughing about.

[Female, 40, Nonprofessional]

She had the same sense of humor and we decided that humor was an excellent defense.

[Female, 52, Professional]

There was a certain glib tone in the air much of the time, and she appreciated it and that was nice, to feel that I could say something that was funny and smart and she would appreciate it.

[Male, 52, Nonprofessional]

Sometimes the therapist will do or say something wonderful.

I had a very creative therapist, who used hands-on activities. Once he took a cup that had a hole in the bottom, and he talked about how I couldn't accept positive stuff and it was always dripping out the bottom and I always needed more. He had a tray and water. He also had a cassette tape, and on it he wrote all the things I would whine about, like "No one loves me," or whatever, and he put it in the tape player and turned up the volume, and of course it was all static, and he said, "These are your mantras, and you can't hear anything else." And he asked me to carry the tape around with me.

[Female, 48, Nonprofessional]

A few people said that therapy was never fun.

There's no fun in therapy!

[Female, 41, Nonprofessional]

There wasn't much fun.

[Male, 44, Professional]

I don't really find it fun.

[Female, 28, Nonprofessional]

NUMERICAL DISTRIBUTION

Professionals: Six people said the most fun was laughing and discussing something with the therapist; 4 said discovery or insight; 5 said seeing the results; 2 said the freedom of the process; 1 said the education; 1 said being the center of attention. One person said nothing was fun.

Nonprofessionals: Ten people said the most fun was laughing and discussing something with the therapist; 9 said discovery or insight; 8 said seeing the results and feeling better; 6 said the relationship with the therapist; 2 said the freedom of the process; 1 said the education; 1 said being the center of attention; 1 mentioned a specific technique of the therapist. Two people said nothing was fun.

COMMENTS

Again, both groups gave similar responses. In spite of the public image of dark solemnity, most people have fun at some time in therapy. Being able to laugh at oneself is a good indicator of mental health. The excitement of discovery can feel exhilarating.

As the therapist, I share in patients' fun when we work with dreams, or when they learn something about themselves that turns out to be liberating. Sharing a good laugh is a wonderful connection. Knowing there will be such moments makes the dark times easier to tolerate.

As the patient, I need a therapist who can have fun with me without thinking that I'm not being serious about the therapy. I'll work hard when I need to if I can have the freedom to enjoy the relationship and the process.

RELATED READING

Ehrenberg, D. B. (1991). Playfulness and humor in the psychoanalytic relationship. *Group* 15(4):225–233.

Johnson, C. (1995). A statement about play and adults in analytic psychotherapy. *Free Associations* 5(3, pt. 1):103–110.

Saper, B. (1988). Humor in psychiatric healing. *Psychiatric Quarterly* 59(4):306–319.

Squier, H. A. (1995). Humor in the doctor–patient relationship. *Family Systems Medicine* 13(1):101–107.

🔊🔊🔊🔊

Question 95: How did your expectations of therapy match up with the actual experience?

Most patients start therapy with specific complaints and dissatisfactions, and corresponding expectations about the effects of therapy on those complaints. Some expectations may be unconscious (for example, the wish for a magical transformation), but this question explores the conscious ones.

Most people said they had expected something when they began treatment. These expectations were sometimes met.

> I was hoping to get some help with some problems and I did.
> [Male, 45, Nonprofessional]

> They matched up well. What I saw in the workshop was what I got.
> [Female, 59, Professional]

> I went into it with a very specific goal and I came out with what I wanted.
> [Female, 44, Nonprofessional]

Even when patients have been disappointed in previous treatments, they may still have some hope.

> I had seen a variety of therapists from a variety of schools. I would have to take a moment to count up all the therapists I've seen. And

I was ill-served by many of them, and that was one of the things she was very good about, that is, sympathizing with my ill treatment at the hands of prior therapists. Despite that, for whatever reason, I was still optimistic that therapy was of value. This was the first therapy that I felt actually fulfilled my hopes for it.

[Male, 48, Nonprofessional]

Sometimes what the patient gets feels like neither less nor more, just different from what was expected.

It was quite different: long and integrated with the rest of my life.

[Female, 52, Nonprofessional]

It was different in that I had thought that I would lay out my problem and the therapist would say, "Oh, it's because of this," and I would be a transformed person. It doesn't work that way. I do feel like a different person, but it's more like I'm the same person differently.

[Female, 39, Nonprofessional]

I discovered that my fantasy that therapy would "fix" me so that I would never again do what I had done (which was my terrible fear at that point) was not what was going to happen in therapy.

[Female, 48, Nonprofessional]

It was more subtle than I expected. Rather than getting fixed, I think my soul got healed.

[Female, 46, Nonprofessional]

Often the therapy exceeded the expectations.

It completely surpassed my expectations. It was completely different from what I thought it would be—much more in-depth.

[Female, 45, Professional]

I wasn't sure what I expected, but I felt it all turned out much better than I had hoped for.

[Male, 52, Nonprofessional]

It was much more than I ever expected.

[Male, 50, Professional]

I don't expect miracles, but the work I did with him allowed me to have miracles.

[Male, 46, Nonprofessional]

I ended up feeling better than I would have believed possible.
> [Female, 50, Professional]

It was better. My expectation was to break the depression, but I never thought I'd get rid of the panic attacks. She was very optimistic and encouraging that they would stop, and they did.
> [Female, 51, Professional]

I got much, much more than I expected. I had no idea when I started what was possible.
> [Female, 51, Professional]

I had a fear that therapy was going to "normalize" me, and she was very good at convincing me that that wasn't the point, that the point of therapy was to help me live with who I am. The experience was far better than I expected.
> [Male, 50, Nonprofessional]

Some people were disappointed.

I don't think I got anything out of it.
> [Female, 48, Nonprofessional]

I believe I had a failed analysis.
> [Female, 57, Professional]

I expected to do some work, and I did nothing. It was a waste of time and money.
> [Female, 48, Nonprofessional]

Even when the treatment has been useful overall, the patient may still feel disappointed in some ways.

It wasn't as profoundly transforming as I thought it might be, as my fantasy was. It was quite substantially helpful, but not as transforming.
> [Male, 42, Professional]

My experience was good but it didn't live up to my expectations that I would find the master key to self-understanding.
> [Male, 49, Nonprofessional]

Compared to the previous therapist, it was an improvement: she wasn't controlling, she wasn't intrusive, she was smart, she did give input. It was useful, but it didn't go the extra step. I feel greedy because I wanted so much more.

[Female, 50, Professional]

I expected it to be a quicker fix than it was.

[Male, 48, Nonprofessional]

NUMERICAL DISTRIBUTION

Professionals: Seven said the experience exceeded their expectations; 5 said it met their expectations; 2 said it was much less than they expected. Five people said it was both more than and less than they expected. One person said she had no expectations.

Nonprofessionals: Eleven said the experience exceeded their expectations; 20 said it met their expectations; 5 said it was much less than they expected. One person said it was both more than and less than she expected. Three people said they had no expectations.

COMMENTS

Many of the people in both groups had a number of therapies prior to the one discussed here, and so they were relatively sophisticated about what to expect. Many of those in their first therapy found it exceeded their expectations.

As the therapist, I welcome someone with high expectations. I want to work with someone who expects a lot from the treatment, because she will probably be more likely to work hard and push both herself and me to get there. I don't mind surprising someone with more than he expected, especially if that motivates him to try for more. So many people settle for less than they can have.

As the patient, I want a lot from therapy. I'm spending my time and my money, usually a significant portion of my income, and I want to see results. I want to know that my therapist believes in the possibilities too, because that makes them seem more attainable.

RELATED READING

Conte, H. R., Ratto, R., Clutz, K., and Karasu, T. B. (1995). Determinants of outpatients' satisfaction with therapists: relation to outcome. *Journal of Psychotherapy Practice and Research* 4(1):43–51.

Johnson, L. D., and Shaha, S. (1996). Improving quality in psychotherapy. *Psychotherapy* 33(2):225–236.

Mash, E. J., and Hunsley, J. (1993). Assessment considerations in the
identification of failing psychotherapy: bringing the negatives out
of the darkroom. *Psychological Assessment* 5(3):292–301.

Perreault, M., Leichner, P., Sabourin, S., and Gendreau, P. (1993). Patient satisfaction with outpatient psychiatric services: qualitative
and quantitative assessments. *Evaluation and Program Planning* 16(2):
109–118.

🔒🔒🔒🔒

Question 96: What have been the benefits of therapy?

I'm sure that most therapists could articulate at great length all the
benefits of the therapeutic experience, but what do the patients say
about it?

Some people said they were more satisfied and happier in life.

> I feel I've become less detached, more emotionally present.
>
> [Female, 59, Professional]

> I feel like my soul was healed.
>
> [Female, 46, Nonprofessional]

Some said they saw more choices available to them.

> It really enabled me to look at myself and my relationships with other
> people in a way that made me understand that I had a lot of choices
> and didn't have to react to everything, didn't have to buy into every-
> thing. I really felt these benefits after I stopped. It was in reflection
> that it came full circle for me.
>
> [Female, 45, Nonprofessional]

> There is an exploration of inner space, and you will have so many
> more options in your life that you've never dreamed of. It opens up
> your world so you can make much better choices in vocation and
> relationship and every other way.
>
> [Female, 57, Professional]

> It allowed me to see that there are different ways to be in this world,
> and I chose one way for a very long time. I found more options, and
> greater insight.
>
> [Female, 47, Nonprofessional]

Some said they had become more themselves.

> I'm more in touch my feelings. I'm more at ease with being a professional and a woman. I'm more at ease with being who I am rather than trying to be something else.
>
> [Female, 50, Nonprofessional]

> I have so much more of myself.
>
> [Female, 45, Professional]

> I feel like a real person.
>
> [Male, 48, Nonprofessional]

> I don't think I'm as neurotic, I'm no longer bulimic, I understand a lot better my family dynamics and where things came from, and have been able to change those things, do it differently and break some of the family patterns and roles that I was expected to play. I'm much more me.
>
> [Female, 45, Professional]

Others said they had come to know and understand themselves better.

> I was able to develop some compassion for myself as a child, and hopefully that carries over to today. Until you can do that, it's very hard to be a parent and to be a person.
>
> [Female, 46, Nonprofessional]

> It was such a real opportunity to explore yourself in real depth, stuff that otherwise you just never get to, you just always put it off.
>
> [Female, 48, Professional]

> I got more of an understanding of why I do what I do. I've become more aware of how I am, changes that I've made.
>
> [Female, 48, Nonprofessional]

Some said they were functioning better, and had more confidence.

> I cleared away all my shit, and I'm very different from what I used to be. I'm not obsessed with self-doubt, and I'm a pretty well-functioning person.
>
> [Female, 62, Professional]

She helped me get on with life—she helped me sort through things I wanted to deal with and things I never dreamt of dealing with.

[Female, 42, Nonprofessional]

When I started therapy, I was pretty fragmented inside, and marginal in terms of being able to be with and understand myself. I've gotten a life.

[Male, 50, Professional]

I've got a hard life, but I've developed a confidence in myself that I can deal with this stuff in ways that I never could before. It's tough but it's manageable.

[Male, 49, Nonprofessional]

It takes down rigid, obsessive personality features and loosens people up. It gets people more in touch with their core essences, and spontaneity, their true self, getting more authentic. For someone who is not well put together, it's building an ego, becoming more functional, adapting.

[Male, 30, Professional]

Several people said their relationships to other people had improved.

It allowed me to break the pattern of coldness and abandonment that was my father's approach to fatherhood and to marriage, and do it with awareness so I don't cause as much damage. To love the people I love more deeply.

[Male, 46, Nonprofessional]

I've been much more available to people who I'm willing to be available to, and not available to people I don't want to be available to. It's been much easier to know the difference between those two situations. It's allowed me to have a long-term relationship with one person, and it's been very fulfilling.

[Male, 52, Nonprofessional]

I found improved interpersonal relationships, at all different levels, and the ability to sustain an intimate relationship.

[Female, 42, Nonprofessional]

Others said they had gotten relief from some troubling symptoms.

I'm less anxious when presenting things in public.

[Female, 56, Professional]

I got rid of my depression and my panic attacks.

[Female, 51, Professional]

I got over my fear of flying, both on the real level of getting in the plane and the metaphoric level of taking off and being free.

[Female, 62, Professional]

Several said they had achieved more success, professionally or personally.

I've developed a new career, based in part on identification with her.

[Male, 44, Professional]

I made huge progress in the job area, not only changing jobs but changing careers. And I worked a lot on my relationship with my mother.

[Female, 45, Nonprofessional]

I got a better capacity to love and a better capacity to work. I never had trouble playing so there wasn't much change there.

[Male, 42, Professional]

Others said the therapist had helped them cope through a difficult period.

She really helped me through some very hairy times.

[Female, 50, Nonprofessional]

I came out of the trauma.

[Female, 48, Nonprofessional]

It was an emergency treatment. I was afraid that maybe I would have a nervous breakdown, although I never actually started acting strange, but it made me feel more confident that that wasn't going to happen. I felt that I was taking good care of myself by going.

[Male, 42, Nonprofessional]

NUMERICAL DISTRIBUTION

Professionals: (Some people gave more than one response.) Six people said they had become more themselves; 4 said they had gotten over symptoms of some sort; 4 said they were more satisfied and happier; 3 said they were more successful in work; 3 said they were functioning better; 3 said therapy had helped them over a difficult period; 2 said they had better relationships; 2 said they perceived more options; 2 said therapy had allowed them to explore themselves.

Nonprofessionals: (Some people gave more than one response.) Eight people said they had become more themselves; 7 said they had better relationships; 6 said therapy had helped them over a difficult period; 5 said therapy had allowed them to explore themselves; 4 said they were functioning better; 3 said they perceived more options; 2 said they had become more confident; 3 said they had become more self-accepting; 2 said they had gotten over symptoms of some sort; 2 said they were more satisfied and happier; 1 said he was more successful in work.

COMMENTS

Responses to this question were similar between the two groups. One of Freud's most famous remarks was to note that, if you want to see how someone is doing in life, you look at the areas of love and work. Generally speaking, good therapy improves functioning in all areas: at work, at home, with others, with oneself. Most people got at least some of this from their therapy.

As the therapist, I look for signs of improvement in all these areas, and most patients begin reporting them soon into treatment. Occasionally a patient tells me with some anger or disappointment that there has been no change, no improvement, and these patients usually leave if this continues.

As the patient, I need to see some concrete change happening in my feelings or my circumstances, and the connection to therapy must also be clear. I have to know that I have somehow created the difference. Since I know what the process is capable of achieving, I will attribute a lack of results to the therapist and will almost certainly go elsewhere if something doesn't happen soon.

RELATED READING

Clementel-Jones, C., Malan, D., and Trauer, T. (1990). A retrospective follow-up study of 84 patients treated with individual psychoanalytic psychotherapy: outcome and predictive factors. *British Journal of Psychotherapy* 6(4):363–374.

Hanna, F. J., and Puhakka, K. (1991). When psychotherapy works: pinpointing an element of change. *Psychotherapy* 28(4):598–607.

Haug, U. (1992). Summary of a large-scale psychotherapy study. *Psychoanalytic Psychotherapy* 6(2):169–180.

Johnson, L. D., and Shaha, S. (1996). Improving quality in psychotherapy. *Psychotherapy* 79(2):225–236.

☙☙☙☙

Question 97: Have there been any negative effects of therapy?

We know the potential benefits of therapy, but did any of our interviewees feel that something bad came out of treatment?

Most people said there were no negative effects, even when the therapist was not so good.

> Even with this terrible last therapist I learned a lot about myself and I'm much stronger.
>
> [Female, 57, Professional]

A few people mentioned the expense.

> Sometimes I think about all the money I spend on it, but I tell myself it's an investment for my future.
>
> [Female, 42, Nonprofessional]

> It's cost me a fortune, but who knows how much I've made as a result? It costs time, too.
>
> [Male, 53, Professional]

> I could have put a down payment on a house with what I spent.
>
> [Female, 44, Nonprofessional]

When the therapy was not helpful, it sometimes felt detrimental.

> I think it's left me a little mistrustful of therapists in general.
>
> [Female, 48, Professional]

> The negative effects were while I was seeing her.
>
> [Male, 44, Professional]

I was really a mess when I stopped, and as soon as I stopped I began to feel better.

[Female, 48, Nonprofessional]

Sometimes patients feel that time has been wasted, and resolution of problems delayed.

I couldn't talk to her about a certain issue because she knew the people involved, so there was a whole aspect of who I am that couldn't get brought into the therapy.

[Female, 45, Professional]

I believe that a lot of issues in my marriage would have been dealt with much sooner if we had seen someone else.

[Female, 45, Nonprofessional]

Even when the therapy is working, it can sometimes have a negative impact.

I think there were some years where I was overinvolved to the detriment of my pursuing a life outside of therapy. I'm not sure I was together enough to have done it, though, so I'm not sure.

[Male, 50, Professional]

At times it's made me more depressed. It gets worse before it gets better.

[Male, 30, Professional]

I find that I dislike certain people more than I used to.

[Female, 39, Nonprofessional]

NUMERICAL DISTRIBUTION

Professionals: Fourteen said there were no negative effects; 6 mentioned some negative impact.

Nonprofessionals: Thirty said there were no negative effects; 4 mentioned the expense; 6 mentioned some other negative impact.

COMMENTS

There were no major differences between the two groups in response to this question. About a quarter of both groups reported something they were unhappy about, most often the cost.

As the therapist, I hope that patients feel therapy was worth the expense, and that there were no other problems or damage as a result of being in therapy. The only negative effect of doing therapy that I am aware of is an impatience with the usual level of casual conversation, which can seem so superficial compared to things we discuss in therapy.

As the patient, I don't experience any negative effects from a successful therapy. A bad experience can leave me frustrated, angry, and filled with self-doubt.

RELATED READING

Masson, J. M. (1988). *Against Therapy: Emotional Tyranny and the Myth of Psychological Healing.* New York: Atheneum.

Rachman, S. J. (1973). The effects of psychological treatment. In *Handbook of Abnormal Psychology,* ed. H. J. Eysenck, pp. 805–861. San Diego, CA: EDITS Publishers.

Schofield, W. (1986). *Psychotherapy: The Purchase of Friendship.* New Brunswick, NJ: Transaction.

Sjodin, C. (1994). Quality assurance and quality assessment as integral ongoing aspects of psychoanalysis and psychotherapy. *International Forum of Psychoanalysis* 3(3):183–193.

☙☙☙☙

Question 98: Are you glad you did it?

Are patients glad they went to therapy? Are they satisfied with the results? Do they feel that the problems they began with have been resolved? Do they feel they got their money's worth?

We might assume that the patient who has a good experience in therapy is glad he or she went, and in most cases this turns out to be true.

> At times I questioned while I was going, because I spent so much money on it, always paying out of pocket, but it changed my life.
>
> [Female, 45, Professional]

> It saved my life.
>
> [Female, 48, Nonprofessional]

People will tell you that it saved their lives, but it created my life.
[Male, 49, Nonprofessional]

I had a really good experience, and it makes me feel sorry for those people who didn't. So few people seem to have a good experience.
[Female, 45, Nonprofessional]

Some people thought the experience would have been better if they had been more knowledgeable.

A lot of the work was good work. I just wish I had known more about boundaries.
[Female, 45, Nonprofessional]

I probably would have been happier with it if I had been more active and more confrontational, and not just going along with his way of doing things.
[Female, 58, Professional]

Even when the therapy was not what the patient wanted it to be, some people could still find value in it.

It was useful even though it was not very good because I now know how not to work.
[Female, 57, Professional]

Only a few people in each group were seriously dissatisfied.

It wasn't what I wanted.
[Female, 48, Nonprofessional]

Would I go back to her? Only if I could say to her that I need a different way of intervening.
[Female, 50, Professional]

It only helped a little and it was too expensive.
[Female, 28, Nonprofessional]

NUMERICAL DISTRIBUTION

Professionals: Eighteen said they were glad they did it; 2 said they were not.

Nonprofessionals: Thirty-eight said they were glad they did it; 2 said they were not.

COMMENTS

People don't always know how they feel about therapy until it's over, which is why interviews took place at least 3 months after termination. It can take some time to integrate the work of therapy before results are fully visible, and some of this may occur after treatment has stopped. Here again there was no major difference between the groups: most people are glad they had therapy and happy about the results.

As the therapist, I hope that everyone who leaves my office is glad they were there, both weekly and after therapy is finished. I know this is not always the case, but I think it happens most of the time.

As the patient, I am always glad to be in therapy, even when it's not fabulous, because I am always learning something. Even a bad therapist can be useful in validating what I know and believe and in confirming my strength in leaving.

RELATED READING

Gaston, L., and Sabourin, S. (1992). Client satisfaction and social desirability in psychotherapy. *Evaluation and Program Planning* 15(3): 227–231.

Langs, R. (1989). *Rating Your Psychotherapist.* New York: Henry Hull.

Powell, D. H. (1995). Lessons learned from therapeutic failure. *Journal of Psychotherapy Integration* 5(2):175–181.

Weiss, J. (1993). *How Psychotherapy Works: Process and Technique.* New York: Guilford.

Wilcoxon, S. A. (1991). Clarifying expectations in therapy relationships: suggestions for written guidelines. *Journal of Independent Social Work* 5(2):65–71.

℞℞℞℞

Question 99: How do you think therapy works?

How does talking about problems and experiences lead to personality change? Answers to this question fall primarily into two main categories: one emphasizes the relationship with the therapist—the "corrective emotional experience"—and the other emphasizes insight and understanding.

Let's look first at those responses that highlight the relationship with the therapist.

> A lot of why it works is the relationship. If there were one thing that makes for good or bad therapy it would be that.
>
> [Female, 50, Professional]

> It's the relationship between the patient and the therapist. It's an undoing of the early childhood trauma, with the help of the therapist as facilitator. You relate to another human being in a different way, and that changes the psychic structure inside of you.
>
> [Female, 57, Professional]

> It's developing a relationship that's purer than other relationships, and that enables you to have a better sense of yourself. You get a different framework, a different point of reference. He became my point of reference, and I always say he brought me up.
>
> [Female, 52, Nonprofessional]

> You get a chance to be yourself with somebody who cares about you, and you get a chance to look at all the scary stuff inside with someone who believes in you and cares about you and makes it possible for you to start growing up again.
>
> [Male, 50, Professional]

> I used to think of it as a kind of "talking cure"—I would talk and somehow I'd get better. Now I think that a lot of it has to do with being able to work out a lot of relationships through the transference with the therapist, undoing the childhood damage. You establish the relationship and have to be aware that this is what the relationship is going to do. The most important part is talking about the relationship with the therapist.
>
> [Female, 45, Nonprofessional]

> It's somebody listening. I believe if everybody had one person who listened to them and accepted them, people wouldn't distort and get messed up. Therapy is an opportunity to get that kind of support, and somebody to listen to you and take an interest in your life, and be with you while you grow.
>
> [Female, 51, Professional]

It works because of the relationship that's formed between the patient and the therapist. The act of two people being in a room and talking, and having one person there for you with very set guidelines. It's a sort of controlled relationship.

[Female, 42, Nonprofessional]

It sounds like a cliché but it's primarily the relationship. Being joined and then having a corrective emotional experience with someone else. I believe less and less that theory matters.

[Female, 52, Professional]

It works by remodeling your relationships with people who are intimate with you. If the relationship with the analyst is successful, you learn a different model from the ones you had as a child, one that's a lot healthier. It gives you a tapestry of interactions that you can use outside. It's rebuilding the original close intimate relationships that should have occurred with your family in a healthy way.

[Female, 45, Nonprofessional]

The relationship does it. The objective of the therapist is to figure out what the belief system is and what the experiences were that formed the belief system, what the person holds true about themselves that is debilitating, and through the relationship to rework those beliefs so they are in line with reality.

[Female, 50, Professional]

When it works, it has to do with how I feel about the person, and if I like the person I'm willing to be a lot more open to the process, and that alone is how it works. You have to be ready for it. You have an advocate and somebody to trust, and to know that person is there for you is wonderful.

[Female, 42, Nonprofessional]

It provides a relationship in which you can learn and enact a new way of relating to another person. It's only in relation to other people that you become who you are.

[Male, 48, Nonprofessional]

I think it's magic. It's about the contact between two lives, and something divine happens that's healing. It's very spiritual.

[Female, 45, Professional]

Some people said that the most significant aspect of the relationship was the mirroring, the reflection back to the patient of a new self-
concept.

> Reflecting neutrally and consistently back to the patient over time is
> how therapy really works. Parents provide distorted mirrors to people
> of who they are, and the therapist over time repeatedly keeps re-
> flecting back a more accurate picture.
>
> [Female, 45, Professional]

> You can look at it two different ways: it's a way of reflecting your
> feelings and experiences back onto yourself by hearing them spoken
> and by having them reflected by another person, which helps you
> look at them differently. Also, you look to the person you're talking
> to to change your way of thinking, by questioning some of the things
> you believe.
>
> [Female, 53, Nonprofessional]

> It's an interaction with someone else that's a helpful mirror on the
> self, and offers positive self-reflection. The therapist can create a much
> more consistent empathic early mother, and can mirror back a more
> positive self-image.
>
> [Female, 59, Professional]

Several people emphasized the safety that the therapist creates.

> It's having someone accept you, whatever you're saying, without
> judgment, that allows you to accept yourself.
>
> [Female, 44, Nonprofessional]

> Another person hears all my stuff, and I see it filtered through her
> mind and her feelings, and she accepts me, which allows me to accept
> myself. I air out all my secrets and demons and I'm not afraid of my
> inner self anymore.
>
> [Female, 62, Professional]

> It provides people a safe and supportive place, person, and atmo-
> sphere to experience in a full way some of the real stuff that's going
> on, instead of covering it up, as in their normal lives, with a lot of
> nonsense and diversions. It gives you the support to face who you
> really are. The ways that helps is, if you can really know yourself, you
> get to know the good parts.
>
> [Male, 46, Nonprofessional]

It gives you the chance to confront things that you're afraid to confront on your own.

[Male, 42, Nonprofessional]

Part of it was an intellectual process, but the more important part was letting it all rise up from below the surface so that I could see it. She was the perfect analyst for me because she made it safe enough to do that. She was a catalyst, in that she didn't interfere in it and she didn't get transformed herself. I knew all this beforehand, but it was surprising to me that it actually happened. It was a real experience rather than an idea.

[Male, 52, Nonprofessional]

Other people emphasized the insight, the "aha" experience, that flash of understanding in which all becomes clear and the meanings shift.

When the patient "gets" something, it becomes more alive for her. I remember an early therapist talking about how crazy my father was. I had never thought of my father as being crazy, and it felt like it instantly reframed everything. It's that reframing that empowers you to see things in a new way.

[Female, 58, Professional]

Therapy is not supposed to make you happy, it's supposed to help you understand why things are happening the way they are, why you do what you do. It works by developing your understanding of your own dynamics.

[Female, 50, Nonprofessional]

It works by allowing someone to internalize certain ideas that they can grasp intellectually, but it takes a process to internalize it to the point where they're willing to make it part of their lives.

[Female, 55, Professional]

It works by a kind of education: a little bit of unlearning, and relearning what have become well-worn synaptic paths, and getting those vesicles to open up at other synapses, which is hard to do consciously. That's why it takes a while.

[Male, 51, Nonprofessional]

A big part of it for me was the dream work. The "aha" experience, the understanding, is something that's very hard to get by yourself.

Not that it can't happen, but you need time to relate the dream, an hour or even more, to begin to plumb the depths of the dream. I don't know that you can do that yourself without having someone listening, the combination of the listening and the comment or question. Or maybe it's just having the time and the space and someone saying this is important enough to do. Those things do plug you into and make you find out who you were and what you were feeling in a way that nothing else can do.

[Female, 46, Nonprofessional]

The first step was to figure out why certain patterns got established, but it's not enough to know it intellectually, you have to know it in your gut.

[Female, 39, Nonprofessional]

Several people said that the combination of both the relationship and the insight was crucial, that both elements were necessary.

It's about love and truth. Love refers to the connection, the empathy, the caring, the transference, the relationship factors. Truth refers to the interpretation, the behavioral skills, the concrete insights.

[Male, 30, Professional]

It provides people with new experiences, and therefore with options they haven't had before. It's a corrective experience, both emotionally and cognitively.

[Female, 56, Nonprofessional]

Some people said it was the reworking of the personal narrative that creates a new story with new meanings.

It works by opening up ways of talking about things, and because the pressure to put things into language requires an imaginative and emotional engagement with them that recasts them. It doesn't necessarily get you to the truth, but it gives you articulated vantage points on things that you otherwise wouldn't have had. It obliges you to bring things out into the shared arena of human interaction, and the therapist becomes a kind of symbolic stand-in for lots of others. Once you've done that, you can turn to those real others and engage better. It provides some real paradigms and real ideas.

[Male, 50, Nonprofessional]

People re-tell their stories and change their personal narrative, and get a chance to rework them, and tell themselves a narrative that's more acceptable—one that makes them feel better.

[Female, 51, Professional]

Therapy works by talking about the issues in a therapeutic setting, working through them, so the poison doesn't have the same effect on you. You can't exorcise the things that are troublesome and the problems that you've had in your childhood and your relationships, but you can make them a part of you, so that it's no longer a liability. It's an asset, because you can understand yourself and therefore understand and empathize with other people.

[Female, 41, Nonprofessional]

Several people emphasized the motivation and engagement of the patient.

I think a lot of it comes from yourself. You probably already know a lot of the answers, and maybe you just need someone to make you aware of that.

[Male, 45, Nonprofessional]

It only does what it does if you're willing to try to change, or accept what the therapist is telling you. The therapist is like a coach, and if you want to play the game and win, then you follow what the coach says. If you don't, you're wasting your time.

[Male, 52, Nonprofessional]

I've thought a lot about that. There's the old joke about how it takes a long time and the light bulb has to want to change. That's pivotal—you have to be motivated and really want to roll up your sleeves and roll around in the mud. It works by helping you explore issues in your past that impact on your present, bringing them up, dealing with them. The tools from your past don't necessarily work in the present, so you need to learn a new set of tools, a new set of expectations, and a new understanding of what's normal and what you're entitled to and what you deserve, and what you have control over. The pivotal thing is that you really have to be willing to get down and do the work.

[Female, 41, Nonprofessional]

It works when you're ready to have it work. When you're ready to move the mountain it'll move. It's a combination of the expertise and training of the therapist and the willingness of the patient and the interaction between the two.

[Female, 39, Professional]

It's so much dependent on the person herself figuring out what it is that's there and what the problem is. The therapist might do some pointing out, but it's a lot of work on the patient's part.

[Female, 50, Nonprofessional]

A few people were skeptical about whether therapy works at all.

I feel like it's mostly a crutch, just knowing that there's next week, and maybe there's that answer and maybe they'll tell it to you, they'll cure you, like some kind of miracle cure. It works in the sense that they're promising, or suggesting, that you're going to get better, and just the feeling that you're going to get better, that's the cure.

[Female, 28, Nonprofessional]

I'm not sure I think that it does work. It can get you through a rough moment and make you feel a little more comfortable, but it doesn't actually release people from the stuff that they have, because that's ongoing. You just have to notice it and be objective about it. I don't believe that people are freed from things by analyzing them.

[Female, 48, Nonprofessional]

Because the therapist is receptive, and doesn't have his or her own agenda, except to help you, it's a neutral situation, and as long as you pay your money and go when you should, the therapist is willing to listen and give you positive support and feedback. You're supposed to interact with the therapist, and that's supposed to be a reprogram-ming of the way you interact with people. It's a somewhat artificial situation because of the money involved, in that the therapist cares about you as long as you pay your money, but if you can't pay your money, that's the end of that.

[Female, 50, Nonprofessional]

NUMERICAL DISTRIBUTION

Professionals: (Some people gave more than one response.) Twelve people said therapy works through the relationship; 10 said specifically that it is a corrective emotional experience; 6 said through insight or understanding; 2 said the ongoing self-disclosure; 1 said the technical aspects, interventions, and concrete techniques; 1 said the continuity and regularity of the process; 1 said from learning new skills.

Nonprofessionals: (Some people gave more than one response.) Twenty people said therapy works through insight or understanding; 18 people said therapy works through the relationship; 5 said through the ongoing self-disclosure; 5 mentioned the skills of the therapist; 4 said through the freedom of the process; 4 said the motivation of the patient is crucial; 3 said by learning new skills; 3 mentioned the support of the therapist. One person said therapy doesn't work.

COMMENTS

More professionals think therapy works via the relationship, while nonprofessionals are more likely to emphasize insight and understanding. It's interesting to see that the professionals are not significantly better at articulating how therapy works than the nonprofessionals.

As the therapist, I believe in keeping the primary focus on the relationship between the patient and me, although not all patients will accept this or allow it. It can feel dangerous to some patients to work so closely with me, while others see it as a diversion and distraction from their own issues.

As the patient, I may not always see the connection to what is happening between me and the therapist, but I will usually consider the possibility, especially if the therapist has built up credibility and trust with me. I have some suspicion, though, of the therapist who never addresses our relationship, brushing it off, as one previous therapist did, with the explanation that he didn't "work that way."

RELATED READING

Curtis, R. C., and Stricker, G., eds. (1991). *How People Change: Inside and Outside Therapy.* New York: Plenum.

Dinnage, R. (1988). *One to One: The Experience of Psychotherapy.* London: Viking/Penguin.

Mendelsohn, R. M. (1992). *How Can Talking Help? An Introduction to the Technique of Analytic Therapy.* Northvale, NJ: Jason Aronson.

Mohr, D. C. (1995). Negative outcome in psychotherapy: a critical review. *Clinical Psychology Science and Practice* 2(1):1–27.

Rothstein, A., ed. (1988). *How Does Treatment Help? On the Modes of Therapeutic Action of Psychoanalytic Psychotherapy.* Madison, CT: International Universities Press.

Conclusions and Recommendations

We have now reviewed a tremendous amount of material. What does it mean? What are the implications for the practice of psychotherapy? How can therapists better serve their patients? I think the responses in the book indicate several things.

OBSERVATIONS

First, they suggest that many patients are undereducated about what to expect in therapy, how the process works, and how the therapist will behave. Many new patients don't know what their own participation and contribution is supposed to be. They don't know when the therapist is doing what he is supposed to do or when he is deviating from commonly accepted practice.

A good example can be seen in Question 40, in which people were asked if the relationship with the therapist was a regular topic of discussion. A significant portion (55 percent) of the nonprofessional group said that they seldom or never had such discussions. In many modern therapies, the relationship between patient and therapist is the central part of the treatment, and patients need to know these kinds of things to be able to evaluate their therapist's effectiveness.

Another example can be found in Question 79, in which one woman describes her therapist "warning" her about a friend of hers who is also his patient. While she says that she appreciated the warning, why doesn't she know that the therapist's behavior is a clear violation of basic ethical principles? Didn't she wonder what he was telling her friend about her?

Second, these interviews indicate that patients who are angry or unhappy or uncertain about what the therapist is doing don't always say so. In dealing with such issues as the waiting room, the office, the fee, the cancellation policy, eating and smoking, answering the phone, and many others, a large group of patients acknowledge that they don't necessarily tell the therapist of their dissatisfaction, but may fall silent, conceal material, avoid topics, and eventually leave treatment instead.

Third, a significant number of people in both groups were unhappy and dissatisfied with their treatment in individual, couples, and family therapy. Why are these percentages so high? If we offer those treatments, do we really know what we're doing? Or did we just decide to add that modality to our practice because it would bring additional income? Or because we think it might be fun to try? We have all known for a long time that credentials and experience are no guarantee of quality treatment. So how do we ensure that patients get what they need? We must wonder why so many people had an unsatisfactory experience.

RECOMMENDATIONS

There are some things we can do, as therapists and as patients, to improve the situation.

Therapists

Therapists need to examine what they are doing and their justifications for doing it. Therapists who answer the phone during a session, or charge patients for sessions while they are in the hospital, or tell a married patient to go out and have an affair, need to look long and hard at these behaviors, and think about how they would feel about such behavior if they themselves were the patient.

Based on the responses in the interviews, the following behaviors are questionable and require explanation and rationale.

- Not taking a break between appointments
- Starting and/or finishing sessions late
- Taking notes during the session
- Eating, drinking, or smoking during the session
- Answering the phone during the session
- Talking about a patient to another patient, or other breaks in confidentiality
- Getting into an argument with a patient
- Trying to control the patient
- Revealing a lot of personal information about the therapist to the patient
- Charging fees for sessions missed when the patient is hospitalized or otherwise unable to attend

This is not meant to be an exhaustive list. The therapist needs to re-examine and reconsider any behavior or requirement to which a patient has a strong negative reaction. Let me make it clear that I am not advocating immediate or automatic concession by the therapist. I am saying that we need to look carefully at our rules and positions, and try to see the validity of whatever the patient may be telling us about our own behavior.

On a more general level, therapists need to avoid rigidity. One way of conceptualizing neurotic behavior is that it is a rigid (that is, repetitive) response to changing conditions, so an inflexible and arbitrary therapist is a poor role model for any patient. Questioning the rules and examining the exceptions is an important part of therapy for both patient and therapist.

Therapists also need to acknowledge their areas of ignorance. For example, many practitioners go from graduate school to social service agency to private practice, and know little of the business world. These therapists should perhaps refrain from giving patients advice about how to behave at work. Therapists who have no experience raising children should admit that, and those who have never been married should, for example, avoid suggestions to have an affair.

One of the most common complaints of the subjects of these interviews was that the therapist didn't listen, didn't seem to want to understand the point of view and experience of the patient in regard to a dispute or disagreement with the therapist. Perhaps what therapists need here is less anxiety about having their authority challenged, and more confidence about the good will of the patient. If the patient has a position that conflicts with the therapist's, perhaps there is some validity to it.

My experience with my colleagues suggests to me that many therapists fear being somehow controlled by the patient, having their authority usurped, losing the upper hand; and this fear leads them to take a stand that creates a power struggle with the patient. But when that patient quits treatment, little has been gained by either party. If we could all be a little more calm and confident, knowing that we are in charge no matter what the patient may say, we could listen more easily to what the patient is reporting and react in a way that feels good to both of us.

Many inexperienced patients may not know how to object, or what to object to, and we need to find a way to inform patients that this is acceptable and to encourage them to tell us what is bothering them about us. What better role model could we provide than an authority figure who listens to criticism and feedback?

Patients

Patients need to educate themselves: to read books and articles about other people's experiences in therapy, to talk to friends who have experience in therapy, to have a consultation with another therapist if they can't get an acceptable explanation from the therapist they're seeing. Patients need to take a more active role in finding a good therapist, and to make sure that the treatment is what they need it to be.

It may be easy for inexperienced patients to assume that any problems in the therapy are their fault—after all, the therapist is the expert and the authority. But patients need to know that it is not only permitted to question the authority and the behavior of the therapist when they need to, but also an important part of the therapy. And to know also that if they do speak up and the therapist argues and defends and ignores the feedback then there is a serious problem.

Patients need to question any therapist who requires that they not read books in the field, or who tells patients what choices to make, or who pressures them to behave in a particular way. Everyone has become aware that a sexual relationship between patient and therapist is forbidden, but patients need to know that the therapist who has any kind of dual relationship with the patient (that is, who has a social or business connection outside the office) is also violating basic ethical principles.

Patients also need to know that every therapist has blind spots and areas in which his or her own issues may interfere with the patient's progress. Seeing more than one therapist can be extremely useful in catching these deficits. While these interviews focused on only the most recent therapy, many people referred to previous therapies, saying that they did certain work with one therapist and only got to certain other issues with another therapist.

In General

Doing psychotherapy is a wonderful way to spend a professional life. After almost 20 years I still look forward to going to the office each day. Many of my friends envy the enthusiasm I have for my job. The work remains fresh and meaningful, and each new patient brings an unknown universe to explore and understand. What we do together in the course of therapy changes people's lives for the better, shows them new options, and makes skills and energies newly available to them.

But there are problems in the profession. *Shrink Rap* discusses at length what these problems are: many practitioners are less than effective, some are inept, a few are actually unethical; managed care and the medical model threaten to take over the field and limit treatment to a few sessions and a course of psychopharmacological medication; a proliferation of techniques and theoretical approaches puts the field in confusion about what works best and what fails to work at all. Both therapist and patient must bear the responsibility for making any particular treatment work, but the solution for the problems of the field of psychotherapy must come from the professionals who practice it.

ABOUT THE AUTHOR

Lee D. Kassan received an M.A. in psychology from the New School of Social Research in New York. He is a Fellow of the American Institute for Psychotherapy and Psychoanalysis, where he was also a supervisor. Former Director of the Adolescent Program at Odyssey House, a therapeutic community treating substance abuse, he is the author of *Shrink Rap: Sixty Psychotherapists Discuss Their Work, Their Lives, and the State of Their Field*. Mr. Kassan is in private practice in New York City, working with adolescents and adults in individual, group, and couples therapy. He is a Certified Group Psychotherapist, and his weekly group has been meeting for nearly twenty years.